BIOLOGY OF RADIATION CARCINOGENESIS

Biology of Radiation Carcinogenesis

Editors

John M. Yuhas, Ph.D

Associate Director for Biology
Cancer Research and Treatment Center
and
Chief of Radiobiology
Department of Radiology
University of New Mexico
Albuquerque, New Mexico

Raymond W. Tennant, Ph.D

Biology Division
Oak Ridge National Laboratory
Oak Ridge, Tennessee

James D. Regan, Ph.D

Biology Division
Oak Ridge National Laboratory
Oak Ridge, Tennessee

Raven Press • New York

Raven Press, 1140 Avenue of the Americas, New York, New York 10036

Made in the United States of America

International Standard Book Number 0–89004–010–9
Library of Congress Catalog Card Number 74–14486

Preface

Society-at-large has been, and will continue to be, exposed to minute doses of ionizing radiation, the major potential hazard of which is the induction of cancer. With the exception of military applications, each type of exposure is an unwanted by-product of some beneficial application of technology, e.g., medical diagnostics and treatment, energy production, etc., and judgments must be made as to whether the benefits obtained offset the risk involved. Clearly, it is impossible to observe the effects of minute doses of radiation in the laboratory, as the experimental sample sizes are beyond the scope of even the largest animal facilities.

It is likely, however, that the effects of minute doses of radiation can be predicted, if the mechanisms involved are completely understood. Toward this end, scientists from a variety of disciplines met in Gatlinburg, Tennessee in April 1975 in the hope of providing a complete understanding of this complex problem.

In contrast to previous works on the subject, this volume, which is based on that symposium, is concerned not with description of empirical facts, but rather with an analysis of the mechanisms involved. Throughout the book, the point is made that a rational prediction of potential hazards to man can only be made if a complete understanding of the mechanisms involved is at hand. Six levels of organization have been included in this survey: molecular, genetic, viral, cellular, intercellular, and population. These categories are somewhat arbitrary, as most of the contributions span more than a single level.

This book is concerned specifically with radiation; however, through a comparison of radiation with other carcinogens the contributors have developed an up-to-date summary of carcinogenesis in general. The book therefore describes not only what we do know with regard to carcinogenesis, but perhaps more importantly what we do not know.

Although a final resolution of this problem remains elusive, the data presented by each contributor have completed a portion of the puzzle, and have indicated that, with continued effort, The Biology of Radiation Carcinogenesis will be resolved. This publication will be of interest to oncologists in general, and to health physicists, radiation therapists, radiation biologists, virologists, and nucleic acid biochemists.

John M. Yuhas
Raymond W. Tennant
James D. Regan
(*June 1975*)

Acknowledgments

The editors are indebted to the following for their help in organizing and running the symposium on "The Biology of Radiation Carcinogenesis": Drs. H. I. Adler (ORNL), A. Hollaender (ORAU), and J. Miller (U. of Wisc.), members of the organizing committee; Drs. M. Elkind (ANL), C. Heidelberger (U. of Wisc.), R. B. Setlow (BNL), A. Girardi (ETCRC), members of the program committee; and Drs. J. B. Storer (ORNL), R. B. Setlow (BNL), H. S. Kaplan (Stanford), M. Elkind (ANL), A. Girardi (ETCRC), and C. Heidelberger (U. of Wisc.); and Mary Jane Loop and Charles Normand, who took care of everything else.

ORNL = Oak Ridge National Laboratory
ORAU = Oak Ridge Associated Universities
ANL = Argonne National Laboratory
BNL = Brookhaven National Laboratory
ETCRC = East Tennessee Cancer Research Center

Contents

Viral Studies

Cellular Studies

Contributors and Participants

Phillip M. Achey
Radiation Biology Laboratory
Nuclear Sciences Center
University of Florida
Gainesville, Florida 36211

Howard I. Adler
Biology Division
Oak Ridge National Laboratory
P. O. Box Y
Oak Ridge, Tennessee 37830

Kathleen R. Ambrose
Department of Microbiology
University of Tennessee
Knoxville, Tennessee 37919

Ernest C. Anderson
Los Alamos Scientific Laboratory
P. O. Box 1663
Los Alamos, New Mexico 87544

Jeffrey L. Anderson
National Cancer Institute
Bethesda, Maryland 20014

Alan D. Andrews
Dermatology Branch
National Cancer Institute
Bethesda, Maryland 20014

William M. Baird
The Wistar Institute
36th Street at Spruce
Philadelphia, Pennsylvania 19104

W. E. Barnett
Biology Division
Oak Ridge National Laboratory
P. O. Box Y
Oak Ridge, Tennessee 37819

Margaret H. Barrington
Scripps Clinic and Research Foundation
La Jolla, California 92037

Bengt Berlin
Statistical Laboratory
Department of Statistics
University of California
Berkeley, California 94720

Daniel Billen
Biology Division
Oak Ridge National Laboratory
P. O. Box Y
Oak Ridge, Tennessee 37830

Paul H. Black
Massachusetts General Hospital
Fruit Street
Boston, Massachusetts 02114

James Blakeslee
Department of Veterinary Pathology
The Ohio State University
1900 Coffey Road
Columbus, Ohio 43085

Lawrence R. Boone
806 Maplehurst Park, Apt. 1
Knoxville, Tennessee 37902

Carmia Borek
Department of Radiology
College of Physicians & Surgeons
Columbia University
New York, New York 10032

Donald C. Borg
Medical Research Center
Brookhaven National Laboratory
Upton, New York 11973

John M. Boyle
Paterson Laboratories
Christie Hospital & Holt Radium Institute
Wilmslow Road
Manchester, England M20 9BX

Blaine Bradshaw
Biology Division
Oak Ridge National Laboratory
P. O. Box Y
Oak Ridge, Tennessee 37830

Emily T. Brake
Biology Division
Oak Ridge National Laboratory
P. O. Box Y
Oak Ridge, Tennessee 37830

Richard Brake
UT–Oak Ridge Graduate School of Bio-
    medical Sciences
Biology Division
Oak Ridge National Laboratory
P. O. Box Y
Oak Ridge, Tennessee 37830

Patricia C. Brennan
Argonne National Laboratory
9700 S. Cass Avenue
Argonne, Illinois 60439

Arthur Brown
Department of Zoology and Entomology
Oak Ridge National Laboratory
Oak Ridge, Tennessee 37830

Stuart Brown
Laboratory of Biochemical Genetics
National Heart and Lung Institute
Bethesda, Maryland 20014

L. K. Bustad, Dean
College of Veterinary Medicine
Washington State University
Pullman, Washington 99163

Lucia H. Cacheiro
Biology Division
Oak Ridge National Laboratory
P. O. Box Y
Oak Ridge, Tennessee 37830

Edrick L. Candler
MAN Program
Oak Ridge National Laboratory
P. O. Box P
Oak Ridge, Tennessee 37830

W. L. Carrier
Biology Division
Oak Ridge National Laboratory
P. O. Box Y
Oak Ridge, Tennessee 37830

S. F. Carson
Biology Division
Oak Ridge National Laboratory
P. O. Box Y
Oak Ridge, Tennessee 37830

Peter A. Cerutti
Department of Biochemistry
College of Medicine
University of Florida
Gainesville, Florida 32601

Sisir K. Chattopadhyay
Department of Dermatology

Yale–New Haven Hospital
174 Linden Street
New Haven, Connecticut 06511

Nelwyn T. Christie
UT–Oak Ridge Graduate School of Bio-
    medical Sciences
Biology Division
Oak Ridge National Laboratory
P. O. Box Y
Oak Ridge, Tennessee 37830

N. K. Clapp
Biology Division
Oak Ridge National Laboratory
P. O. Box Y
Oak Ridge, Tennessee 37830

Carlo M. Croce
The Wistar Institute
36th & Spruce Streets
Philadelphia, Pennsylvania 19104

Shishir Kumar Das
UT–Oak Ridge Graduate School of Bio-
    medical Sciences
Biology Division
Oak Ridge National Laboratory
P. O. Box Y
Oak Ridge, Tennessee 37830

J. P. Daugherty
Biology Division
Oak Ridge National Laboratory
P. O. Box Y
Oak Ridge, Tennessee 37830

K. A. Davidson
Biology Division
Oak Ridge National Laboratory
P. O. Box Y
Oak Ridge, Tennessee 37830

Rufus Day
National Cancer Institute
Bldg. 37, Room 3C24
Bethesda, Maryland 20034

Alain Declève
Department of Radiology
Stanford University
School of Medicine
Stanford, California 94305

Joseph A. DiPaolo
Biology Branch
National Cancer Institute
Bethesda, Maryland 20014

Frank J. Dixon
Scripps Clinic and Research Foundation
La Jolla, California 92037

D. G. Doherty
Biology Division
Oak Ridge National Laboratory
P. O. Box Y
Oak Ridge, Tennessee 37830

J. F. Duplan
Fondation Bergonie
Unite de Recherche 117
180 Rue de Saint-Genes
Bordeaux, France 33076

Leon Dure
Department of Biochemistry
University of Georgia
Athens, Georgia 30602

Rosalie K. Elespuru
UT–Oak Ridge Graduate School of Bio-
    medical Sciences
Biology Division
Oak Ridge National Laboratory
P. O. Box Y
Oak Ridge, Tennessee 37830

Mortimer M. Elkind
Division of Biological and Medical Re-
    search
Argonne National Laboratory
Argonne, Illinois 60439

John J. Elmore, Jr.
Medical Department
Brookhaven National Laboratory
Upton, New York 11973

J. L. Epler
Biology Division
Oak Ridge National Laboratory
P. O. Box Y
Oak Ridge, Tennessee 37830

Bill Farmerie
Bio. Sci. Unit I
Florida State University
Tallahassee, Florida 32306

J. G. Farrelly
Biology Division
Oak Ridge National Laboratory
P. O. Box Y
Oak Ridge, Tennessee 37830

F. M. Faulcon
Biology Division

Oak Ridge National Laboratory
P. O. Box Y
Oak Ridge, Tennessee 37830

Miriam P. Finkel
Argonne National Laboratory
Argonne, Illinois 60439

Farrel Fort
Department of Biochemistry
University of Florida
Gainesville, Florida 32611

D. W. Fountain
Biology Division
Oak Ridge National Laboratory
P. O. Box Y
Oak Ridge, Tennessee 37830

A. A. Francis
Biology Division
Oak Ridge National Laboratory
P. O. Box Y
Oak Ridge, Tennessee 37830

Mary W. Francis
Biology Division
Oak Ridge National Laboratory
P. O. Box Y
Oak Ridge, Tennessee 37830

Herbert A. Freedman
Department of Genetics
Albert Einstein College of Medicine
1300 Morris Park Avenue
Bronx, New York 10461

R. J. Michael Fry
Argonne National Laboratory
9700 South Cass Avenue
Argonne, Illinois 60439

Mary Esther Gaulden
Radiology Department
Southwestern Medical School
5323 Harry Hines Boulevard
Dallas, Texas 75235

E. Gelmann
Department of Radiology
Stanford University
School of Medicine
Stanford, California 94305

Anthony Girardi
East Tennessee Cancer Research
    Center
IBM Bldg., Suite 201
904 Executive Park Drive
Knoxville, Tennessee 37919

M. Goldman
Laboratory of Radiobiology
University of California at Davis
Davis, California

David A. Goldthwait
Department of Biochemistry
Case Western Reserve University
2109 Adelbert Road
Cleveland, Ohio 44106

Joan W. Goodman
Biology Division
Oak Ridge National Laboratory
P. O. Box Y
Oak Ridge, Tennessee 37830

C. F. Gottlieb
Biology Division
Oak Ridge National Laboratory
P. O. Box Y
Oak Ridge, Tennessee 37830

Peter Groer
Argonne National Laboratory
9700 South Cass Avenue
Argonne, Illinois 60439

Dezider Grunberger
Institute for Cancer Research
College of Physicians and Surgeons
Columbia University
99 Fort Washington Avenue
New York, New York 10032

Antun Han
Argonne National Laboratory
9700 South Cass Avenue
Argonne, Illinois 60439

Philip C. Hanawalt
Department of Biological Sciences
Stanford University
Stanford, California 94305

R. E. Hand, Jr.
Biology Division
Oak Ridge National Laboratory
P. O. Box Y
Oak Ridge, Tennessee 37830

M. G. Hanna
Basic Cancer Research Program
NCI–Frederick Cancer Research Center
Frederick, Maryland 21701

Nechama Haran-Ghera
Department of Chemical Immunology
The Weizmann Institute of Science
Rehovot, Israel

P. V. Hariharan
The Hillis Miller Health Center
Department of Biochemistry
University of Florida
Gainesville, Florida 32610

Alice A. Hardigree
Biology Division
Oak Ridge National Laboratory
P. O. Box Y
Oak Ridge, Tennessee 37830

Helga Harm
University of Texas at Dallas
P. O. Box 30365
Dallas, Texas 75230

Walter Harm
University of Texas at Dallas
P. O. Box 30365
Dallas, Texas 75230

Mildred G. Hayes
Biology Division
Oak Ridge National Laboratory
P. O. Box Y
Oak Ridge, Tennessee 37830

Charles Heidelberger
McArdle Memorial Laboratory
University of Wisconsin
Madison, Wisconsin 53706

G. P. Hirsch
Biology Division
Oak Ridge National Laboratory
P. O. Box Y
Oak Ridge, Tennessee 37830

Ti Ho
Biology Division
Oak Ridge National Laboratory
P. O. Box Y
Oak Ridge, Tennessee 37830

Alexander Hollaender
% Associated Universities, Inc.
1717 Massachusetts Avenue, N.W.
Washington, D.C. 20036

J. M. Holland
Biology Division
Oak Ridge National Laboratory
P. O. Box Y
Oak Ridge, Tennessee 37830

Clayton F. Holoway
Health Physics Division
Oak Ridge National Laboratory
P. O. Box X
Oak Ridge, Tennessee 37830

Irene S. Holoway
Freelance Translations
929 Green Hills Road
Knoxville, Tennessee 37919

A. W. Hsie
Biology Division
Oak Ridge National Laboratory
P. O. Box Y
Oak Ridge, Tennessee 37830

Ih-Chang Hsu
Biology Division
Oak Ridge National Laboratory
P. O. Box Y
Oak Ridge, Tennessee 37830

James N. Ihle
Basic Cancer Research Program
NCI–Frederick Cancer Research Center
Frederick, Maryland 21701

Eugene Joiner
Medical Division
Oak Ridge Associated Universities
P. O. Box 117
Oak Ridge, Tennessee 37830

M. Helen Jones
Biology Division
Oak Ridge National Laboratory
P. O. Box Y
Oak Ridge, Tennessee 37830

Henry S. Kaplan
Department of Radiology
Stanford University School of Medicine
Stanford, California 94305

Albrecht M. Kellerer
Department of Radiology
College of Physicians and Surgeons
Columbia University
New York, New York 10032

F. T. Kenney
Biology Division
Oak Ridge National Laboratory
P. O. Box Y
Oak Ridge, Tennessee 37830

J. O. Kiggans, Jr.
Department of Microbiology
University of Tennessee
Knoxville, Tennessee 37916

R. F. Kimball
Biology Division
Oak Ridge National Laboratory
P. O. Box Y
Oak Ridge, Tennessee 37830

Carole A. King
Biology Division
Oak Ridge National Laboratory
P. O. Box Y
Oak Ridge, Tennessee 37830

Dollie M. Kirtikar
Biochemistry Department
Case Western Reserve University
2109 Adelbert Road
Cleveland, Ohio 44106

Joosje C. Klein
Radiobiological Institute TNO
Lange Kleiweg 151
Rijswijk (ZH), The Netherlands

Kenneth H. Kraemer
Dermatology Branch
National Cancer Institute
Bethesda, Maryland 20014

G. C. Lavelle
Biology Division
Oak Ridge National Laboratory
P. O. Box Y
Oak Ridge, Tennessee 37830

Philip D. Lawley
Chester Beatty Research Institute
Pollards Wood Research Station
Nightingales Lane
Chalfont St. Giles
Buckinghamshire, HP 8 4SP, England

J. C. Lee
Basic Cancer Research Program
NCI–Frederick Cancer Research Center
Frederick, Maryland 21701

Mary S. Leffell
Department of Microbiology
University of Tennessee
Knoxville, Tennessee 37916

Richard A. Lerner
Department of Immunopathology
Scripps Clinic and Research Foundation
La Jolla, California 92037

Richard L. Levy
Department of Immunopathology
Scripps Clinic and Research Foundation
La Jolla, California 92037

Carol W. Lewis
Department of Bacteriology and Immunology
University of North Carolina
Chapel Hill, North Carolina 27514

Albert P. Li
*UT–Oak Ridge Graduate School of Bio-
medical Sciences*
Biology Division
Oak Ridge National Laboratory
P. O. Box Y
Oak Ridge, Tennessee 37830

Anna Tai Li
*UT–Oak Ridge Graduate School of Bio-
medical Sciences*
Biology Division
Oak Ridge National Laboratory
P. O. Box Y
Oak Ridge, Tennessee 37830

M. Lieberman
Department of Radiology
Stanford University
School of Medicine

Frank Lilly
Department of Genetics
Albert Einstein College of Medicine
Bronx, New York 10461

John B. Little
Harvard School of Public Health
665 Huntington Avenue
Boston, Massachusetts 02115

Elizabeth Lloyd
Argonne National Laboratory
9700 South Cass Avenue
Argonne, Illinois 60439

Paul H. M. Lohman
Medical Biological Lab. TNO
139 Lange Kleiweg
Rijswijk (ZH), The Netherlands

Mary Jane Loop
Biology Division
Oak Ridge National Laboratory
P. O. Box Y
Oak Ridge, Tennessee 37830

Douglas R. Lowy
Department of Dermatology
Yale–New Haven Hospital
174 Linden Street
New Haven, Connecticut 06511

Judith Rae Lumb
Atlanta University
223 Chestnut Street, S.W.
Atlanta, Georgia 30314

C. C. Lushbaugh, M.D.
Oak Ridge Associated Universities
P. O. Box 117
Oak Ridge, Tennessee 37830

Linda B. Lyons
National Cancer Institute
Bldg. 37, 4C09
Bethesda, Maryland 20014

Lloyd E. MacAskill
*UT–Oak Ridge Graduate School of
Biomedical Sciences*
Biology Division
Oak Ridge National Laboratory
P. O. Box Y
Oak Ridge, Tennessee 37830

J. Justin McCormick
Michigan Cancer Foundation
4811 John R. Street
Detroit, Michigan 48201

Veronica M. Maher
Michigan Cancer Foundation
4811 John R. Street
Detroit, Michigan 48201

D. D. Mahlum
Biology Department
Battelle-Northwest
Richland, Washington 99352

R. G. Martin
National Cancer Institute
Bethesda, Maryland 20014

Peter Mazur
Biology Division
Oak Ridge National Laboratory
P. O. Box Y
Oak Ridge, Tennessee 37830

Charles G. Mead
Biology Division
Oak Ridge National Laboratory
P. O. Box Y
Oak Ridge, Tennessee 37830

Asher Meshorer
Lobund Laboratory
University of Notre Dame
Notre Dame, Indiana 46556

V. S. Mierzejewski
Biology Division
Oak Ridge National Laboratory
P. O. Box Y
Oak Ridge, Tennessee 37830

Don Ray Miller
UT–Oak Ridge Graduate School of Bio-
medical Sciences
Biology Division
Oak Ridge National Laboratory
P. O. Box Y
Oak Ridge, Tennessee 37830

Elizabeth C. Miller
McArdle Memorial Laboratory
University of Wisconsin
Madison, Wisconsin 53706

James A. Miller
McArdle Memorial Laboratory
University of Wisconsin
Madison, Wisconsin 53706

Robert W. Miller
Epidemiology Branch
A-521 Landow Building
National Cancer Institute
Bethesda, Maryland 20014

George E. Milo, Jr.
College of Veterinary Medicine
The Ohio State University
1900 Coffey Road
Columbus, Ohio 43210

Magda H. Morales
UT–Oak Ridge Graduate School of Bio-
medical Sciences
Biology Division
Oak Ridge National Laboratory
P. O. Box Y
Oak Ridge, Tennessee 37830

J. E. Morris
Battelle-Northwest
P. O. Box 999
Richland, Washington 99352

F. E. Myer
Biology Division
Oak Ridge National Laboratory
P. O. Box Y
Oak Ridge, Tennessee 37830

W. Roger Ney
National Council on Radiation Protection and Measurements
7910 Woodmont Avenue, Suite 1016
Bethesda, Maryland 20014

J. Neyman
Statistical Laboratory
University of California
Berkeley, California 94720

Ohtsura Niwa
Department of Radiology
Stanford Medical Center
Stanford, California 94301

M. G. Ormerod
Chester Beatty Institute
Royal Cancer Hospital
Laboratories at Clifton Avenue
Belmont, Sutton, Surrey Sm2 5px
England

T. T. Odell
Biology Division
Oak Ridge National Laboratory
P. O. Box Y
Oak Ridge, Tennessee 37830

J. A. Otten
Biology Division
Oak Ridge National Laboratory
P. O. Box Y
Oak Ridge, Tennessee 37830

Robert B. Painter
Laboratory of Radiobiology
University of California, San Francisco
San Francisco, California 94143

B. C. Pal
Biology Division
Oak Ridge National Laboratory
P. O. Box Y
Oak Ridge, Tennessee 37830

Nelson H. Pazmino
Frederick Cancer Research Center
Frederick, Maryland 21701

G. M. Peterman
Biology Division
Oak Ridge National Laboratory
P. O. Box Y
Oak Ridge, Tennessee 37830

Diana M. Popp
Biology Division
Oak Ridge National Laboratory
P. O. Box Y
Oak Ridge, Tennessee 37830

R. A. Popp
Biology Division
Oak Ridge National Laboratory
P. O. Box Y
Oak Ridge, Tennessee 37830

James R. Prine
H-4 MS 880
Los Alamos Scientific Laboratory
P. O. Box 1663
Los Alamos, New Mexico 87544

Judith O. Proctor
Department of Bacteriology and Im-
munology
University of North Carolina
Chapel Hill, North Carolina 27514

J. M. Quarles, Jr.
Biology Division
Oak Ridge National Laboratory
P. O. Box Y
Oak Ridge, Tennessee 37830

R. O. Rahn
Biology Division
Oak Ridge National Laboratory
P. O. Box Y
Oak Ridge, Tennessee 37830

Ralph J. Rascati
Biology Division
Oak Ridge National Laboratory
P. O. Box Y
Oak Ridge, Tennessee 37830

James D. Regan
Biology Division
Oak Ridge National Laboratory
P. O. Box Y
Oak Ridge, Tennessee 37830

Chris A. Reilly, Jr.
Argonne National Laboratory
9700 South Cass Avenue
Argonne, Illinois 60439

Joyce F. Remsen
Department of Biochemistry
College of Medicine
University of Florida
Gainesville, Florida 32601

Richard J. Reynolds
UT–Oak Ridge Graduate School of Bio-
medical Sciences
Biology Division
Oak Ridge National Laboratory
P. O. Box Y
Oak Ridge, Tennessee 37830

Jay H. Robbins
Dermatology Branch
National Cancer Institute
Bethesda, Maryland 20014

Philip Rosen
Department of Physics
University of Massachusetts
Amherst, Massachusetts 01002

Leon Rosenblatt
Laboratory of Radiobiology
University of California at Davis
Davis, California

Shigeru Sakonju
UT–Oak Ridge Graduate School of Bio-
medical Sciences
Biology Division
Oak Ridge National Laboratory
P. O. Box Y
Oak Ridge, Tennessee 37830

Stefan O. Schiff
Department of Biology
George Washington University
21st and G Streets, N.W.
Washington, D.C. 20006

Elizabeth L. Scott
Department of Statistics
University of California
Berkeley, California 94720

R. B. Setlow
Biology Department
Brookhaven National Laboratory
Upton, New York 11973

Claire J Shellabarger
Medical Department
Brookhaven National Laboratory
Upton, New York 11973

Esther Sid
Department of Statistics
Statistical Laboratory
University of California
Berkeley, California 94720

C. B. Skov
Biology Division
Oak Ridge National Laboratory
P. O. Box Y
Oak Ridge, Tennessee 37830

David M. Smith
H-4, MS 880
Los Alamos Scientific Laboratory
P. O. Box 1663
Los Alamos, New Mexico 87544

James Marshall Smith
College of Medicine
University of Utah
Salt Lake City, Utah 84132

L. H. Smith
Biology Division
Oak Ridge National Laboratory
P. O. Box Y
Oak Ridge, Tennessee 37830

George E. Stapleton
Division of Biomedical and
    Environmental Research
Energy Research and Development
    Administration
Washington, D.C. 20545

Diane Stassi
Biol. Sci. Unit I
Florida State University
Tallahassee, Florida 32306

Richard A. Steeves
Albert Einstein College of Medicine
1300 Morris Park Avenue
Bronx, New York 10803

Andrew Stehney
Argonne National Laboratory
9700 South Cass Avenue
Argonne, Illinois 60439

Zenon Steplewski
Wistar Institute
36th and Spruce Streets
Philadelphia, Pennsylvania 19104

John B. Storer
Biology Division
Oak Ridge National Laboratory
P. O. Box Y
Oak Ridge, Tennessee 37830

Natalie Teich
Department of Dermatology
Yale–New Haven Hospital
174 Linden Street
New Haven, Connecticut 06511

Raymond W. Tennant
Biology Division
Oak Ridge National Laboratory
P. O. Box Y
Oak Ridge, Tennessee 37830

Margaret Terzaghi
Department of Physiology
Harvard University
665 Huntington Avenue
Boston, Massachusetts 02115

J. R. Totter
Biology Division
Oak Ridge National Laboratory
P. O. Box Y
Oak Ridge, Tennessee 37830

R. L. Ullrich
Biology Division
Oak Ridge National Laboratory
P. O. Box Y
Oak Ridge, Tennessee 37830

Mayo Uziel
Biology Division
Oak Ridge National Laboratory
P. O. Box Y
Oak Ridge, Tennessee 37830

D. W. van Bekkum
Radiobiological Institute TNO
Rijswijk (ZH), The Netherlands

Elliot Volkin
Biology Division
Oak Ridge National Laboratory
P. O. Box Y
Oak Ridge, Tennessee 37830

Anita E. Walker
Biology Division
Oak Ridge National Laboratory
P. O. Box Y
Oak Ridge, Tennessee 37830

Raymond Waters
Biology Division
Oak Ridge National Laboratory
P. O. Box Y
Oak Ridge, Tennessee 37830

I. Bernard Weinstein
Institute for Cancer Research
College of Physicians and Surgeons
Columbia University
99 Fort Washington Avenue
New York, New York 10032

Virginia P. White
Graduate School and University Center
The City University of New York
33 West 42 Street
New York, New York 10036

Steven Wiley
UT–Oak Ridge Graduate School of
  Biomedical Sciences
Biology Division
Oak Ridge National Laboratory
P. O. Box Y
Oak Ridge, Tennessee 37830

M. Margaret Williams
Biology Division
Oak Ridge National Laboratory
P. O. Box Y
Oak Ridge, Tennessee 37830

William Winton
Biology Division
Oak Ridge National Laboratory
P. O. Box Y
Oak Ridge, Tennessee 37830

W.-K. Yang
Biology Division
Oak Ridge National Laboratory
P. O. Box Y
Oak Ridge, Tennessee 37830

Ronald Yasbin
Laboratory of Biochemical Genetics
National Heart and Lung Institute
Bldg. 36, Room 1C08
Bethesda, Maryland 20014

Kenjiro Yokoro
Research Institute for Nuclear Medicine
  and Biology
Hiroshima University
Kasumi-cho
Hiroshima, Japan

John M. Yuhas
Biology Division
Oak Ridge National Laboratory
P. O. Box Y
Oak Ridge, Tennessee 37830

Introduction

D. W. van Bekkum*

Radiobiological Institute TNO, Rijswijk, The Netherlands

It is interesting to note that general concern over the health hazards of ionizing radiation has shifted during the past years from its genetic effects to its somatic effects—notably, tumor induction or carcinogenesis. One reason for this change in emphasis has been, no doubt, new scientific information on increased incidence of tumors, notably of the female breast and of the thyroid gland, in humans exposed to doses of radiation below the level that was previously thought to be carcinogenic.) Furthermore, the unprecedented efforts presently being made under the National Cancer Program in the United States have focused attention on cancer, in general, and on factors that increase its incidence, including ionizing radiation.

Whatever the reasons, the practical questions that have to be answered concern estimates of the increase in tumor incidence following relatively low doses of radiation, in much the same way that genetic hazards have been evaluated previously. Even in rodents, we cannot hope to measure directly the increase in tumor incidence that is associated with doses of the order of 1 rad/year or less, so that extrapolations will have to be made from higher dose levels, on which data are already available or can be obtained in the foreseeable future. These extrapolations will of necessity be performed over a broad range, i.e., from doses of the order of hundreds of rads per year down to 1 rad/year or even lower. Actually, such extrapolations should be termed predictions, and the only way by which these predictions can obtain reliability is to base them on a demonstrated knowledge of the mechanisms involved in the induction of tumors by ionizing radiation. It was therefore highly appropriate that the organizers of the 1975 Gatlinburg symposium selected as their topic "The Biology of Radiation Carcinogenesis," and by their choice of speakers have focused on furthering our understanding of the processes that occur between the impact of the radiation itself and the occurrence of a measurable tumor mass. From that stage onward, the processes that take place are becoming better understood every day, because they can be analyzed by better and better methods, from the point of view of the tumor growth itself as well as the reactions to the tumor that occur in the tumor bearer.

With regard to the description of the carcinogenic process itself, it seems

* Presently Fogarty Scholar in Residence, National Institutes of Health, Bethesda, Maryland.

advisable to distinguish two stages—the first one ending with the occurrence of one or more transformed cells, with the property of unlimited and uncontrolled proliferation, the second one being the proliferation of these transformed cells into a clinically detectable tumor mass. The 1975 Gatlinberg symposium was primarily concerned with the first stage, that is, the transformed cell, as defined above, was the end point of most of the discussions.

The pathway by which the carcinogenic process occurs, following irradiation, seemed to have a number of recognizable cornerstones when the symposium started, at least in the mind of the author. It was understood that specific viruses play an essential role in the induction of some tumors by ionizing radiation. Many animal tumors can be evoked by the action of viruses on cells, and in certain cases of radiation-induced tumors, such as the lymphomas that follow fractionated irradiation of C57BL mice and the osteosarcomas of mice, a virus has indeed been isolated from the irradiated tissues or from the tumor itself and has been shown to induce tumors in unirradiated animals.

It was known that many tumor cells carry either abnormal numbers of chromosomes or characteristic aberrant chromosomes, or both, but these features did not seem to have a special significance in uninhibited growth. Also, evidence seemed to be accumulating in favor of an indirect mechanism of transformation, one that involved the transfer of genetic materials from one cell to another. Furthermore, active DNA synthesis, be it during normal duplication or duplication during the repair of radiation-induced lesions, was required for the cells to undergo transformation. The consequence of the latter mechanism could be an increased incidence of transformations following increased opportunities for repair, such as occur with fractionated irradiation. Such observations had been reported for transformation of cells *in vitro* by fractionated doses of X-rays.

It became clear from this Gatlinburg symposium, in which these issues and others were dealt with in depth, that the relevance of all of these points must be critically reconsidered. The causative role of radiation leukemia virus in radiation lukemogenesis was questioned by the same investigators who discovered the virus and described its role more than a decade ago. New and exciting evidence was provided from work with somatic cell hybrids in favor of the specific involvement of one human chromosome coding for the transformation of a tumorigenic phenotype. With regard to the effects of split versus single doses of ionizing radiation, it became evident from the presentations and the subsequent discussions that scoring of transformed cells *in vitro* might yield different results than the results obtained from scoring tumors *in vivo*. As was pointed out by one of the organizers of the symposium upon which this volume is based, different experimental systems and conditions seem to provide us with different answers, and, from all of these seemingly conflicting data, we must derive the main mechanisms of the carcinogenic process.

A great deal of effort has been exerted world-wide in the study of the carcinogenic effects of radiation, viruses, and chemical agents. It is becoming more apparent that each of the other agents can itself prove to be useful in unraveling the mechanisms of radiation carcinogenesis. In addition, many new and more sophisticated methods are being generated by chemists, cell biologists, virologists, and immunologists, methods that can be used to study the interaction of carcinogenic agents with living cells as well as measure the biologic properties of the products of the interaction. With all these advances, it seems that the coming years will show great activity in this field and equal rewards in terms of increased knowledge. The symposium upon which this volume is based has provided much stimulation to its participants to pursue their attempts to unravel the mechanisms of radiation carcinogenesis. The Proceedings may serve to confirm this spirit and perhaps transfer some of it to those readers who could not attend.

Biology of Radiation Carcinogenesis, edited by
J. M. Yuhas, R. W. Tennant, and J. D. Regan.
Raven Press, New York © 1976.

Microdosimetry and Its Implication for the Primary Processes in Radiation Carcinogenesis

Albrecht M. Kellerer

Department of Radiology, Radiological Research Laboratory, College of Physicians and Surgeons, Columbia University, New York, New York 10032

Carcinogenesis has many aspects, and a variety of these aspects are discussed and compared in this conference. In a complex situation, one is naturally forced to simplify. Although this is often necessary and desirable, it can also lead to erroneous interpretation of experimental data and to distorted comparisons. This is particularly true with regard to basic biophysical concepts, such as absorbed dose, relative biologic effectiveness, and the time factor.

The following remarks deal with these three concepts and their relation to radiation carcinogenesis. The first problem is that of absorbed dose and of its inadequacy when applied to cellular or subcellular structures. The second problem is that of the relative biologic effectiveness (RBE) and its change with absorbed dose. The third problem is that of the dependence of the time factor on absorbed dose. Not only the complexities of these factors but also their interrelation and their connection to microdosimetry will be considered.

ABSORBED DOSE AND SPECIFIC ENERGY

All ionizing radiations work essentially by the same mechanism. Ionizing particles as different as photons, electrons, neutrons, heavy ions, and mesons produce the same primary alterations, namely ionization and excitation. Furthermore, the various radiations produce about the same number of such alterations per unit energy imparted to the irradiated medium. This is the justification for applying the same quantity, absorbed dose, $D,$ to all ionizing radiations. The quantity is defined as the energy imparted to an irradiated medium per unit mass.

Equal absorbed doses of different radiations do not, however, produce equal effects. The differences are, as stated, not due to differences in the primary radiation products; they are due to the different microscopic distribution of ionization and excitation in charged particle tracks. Such radiations as α particles, or the heavy recoils of neutrons, that produce ionizations closely spaced along their tracks cause considerably more cellular damage per unit of absorbed dose than do sparsely ionizing radiations.

The fact that the cellular effect depends strongly on the microscopic pattern of energy distribution implies that absorbed dose is not a meaningful concept if one deals with small sites that may be traversed by only one or a few charged particles. Absorbed dose determines only the mean value, or statistical expectation, of the imparted energy; the actual energy in the microscopic region may differ greatly from the expectation value. This is the reason why the quantity specific energy, z, has been introduced (Rossi, 1967; ICRU, 1971). Specific energy is the statistical counterpart of absorbed dose; it is defined as energy actually imparted, divided by the mass of the region.

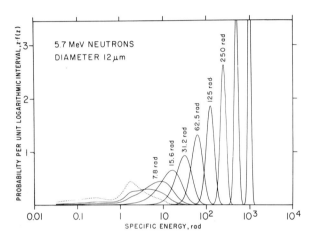

FIG. 1. Probability per unit logarithmic interval of specific energy, z, at various doses of 5.7 MeV neutrons in a spherical tissue region of diameter 12 μm. The distribution of the increments of z produced in single events is shown (– – –). (Rossi and Kellerer, 1975.)

The statistical fluctuations, i.e., the differences between z and D are most important for small volumes, for small doses, and for densely ionizing radiation. Microdosimetry is the extension of classic dosimetry to those situations for which the concept of absorbed dose is not applicable. Its object is therefore the experimental and theoretical determination of specific energy in cellular and subcellular regions. Since specific energy is a random variable, and not a single valued quantity, such as absorbed dose, one can only give probability distributions of its possible values. Figure 1 represents such distributions, namely, the probability distribution of specific energy in regions of approximately cellular dimension upon exposure to monoenergetic neutrons. One notes that the relative fluctuations are very large at small doses, and less at higher doses. Accordingly, absorbed dose is a meaningful concept only if it is sufficiently high in value. The figure is merely an illustrative example; a detailed discussion of microdosimetric concepts relevant to radiation carcinogenesis can be found elsewhere (Rossi and Kellerer, 1975).

In order to obtain a practical criterion for the applicability of absorbed dose, one must determine the range of site diameters and of absorbed doses where the mean deviation of specific energy from absorbed dose is less than a specified value, for example 20%. In Fig. 2, three different radiations are considered, namely, α particles, 430 keV neutrons, and cobalt γ-rays. The ranges of site diameters and absorbed doses for which the mean deviation of specific energy from absorbed dose exceeds 20% are shaded. Above the shaded areas, the quantity, absorbed dose, can be applied directly; within the shaded areas, one must consider specific energy instead of absorbed dose.

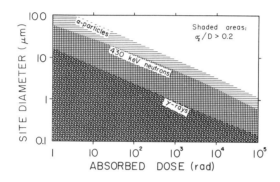

FIG. 2. Diagram of site diameters and absorbed doses for which the specific energy, z, must be distinguished from absorbed dose, D, for three different radiations. Those areas where the mean deviation of z from D exceeds 20% are indicated by shading.

Even without going into the details of microdosimetry, one can make general statements relevant to radiation carcinogenesis at low doses. This will be the subject of the remainder of this section.

Consider the case in which isolated mammalian cells are exposed to an absorbed dose of 1 rad of α particles. Then, 99% of the cell nuclei are entirely free of energy deposition by particles; they are not traversed by even a single charged particle. But 1% of all cell nuclei are traversed by one α particle. This single α particle produces specific energies in the nucleus, of the order of 100 rad. The probability that more than one α particle appears in the nucleus is only 10^{-4} and can therefore be neglected. In this situation, the dose-effect curve must be linear. This follows from the fact that only those cells that are traversed by a charged particle can be affected and that the number of cells actually traversed is proportional to absorbed dose. One may use the term *small dose* to designate the cases in which the event frequency in the nucleus of the cell is much smaller than one. Regardless of the cellular mechanisms one can then state that the dose-effect curve for any action of ionizing radiation on individual cells must be linear; it follows equally that there is no dependence on dose rate, since all effects are produced by individual particles.

At the same absorbed dose, the event frequencies are much larger for sparsely ionizing radiations than for densely ionizing radiations. Figure 3 illustrates the differences for the same radiations which have been compared in Fig. 2. In the figure, those ranges of site diameter and absorbed dose are shaded in the area where the mean number of particle traversing a given cell region is less than one. Whenever one deals with critical sites, and with absorbed doses that correspond to a point substantially inside the shaded regions, the dose-effect curve must be linear. On the other hand if, as in the results of Shellabarger et al. (1974) and Vogel (1969) on the induction of mammary tumors in the Sprague-Dawley rat, one finds nonlinearity at small doses of neutrons, one must conclude that the effect does not reflect

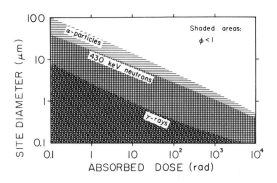

FIG. 3. Diagram of site diameters and absorbed doses for which the mean event frequency, ϕ, is less than one. The areas with ϕ less than one are indicated by shading for three different radiations.

damage to independent cells, but that there is interdependence between damaged cells (Rossi and Kellerer, 1972, 1975).

The statement concerning the linearity of cellular dose-effect relations at small doses is valid regardless of the mechanisms involved in the effect. Linearity, however, may extend to doses higher than the doses that would be predicted by using Fig. 3. There are experimental results on various higher organisms that indicate that this is indeed the case. It will be useful to summarize these results.

The microsimetric analysis of various effects produced in eukaryotic cells by sparsely ionizing radiations and by neutrons has led to the conclusion that the cellular damage is proportional to the square of energy deposited in sensitive sites, which are somewhat smaller than the nucleus of the cell (Kellerer and Rossi, 1972):

$$\epsilon(z) = k\,z^2 \tag{1}$$

A quadratic dependence on specific energy will not result in a quadratic dependence on absorbed dose. The reason is that even at smallest absorbed doses considerable energy concentrations occur in those cells traversed by a charged particle. This results in the linear component discussed above. One can formulate this quantitatively, and finds that the quadratic dependence on specific energy corresponds to a linear-quadratic dependence on absorbed dose:

$$\epsilon(D) = k(\zeta D + D^2) \tag{2}$$

The coefficient, ζ, in the linear term has a simple microdosimetric interpretation. It is the mean specific energy produced by individual charged particles in the sensitive site. This quantity, ζ, is proportional to the dose average linear energy transfer, $\bar{L}_D$, in those cases where the concept of linear energy trans-

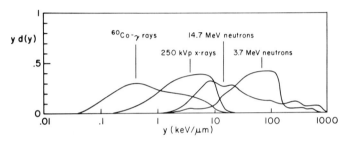

FIG. 4. Distribution of dose in y for single events in spherical tissue regions for various radiations. The curves refer to a diameter of 1 μm (Kellerer and Rossi, 1972). The value of z in rad is equal to 20.4 y.

fer (LET) is applicable. But, the formulation in terms of microdosimetry is more rigorous and accounts for various factors neglected in the LET concept.

Figure 4 gives examples for the actual probability distributions of the energy concentrations produced in a region of 1 μm diameter by individual particles of different radiations. One can express these distributions either in terms of specific energy or in terms of lineal energy, y, which is the microdosimetric analogue of LET (ICRU, 1971). One may note the marked differences between the various radiations, but it is equally interesting to realize that even with one and the same radiation one can have energy distributions that differ by orders of magnitude. In the present context, it is sufficient to point out that the mean value, ζ, of the distributions is the coefficient in the linear term of the dose-effect relation. One can also see, from Eq.(2), that at an absorbed dose equal to ζ the linear component is equal to the quadratic component. Although ζ may be only a few rad for sparsely ionizing radiation, it is equal to hundreds of rad for densely ionizing radiations (Kellerer and Rossi, 1972).

Equation (2) appears to be well established for cellular effects at small doses, such as mutations in plants (Sparrow et al., 1972; Kellerer and Brenot, 1974) or chromosome aberrations in mammalian cells (Schmid et al., 1973; Biola et al., 1971). It furthermore appears that the logarithm of the survival probability in various *in vitro* studies with mammalian cells follows the same linear-quadratic relation (Gray Conf., 1974). The restriction of Eq. (2) is that it does not apply to tissue effects that may depend on complex interactions of damaged cells, partially damaged cells, and undamaged cells. But the analysis of RBE can, as has first been pointed out by Rossi (1970), lead to general statements even in such complex situations.

RBE AS FUNCTION OF ABSORBED DOSE

According to the linear-quadratic dose-effect relation, the RBE of two radiation qualities must be constant in cases when the linear term is dominant for both radiations at very low doses. The asymptotic value of RBE is proportional to the ratio of the mean increments, ζ, for the two radiation qualities, and this ratio can be quite large. Some examples are given below.

The other limiting case is that of large absorbed doses. In this case, the quadratic term dominates for both radiation qualities, and the value of RBE will be equal to one if the constant, k, in Eq. (2) is the same for both radiation qualities. In the intermediate dose range, the RBE will decline as the absorbed dose increases. In the present context, it is sufficient to consider the characteristic dependence of RBE on absorbed dose. But Fig. 5 represents the actual curves from Eq. (2) for different ratios of ζ.

It has been found that these characteristic curves do not only apply to cellular effects but also to effects at the tissue level, including carcinogenesis (Kellerer and Rossi, 1972). This is remarkable as the linear-quadratic, dose-effect relation cannot be postulated for many of these effects. In studies of

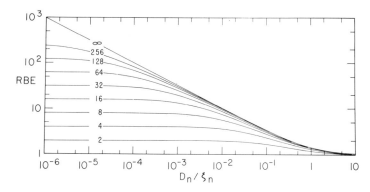

FIG. 5. Relation between RBE and dose resulting from Eq.(2). The dose is given as multiple of the quantity ζ_n; the parameter of the curves is the ratio of ζ_n to the corresponding quantity ζ_x of the reference radiation.

the skin reaction, for example, there is no natural numerical scale of the effect, and the very notion of a linear or a nonlinear, dose-effect relation therefore loses its meaning. In carcinogenesis, one may determine the time to reach a certain incidence, or one may measure the incidence at a specified time; both procedures are meaningful, but they may not lead to the same numerical relations.

The complicating factors that enter into the dose-effect relation are presumably the same, or nearly the same, for different radiation qualities. Accordingly, they cancel if one studies RBE, and this explains the fact that one obtains the characteristic RBE-dose relations even in such complex situations as carcinogenesis.

The induction of mammary tumors in the Sprague-Dawley rat is a particularly clear example of the applicability of RBE-dose analysis. In the studies of the induction of mammary tumors in Sprague-Dawley rats (Shellabarger et al., 1974; Vogel, 1969), the dose dependence of the incidence of tumors up to 11 months after irradiation with neutrons has been found to be highly nonlinear (Rossi and Kellerer, 1972, 1975). The nonlinearity is not of the commonly observed type that corresponds to a quadratic dependence on absorbed dose. Rather, it has been found that the effect is nearly proportional to the square root of the absorbed dose of neutrons. This is the case at small doses of neutrons, in which the fraction of cells traversed by a charged particle is small. One must therefore conclude that the observed effect reflects the interdependence of damaged cells. The nature of this interdependence has not been clarified; it may be related to virus release, to hormonal factors, or it might even be explained by the presence of clusters of sensitive cells, which cannot lead to separate tumors. It is likely that the anomalous dose-effect relation for neutrons is linked to the anomalous nature of the biologic system, i.e., to the high spontaneous incidence of mammary tumors in the Sprague-Dawley rat. More detailed information on this experimental system is presented by Shellabarger (1975) at this conference. The essential point in the present context is that, in spite of physiologic complexities, the RBE depends on absorbed dose in a simple way that can be understood in terms of microdosimetry.

Figure 6 represents the RBE for the induction of mammary tumors by 430 keV neutrons as a function of the neutron dose (Shellabarger et al., 1974). The vertical bars cover those values of RBE excluded on the basis of the statistical analysis. The curve is the best estimate of the neutron RBE. Although these data are based on a preliminary analysis of an experiment just now being terminated, one can already infer extremely large values of RBE at small neutron doses. This means that sparsely ionizing radiations are much less carcinogenic at small doses than are densely ionizing radiations. It also illustrates that it is meaningless to quote values of RBE for a radiation without specifying the level of absorbed dose.

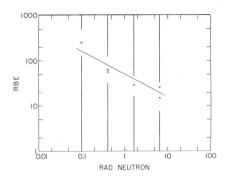

FIG. 6. The RBE of 430 keV neutrons relative to sparsely ionizing radiation for the induction of mammary tumors in the Sprague-Dawley rat (Shellabarger et al., 1974). The vertical bars indicate the ranges of RBE values, which are excluded with statistical significance exceeding 95%.

These considerations are particularly relevant to the problem of the linear extrapolations in radiation protection. The primary mechanisms of radiation carcinogenesis are not sufficiently known to exclude a linear, dose-effect relation for any type of radiation. But we can conclude that linear extrapolations from large to small doses cannot be simultaneously valid for sparsely ionizing radiation and densely ionizing radiation. This follows from the characteristic change of RBE with absorbed dose; if the dose relations for both radiation qualities were linear over a wide dose range, the RBE would have to be constant.

As an example of particular importance one may consider the incidence of leukemia in the survivors of the nuclear explosions in Hiroshima and Nagasaki. A substantial part of the absorbed dose in Hiroshima was due to neutrons, whereas the radiation in Nagasaki was essentially γ-rays. The data on leukemia incidence are not extensive enough to permit a definite statement whether the dose-effect relation in either of the two cities is linear or nonlinear. A nonparametric statistical analysis of the data (Rossi and Kellerer, 1974), however, indicates that the RBE of the radiation in Hiroshima as compared to that in Nagasaki follows the typical dose dependence observed in many other cases. As indicated in Fig. 7, the result is established only on a 86% confidence level. But it cannot be dismissed, since it is in agreement with basic biophysical considerations.

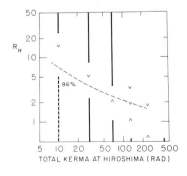

FIG. 7. The RBE of the radiation in Hiroshima for the induction of leukemia compared to that in Nagasaki as a function of kerma in Hiroshima (Rossi and Kellerer, 1974). The bars indicate those values that can be excluded with 95% confidence; the broken bar stands for a level of confidence of 86%. The broken curve is the result of a least-squares fit.

DEPENDENCE OF THE TIME FACTOR ON ABSORBED DOSE

The preceding section has dealt with RBE and its dependence on absorbed dose. An analogous dependence on absorbed dose must apply to the time factor. This will be the object of the present section.

The time factor is defined as the ratio of absorbed doses that produce the same effect at different irradiation times or dose rates. A quantitative treatment of the time factor is complicated by the fact that there is an unlimited number of different temporal distributions of a given absorbed dose. One may compare two dose-effect curves established with two different irradiation times; alternatively, one may compare dose-effect relations established with two different dose rates. The latter method is more commonly applied. The two methods, however, can lead to significantly different results (Kellerer and Rossi, 1972). Further complications arise when one deals with fractionated irradiation. The results presented by Yuhas (*this volume*) illustrate the complexities in the study of the time factor in carcinogenesis. They also illustrate the fact that the time factor depends on absorbed dose and that it is therefore meaningless to quote its value without specifying the absorbed dose. The following remarks will deal with one special case.

Assume that the cellular effect follows the linear-quadratic dependence on absorbed dose expressed in Eq.(2). One may then consider the time factor between irradiation over a short period, during which no recovery of sublethal damage occurs, and irradiation over a long period, during which recovery from sublethal damage is complete, and accordingly, the quadratic component in the absorbed dose can be disregarded. The doses for the short period of irradiation will be designated by D_s, the doses for the long one by D_L. The condition for equal effect is then:

$$\zeta D_L = \zeta D_s + D_s^2 \tag{3}$$

The time factor, *TF*, is equal to D_L/D_s, and therefore one obtains

$$TF = 1 + D_s/\zeta$$

This is represented graphically in Fig. 8. As one would expect, the time factor is largest for sparsely ionizing radiations, i.e., if the mean increment produced by individual charged particles is small. For densely ionizing radiations, where ζ is large compared to the absorbed dose, the time factor is close to one, i.e., the temporal distribution of absorbed dose is of relatively little influence. In all cases, however, the time factor is proportional to absorbed dose. It is therefore meaningless to quote time factors without specifying the effect level or the absorbed dose. Furthermore, one cannot apply time factors observed at high absorbed doses to the small doses that are relevant in radiation protection. Observations at high absorbed doses are relevant to questions of radiation protection only, insofar as they yield information concerning the linear component in the dose-effect relation.

These considerations apply only to cases in which the time factor is due to the recovery of sublethal damage. It has been pointed out that the induction of mammary tumors in the Sprague-Dawley rat involves a more complicated mechanism. The incidence per unit dose decreases with increasing neutron doses, and for X-rays one obtains a nearly linear, rather than a quadratic, dose dependence. A process that counteracts oncogenesis at larger doses should be most effective at short irradiation times. The time factor may therefore be small, or even negative. In fact, Shellabarger (1975) found very little reduction of tumor incidence if a certain X-ray dose is administered over a longer time.

A negative time factor need not always be due to intercellular effects. Borek (*this volume*) presents results to show that even in isolated cells one may deal with a negative time factor. It has been found that the transforma-

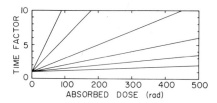

FIG. 8. Time factor for irradiation over a short period versus that over a long period, where complete recovery from sublethal damage occurs. The slope of the lines is proportional to ζ. The values of ζ are: 10, 20, 50, 100, 200, and 500 rads.

tion yield in cloned hamster embryo cells increases if an X-ray dose of 50 or 75 rad is given in two separate fractions instead of a single fraction. There is, as yet, no definite explanation of this interesting phenomenon; but one may surmise that the increased transformation rate at longer irradiation times is due to the fact that misrepair of sublethal damage can then play a greater role.

The occurrence of a negative time factor in the production of bone sarcomas by α particles poses a related problem (Gössner et al., 1975). It is an open question whether, in this case, one deals with intracellular or intercellular mechanisms.

CONCLUSIONS

Three biophysical concepts relevant to radiation carcinogenesis have been considered. Due to the statistical fluctuations of energy deposition on a microscopic scale, the absorbed dose loses its meaning whenever its value is not sufficiently large and whenever one deals with cellular or subcellular regions. Criteria have been given to indicate whether for a given site diameter and a given value of absorbed dose the statistical fluctuations are important. It has been pointed out that, at very small doses, all cellular dose-effect relations must be linear, but that at higher doses, the quadratic term in absorbed dose must be taken into account.

The statistical nature of energy distribution is responsible for the different relative biological effectivenesses of different radiations; it furthermore is responsible for the increase of RBE with decreasing absorbed dose. It has been found that the characteristic dependence of RBE on absorbed dose applies not only to cellular effects, but also to such processes as radiation carcinogenesis, which may depend on the interaction of damaged cells.

Not only RBE but also the time factor depends on absorbed dose. As with RBE, it is therefore meaningless to quote its value for a certain radiation and for a certain biologic system without specifying absorbed dose. The problem of the time factor is in many ways more complicated than the problem of RBE. Microdosimetry permits numerical predictions only as far as one deals with recovery from sublethal damage. Additional cellular and intercellular processes can lead to a negative time factor, i.e., to increased carcinogenesis at the same absorbed dose but at longer irradiation times. These processes are only incompletely understood.

ACKNOWLEDGMENT

This investigation was supported by Contract AT(11–1)3243 from the USAEC and USPHS Research Grant No. CA 12536 from the National Cancer Institute.

REFERENCES

Biola, M. T., LeGo, R., Ducatez, G., and Bourguignon, M. (1971): *Formation de Chromosomes Dicentriques dans les Lymphocytes Humains Soumis In Vitro a un Flux de Rayonnement Mixte (Gamma, Neutrons)*. IAEA, Vienna, pp. 633–645.

Borek, C. (1975): Neoplastic transformations *in vitro* of mammalian cells by X-rays and neutrons. Proceedings of this conference.

Gössner, W., Luz, A., Müller, W. A., and Hug, O. (1974): Bone tumor risk in mice after single and repeated injections of ^{224}Ra. Abstract, *Radiat. Res.*, 59:55 (Nos.).

Gray Conference Proceedings 6th (1974), London. (*In press.*)

ICRU (1971): *Report 19: Radiation Quantities and Units*. International Commission on Radiation Units and Measurements, Washington, D.C.

Kellerer, A. M., and Brenot, J. (1974): On the statistical evaluation of dose-response functions. *Rad. Environ. Biophys.*, 11:1–13.

Kellerer, A. M., and Rossi, H. H. (1972): The theory of dual radiation action. In: *Current Topics in Radiation Research*, Vol. 8, North-Holland, Amsterdam, pp. 85–158.

Rossi, H. H. (1967): Microscopic energy distribution in irradiated matter. I. Basic considerations. In: *Radiation Dosimetry*, Vol. I, Academic Press, New York, pp. 43–92.

Rossi, H. H. (1970): The effects of small doses of ionizing radiation. *Phys. Med. Biol.*, 15:255–262.

Rossi, H. H., and Kellerer, A. M. (1972): Radiation carcinogenesis at low doses. *Science*, 175:200–202.

Rossi, H. H., and Kellerer, A. M. (1974): The validity of risk estimates of leukemia incidence based on japanese data. *Radiat. Res.*, 58:131–140.

Rossi, H. H., and Kellerer, A. M. (1975): Biophysical aspects of radiation carcinogenesis. In: *Cancer, A Comprehensive Treatise*, Vol. 1, pp. 405–439. Plenum Press, New York.

Schmid, E., Rimpl, G., and Bauchinger, M. (1973): Dose-response relation of chromosome aberrations in human lymphocytes after *in vitro* irradiation with 3 MeV electrons. *Radiat. Res.,* 57:228–238.

Shellabarger, C. J., Kellerer, A. M., Rossi, H. H., Goodman, L. J., Brown, R. D., Mills, R. E., Rao, A. R., Shanley, J. P., and Bond, V. P. (1974): *Rat Mammary Carcinogenesis following Neutron or X-radiation. Biological Effects of Neutron Irradiation,* IAEA, Vienna.

Sparrow, A. H., Underbrink, A. G., and Rossi, H. H. (1972): Mutations induced in *Tradescantia* by small doses of X-rays and neutrons: Analysis of dose-response curves. *Science,* 176:916–918.

Vogel, H. H. (1969): Mammary gland neoplasms after fission neutron irradiation. *Nature (London),* 222:1279–1281.

Yuhas, J. M. (1975): Dose-response curves and their alteration by specific mechanisms. Proceedings of this conference.

Biology of Radiation Carcinogenesis, edited by
J. M. Yuhas, R. W. Tennant, and J. D. Regan.
Raven Press, New York © 1976.

Inferences on Radiation Carcinogenesis Revealed by Selected Studies in Animals

Leo K. Bustad, M. Goldman, and L. Rosenblatt

Washington State University, Pullman, Washington 99163 and University of California, Davis, California 95616

During the past two to three decades, we have collectively or independently made many observations on radiation carcinogenesis. We have compared these observations with observations derived from studies of neoplasia in humans, experimental animals, or mammalian tissue culture exposed to various carcinogens. We have selected some of these studies for analysis, in the hope of being enlightened about the complexities and paradoxes that characterize neoplasia. Animal experiments will be emphasized, since human experiences in carcinogenesis are poor "experiments," whether they be studies of the early radiation workers or radiologists, the Hiroshima-Nagasaki survivors, the radium dial painters, the Marshallese, and/or the children exposed to X-irradiation *in utero* or in early life. One common thread characterizing these retrospective studies is that the radiation exposures were generally not well defined.

In most animal experiments, radiation exposure is well defined, and because animals and people exhibit similarity in response, a substantial amount of information about carcinogenesis and the risk of radiation carcinogenesis has been obtained. We selected the experiments we found most familiar and interesting. These studies generally involve heterogeneous populations of animals with long lives exposed to various radionuclides, particularly those related to the nuclear energy fuel cycle. We hope that they will be instructive, relative to the risk of cancer posed by energy-related radiation.

We have selected studies concerned with bone and bone marrow, skin, and thyroid. Before we discuss these studies, however, it may be helpful to review briefly some concepts regarding initiating and promotional events in the neoplastic process. Those of us who have been 39 years old for many years recall the discussions that surrounded the speculations of Berenblum and others regarding the mechanism of carcinogenesis, i.e., two separate components with independent mechanisms that involved initiating and promoting events (Berenblum, 1954). The idea of precarcinogenic action (i.e., initiation) and epicarcinogenic and metacarcinogenic action (i.e., promotion), however, did not originate with Berenblum's reports in 1941 on the carcinogenic action of croton resin and on cocarcinogenic action (Berenblum, 1941a,b). It really appeared earlier when John Hill (1759) suggested that snuff might be an etiologic agent or "bring into action the seeds of the disorder" (i.e., serve as a promoting agent). (This preceded by 16 years, Percivall Pott's report on scrotal cancers in chimney sweeps. Pott, 1775.) Hill stated:

> Whether or not polypusses [cancers], which attend Snuff-takers, are absolutely caused by that custom: or whether the principles of the disorders were there before, and Snuff only irritated the parts, and hastened the mischief, I shall not pretend to determine; but even supposing the latter only to be the case, the damage is certainly more than the indulgence is worth; for who is to say, that the Snuff is not the absolute cause, or that he has not the seeds of such disorder which Snuff will bring into action.

Some of the events that occurred between 1759 and 1941 are interesting to review; Boutwell (1974) referred to these in his recent excellent review of the function and mechanism of promoters of carcinogenesis. Although he addressed the subject in the context of chemical carcinogenesis and skin, his findings are relevant to the subject of radiation-induced carcinogenesis. [See Casarett (1973) for a timely review of radiation carcinogenesis.] The early results of neoplasia induction are similar in both chemical- and radiation-induced cancers, since both examples show a nonlinear dose-response curve. For purposes of discussion, we might consider an initiating step that may require quite small radiation doses and that may never progress to cancer. The promotion step may have both a conversion and a propagation component and probably requires more substantial doses of radiation, either as large single doses or multiple, smaller, yet significant doses of radiation. Propagation involves a regeneration stimulus following either cell-killing doses of radiation or the action of other cytotoxic physical agents or chemicals. Radiation-induced neoplasia of the thyroid and skin in young animals appears to manifest a higher incidence and a shorter latency, although this may not reflect greater sensitivity to the initiating step of neoplasia. The apparent sensitivity may be the result of the remarkable proliferation of cells of the skin and the thyroid (and other tissues) in the very young, which may be sufficient for clone propagation.

BONE-SEEKING, RADIONUCLIDE-INDUCED NEOPLASMS OF BONE AND BONE MARROW

For the past 15 years, University of California–Davis Radiobiology Laboratory personnel have been conducting extensive studies on radiation dose effects in hundreds of dogs fed bone-seeking radiostrontium daily from the onset of fetal ossification to early adulthood (1.5 years old) at seven levels, varying from 0.025 to 36 μCi/day with associated skeletal doses of approximately 0.01 to 13 rads/day. Comparable groups of dogs were given ^{226}Ra in eight intravenous doses from 14 to 18 months of age (Goldman et al., 1969). Other dogs received injections of ^{90}Sr at doses similar to those given the dogs injected at the University of Utah, where an extensive study on radiation dose effects has been conducted over the past 25 years utilizing single injected doses of a number of bone-seeking radionuclides (Mays et al., 1969).

From these studies on bone-seeking radionuclides, and from others performed elsewhere on many species over the past few decades, has evolved an extensive body of knowledge on the onset of neoplasms associated with the bone or bone marrow consequent to chronic radionuclide exposure (Finkel and Biskis, 1968; Bustad et al., 1971; United Nations, 1972; Goldman et al., 1973; Evans, 1974). We have selected studies in which we can compare the effectiveness of low and high linear energy transfer (LET) radiations in producing tissue injury and neoplasia. In order to encourage innovative thinking, we have chosen a method for summarizing dose-effect data. One of the oldest and most used toxicological tools for quantifying dose-effect relationships in nonnuclear carcinogenesis studies is the probit function to linearize the S or sigmoid-shaped response curve following graded exposures (Finney, 1952). Assuming that the deposited radionuclide can be considered a toxicologic agent, and further assuming that the degree of response to the radionuclide need not follow a dose-effect proportionality, i.e., a linear relationship, we have found that the data are better fit by an S-shaped curve and are, therefore, amenable to probit analysis (Rosenblatt and Goldman, 1967).

Following graduated doses of plutonium, radium, or ^{90}Sr in hundreds of beagle dogs at the University of Utah, Dougherty and Rosenblatt (1969), within about a month following the intravenous injection of the radionuclides, noticed that a maximum effect in terms of a depression in the circulating neutrophiles was evident. The relationship of neutropenia to administered dose (microcurie per kilogram injected) was S shaped, and therefore the transformation to a probit model was done with facility. For the first year post-injection, depression of circulating neutrophiles for the three nuclides chosen can be summarized by three parallel lines (Fig. 1). Although the radiation quality and the subsequent microdistribution of the deposited burden vary among the three nuclides, note that, at least initially, the net effect (of injury and repair) in this renewing population of marrow cells is demonstrated by one representative cellular component, that is, the neutrophiles. Similar response curves have been derived for the other cellular elements in circulating blood following bone-seeking radionuclide administration (Bustad et al., 1969; Dougherty and Rosenblatt, 1969). It is significant that despite differences in metabolic pattern and radiation quality, the probit slopes of the response curves are the same. We note that whether the radiation quality is low LET (^{90}Sr), a mixture of low and high LET (^{226}Ra), or high LET (^{239}Pu), the effect on the neutrophile populations of the bone-

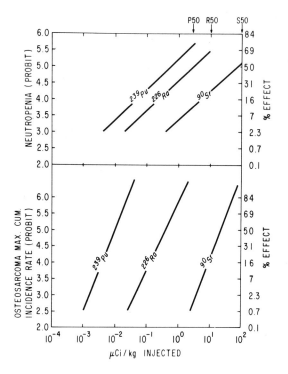

FIG. 1. Peak effect of injected ^{239}Pu, ^{226}Ra, and ^{90}Sr on bone marrow shown as the probit of the neutropenia (upper panel) related to the subsequent estimate of maximum cumulative incidence rate of osteosarcomas in beagles (lower panel). These two effects appear to have parallel slopes independent of radiation qualities.

seeking radionuclides is seen in parallel responses; that is, the incremental increase in dose is nonlinear and the relative effectiveness appears to be the same (Goldman and Rosenblatt, 1975). Obviously, a dose conversion, in rads per microcurie, could rearrange the relative distances between the two parallel curves, but their ranking would remain the same, and the slope would not change regardless of the dosimetric units on the abscissa.

At the University of California–Davis, we have noted a similar parallelism in the index of injury derived from scoring changes in the skeleton as seen by radiographic examination in the case of ^{226}Ra and ^{90}Sr (Williams and Hansen, 1972). Although a qualitative or semiquantitative radiographic scoring of a variety of skeletal lesions and a measure of hematologic alteration in terms of neutropenias or lymphopenias do not necessarily directly measure alterations in *the target* cell population at risk for neoplasm induction, they appear to be reasonable biologic dosimeters that permit a comparison of the three types of radiation under discussion. The effectiveness of the radiation does not appear to be as LET dependent as one might expect from looking at the effects on cells in tissue culture subjected to similar radiation.

Most cell culture studies involve either cloning potential or cellular survival after acute or fractionated high dose-rate exposures. One salient feature of most *in vitro* studies is the derivation of different slopes, i.e., D_0, for cells subjected to high LET versus low LET radiation (Barendsen, 1968). In almost all cases of beta, gamma, or low LET radiation, a shoulder exists at the low-dose end, but such a shoulder is absent following high LET radiation. This suggests that different modalities operate in the mechanisms of cell sterilization as measured by these end points. Largely because of such observations, many workers insist on a linear approach to high LET radiation risk assessment. There are, however, difficulties in linking differences in curves of cell response *in vitro* to varying radiation qualities to predictions of tumor risk. Furthermore, most radiobiologists commonly accept that the traversal of a nucleus by a high LET particle ($\sim 100 \mathrm{kEv}/\mu\mathrm{m}$) almost without exception results in the sterilization of that particular cell, rendering it incapable of successful division. If that is true, then that particular cell cannot be the progenitor of a clone of neoplastic cells. For low LET radiation, particularly at low doses and dose rates, different mechanisms are often postulated, in which a point mutation or an unrepaired single-strand DNA break may be the mechanism (the initiating event) that leads to neoplasia.

A fundamental question to be answered is whether the cell that is irradiated is itself the progenitor of the tumor clone that ultimately is manifested as a cancer. If so, how can one postulate the same mechanism for both types of radiation? Further examination of this question is aided by an examination of Figure 1, in which the probit of the calculated maximum cumulative incidence rate of osteosarcomas in the same dogs, in which the neutropenias were observed earlier, is plotted for the three nuclides of interest. Again, the use of the probit is merely a convenience dictated by the fact that the data themselves determine the shape of the curve. Here we see the final consequences of the cumulative radiation exposure; again note that the three curves for response are parallel, and the relative toxicity (per microcurie) increases in going from ^{90}Sr to ^{226}Ra to ^{239}Pu.

If the analogy derived from tissue culture experiments is correct, one might expect the high and the low LET radiation to be manifested in terms of different slopes for the carcinogenicity of the three radionuclides. The fact that these slopes are parallel leads us to another inference; that is, some common mechanisms may be responsible for the tumorigenicity of the three bone-seeking radionuclides, and these mechanisms appear, to some extent, to be independent of the quality of irradiation. In all three bone-seekers, the distribution of the radiation dose in the tissues at risk is more or less uniform whether the ultimate fate of the radionuclide is a mixture of surface and volume deposition or primarily a deposition on the entire (cellular) surface of the skeletal matrix (i.e., ^{239}Pu) (ICRP, 1967). In all three instances, we may assume that the same kinds of cells are being irradiated with varying degrees of efficiency, and that the "injury" and "repair" that obtain in those microvolumes that ultimately result in neoplasia have common mechanisms. Interestingly, in each of the radionuclides tested, the effects cover a relatively narrow range of dosage; that is, the maximum and minimum effects are almost all obtained within a dosage range of approximately a factor of ten for each radionuclide.

Almost invariably, for most nonnuclear toxic agents that produce neoplasia, if a probit fit to the data appears to obtain, one is forced to reevaluate the relative merits of a possible practical threshold for effect (Evans et al., 1969; Evans, 1974). We do not assume that at levels below this range of a factor of ten in dosage, zero tumor probability exists. We merely suggest that the probability is exceedingly small and may never be mathematically or statistically provable in doses below those shown in Figure 1 for each of the nuclides. It is interesting and perhaps not coincidental that the minimum dosage that appears to be associated with the minimum tumor risk (i.e., incidence) is not too dissimilar from the minimum dosage that produces a neutropenia. This is not to say that neutropenia per se is responsible for tumors, but it is an indirect measure of possible local tissue disruption and injury, and the possibility of a change in a common stem cell may be worth considering. We suggest that the local tissue events associated with attempts at repair of this "injury" might have a higher correlation with tumor risk than the direct radiation effect on cells.

Some further inferences regarding dose rate, site, cell killing, repair, cell density, and appearance and location of bone tumors have been derived from the studies of Nilsson on mice receiving injections of ^{90}Sr (Nilsson, 1970). He measured the number of osteoblasts on the surface of bone trabeculae and noted a nonlinear dose responsiveness in terms of depletion of osteoblasts as a function of dosage and time. At "the most effective" radiation exposures for osteosarcoma production, the osteoblastic concentration per unit length of trabecular surface exhibited recovery following an initial depression, suggesting a renewal or repair of the population followed by a rapid appearance of tumors. One inference from this study might be that an increase in radiation dose rate could be expected to increase the fraction of surviving cells that might be recruited into a "renewal status," and might increase the transit time per cell; but it might have minimal effects on other local factors (Goldman and Bustad, 1972). Nilsson's data provide indirect support for a hypothesis about local tissue environmental change; that is, local tissue destruction is a major factor in radiation carcinogenesis, at least with respect to sarcoma induction following bone-seeking radionuclide exposure.

Another important observation about bone and bone marrow concerns changes in karyotype. In a recent, very helpful review, Pitot (1974) suggested that, except for the Philadelphia chromosome, no specific karyotype pattern has been associated with neoplasia. Relative to this suggestion, we have observed two interesting phenomena in two radiation-induced neoplasms in the dog. The first is an extra chromosome that appeared in two lines of radiation-induced granulocytic leukemia (Shifrine et al., 1973). The other is a hypodiploid alteration in all radiation-induced osteogenic sarcomas (Wolf et al., 1972), as well as in several spontaneous osteogenic sarcomas from dogs from the University of California–Davis Veterinary Teaching Hospital. In all the cells from more than 50 osteosarcomas, a hypodiploid pattern of 45 to 55 chromosomes was observed, 15 to 25 of which were meta or submetacentric chromosomes or a mixed population comprising the hypodiploid line and its tetraploid. This compares with the normal canine karyotype of 78 chromosomes: 38 pair of acrocentric autosomes and two submetacentric sex chromosomes. The appearance of consistently similar karyotypes in both radiation-induced and spontaneously occurring osteosarcomas strongly suggests that the karyotypic alteration is not a primary radiation effect.

NEOPLASIA OF THE SKIN

Skin cancer was one of the first forms of radiation-induced tumors to be described in humans. Cancer appeared with high frequency on the hands, forearms, and faces of early radiologists and technicians whose skin had been damaged and had previously exhibited radiation dermatitis. By 1911, over 50 cases of skin tumors had been described. The incidence of these tumors fortunately decreased as operating personnel recognized radiation hazards and established stringent precautions. But the latency of skin tumors is very long. In humans, it seems to vary from 6 to 56 years, with a suggested average of 13 to 26 years (Henshaw et al., 1951; Van Cleave, 1968). In animals, it is correspondingly less, being somewhat related to their life-span.

Our studies of skin tumor induction have involved mainly the application of beta-emitting sources on or in the skin of rabbits, sheep, and swine at doses in the kilorad range (George and Bustad, 1966). Plutonium-239, too, was injected into over 300 sites on white pigs (Cable et al., 1962; McClellan, 1966), which were maintained up to a decade or more, but no tumors were observed. Only one possible tumor of the skin (an "early squamous cell carcinoma") has ever been observed in our swine, the skin of which was exposed to radiation, and that in one of several exposed to over 19,000 μCi hr from a radioruthenium particle 12.5 years previously (Karagianes et al., 1968).

Although we observed few neoplasms in the limited number of rabbits and sheep the skin of which was irradiated, neoplasms were observed in areas manifesting grossly observable lesions following exposure to 16,000 rads (George and Bustad, 1966). Leith et al. (1973) also thought skin tumors in an experiment involving hundreds of mice probably depended on acute skin damage following helium-ion irradiation.

As has been described by Albert et al. (1967a,b) as well as Leith et al. (1973), the depth of irradiation with heavy particles or electrons is important in tumor induction. Albert et al. (1967a,b) suggested that tumor formation may depend on irreparable damage to the hair follicles; substantial radiation exposure of the basal cell layer of the epidermis and epidermal appendages, in order to block effective repair, is required to produce such damage. With damage or death of cells, the control mechanism between contiguous cells is disturbed.

We do not have a ready explanation for the very low incidence of skin tumors in swine. The latency, however, may approximate (or exceed) their life-span. If a principal source of skin tumors is hair follicle cells, as Albert et al. (1967a,b) suggest, sparsely haired swine may be expected to have a low incidence of skin tumors. The reported incidence of skin tumors in mice and rats is much higher than that in larger animals. For risk assessment, therefore, the rodent may not be a good model, since the incidence of radiation-induced tumors in humans appears to resemble the lower incidence observed in large animals. Enough work, however, has not been done in large animals to select a good model for risk assessment.

RADIATION-INDUCED THYROID NEOPLASIA

For over three decades, radioiodine (chiefly ^{131}I) has been widely used in diagnostic and therapeutic medicine, and thousands of humans and experimental animals have received doses varying from a few microcurie to hundreds of millicurie. As a result of these exposures, as well as of accidental exposures to fallout in the South Pacific (Conard et al., 1970), many thyroid neoplasms have been observed. The most extended study with radioiodine was one using sheep at Hanford Laboratories from 1950 to 1965. Many of the animals were given daily doses of radioiodine for their entire lifetime (up to 11 years). The doses utilized ranged from 0.15 to 1800 μCi/day (Bustad et al., 1957). Single doses in the 5 to 15 mCi range were also utilized (Marks et al., 1962).

The most effective doses for inducing adenomas in sheep seemed to be 1 to 10 rads/day to the thyroid for four to six years, for total thyroid doses of 2,000 rads or more. Shorter-term studies involving single or multiple doses of radioiodine have been conducted in rodents, dogs, pigs, and cows (Bustad et al., 1957; Marks and Bustad, 1963; Garner, 1964; McClellan and Bustad, 1964; Bustad et al., 1965). The preponderance of tumors appear to be adenomas.

The incidence of neoplasms has been very high in sheep and humans (as well as rodents) with single doses of equivalent ^{131}I rads of several thousand rads. The incidence seemed to fall after exposure to severely damaging to ablative doses ($> 10,000$ to 30,000 rads in sheep and humans). It is suggested that, with higher doses of irradiation, cellular damage to the follicular cells is of such magnitude as to preclude extensive proliferation in response to stimuli. With lower, but still damaging levels of irradiation, the cells retain the capacity to respond to stimuli by proliferation (and adenoma production).

It appears that following damaging doses of radioiodine, the life-span of the affected follicular cells (normally very long) may be significantly shortened. These cells, however, may show normal or near-normal thyroid function for a time following damaging doses of radiation as determined by thyroid uptake of tracer doses of [131]I. But, with time, these cells die and appear not to be replaced. This is substantiated by our studies in young adult sheep given single 5- to 15-mCi doses of ^{131}I and then followed for many years. These sheep, which appeared initially euthyroid, eventually manifested signs of hypothyroidism. More recently, this phenomenon has been observed in hyperthyroid humans previously treated with millicurie amounts of radioiodine (Nofal et al., 1966; see also Werner, 1971).

It has been thought for some time that radioiodine probably induces neoplasia by direct irradiation of the follicular cells and subsequent stimulation by thyroid stimulating hormone (TSH). Considerable data substantiate this suggestion; tumors, however, have been observed in animals in which damage to the thyroid may not have been sufficient to increase the normal circulatory level of TSH perceptibly. Perhaps sufficient TSH is normally present to stimulate the cellular proliferation that is necessary for tumor development.

Before we leave the subject of radioiodine and the thyroid, it is well that we address the subject of the Marshallese children (Conard et al., 1970). It is generally known that their reported thyroid dose was less than the several thousands of rads we found so effective in thyroid tumor induction in sheep and rats. Many workers, in discussing the Marshallese, speak of the very high incidence of thyroid neoplasms as examples of tumor induction by low levels of irradiation. The estimate of the highest radiation dose to the thyroids of Marshallese children was 1,400 rads plus approximately 175 to 200 R of whole-body irradiation. This is not, as some would have it, a low dose of radiation; furthermore, it was experienced over a short period of time. Many seem to forget that a major contributor to the thyroid dose was the short-lived radioiodines that emit very energetic beta particles. These radioiodines are more biologically effective than [131]I. On the basis of the very careful work of Walinder et al. (1972), as well as the work of others and ourselves, we are moved to estimate thyroid dose in equivalents of [131]I (Bustad, 1973). It should be recalled that the Marshallese were removed from their residences two days after the detonation, a period in which the short-lived iodines predominated. Assuming that 50 to 75% of the thyroid dose was due to the short-lived radioiodines (Harrison, 1961), which may be at least three times more effective than ^{131}I, and to acute gamma (or x-) irradiation which may be five to ten times as effective as [131]I (McClellan et al., 1963; Saenger et al., 1963), the equivalent rad (in ^{131}I rads) would be over 4,000 rads. This seems to be a more reasonable estimate in view of the effects noted, which included frank thyroid damage. If some children were nursing or sucking on various objects, including their fingers, they probably received an even larger dose. On the basis of extensive animal work with ^{131}I, we could not explain the extensive thyroid damage that occurred in the Marshallese if the thyroid dose were only 1,500 rads. Recalculating the dose establishes the agreement we have come to expect among mammalian species, including humans, on the basis of other comparative studies. Our work with dogs, simulating the Marshallese exposures, also agrees with these suppositions. In dogs exposed to a thyroid dose of approximately 1,500 rads from ^{131}I administered with or without concomitant acute whole-body exposure to 175 R x-irradiation, or to a thyroid dose of 4,500 rads from administered ^{131}I, an effect on thyroid function was observed only in the 4,500 rads group up to 6 years following exposure (Book and Bustad, 1973).

CONCLUSION

The studies reviewed include those having to do with bone, bone marrow, skin and thyroid. The induction of cancers in animals following exposures to a variety of radionuclides deposited with different metabolic patterns regarding retention and dose rate suggests that under conditions of chronic radiation exposure, tissues at risk undergo a sequence of cellular injury and repair, the net effect of which can occasionally be inferred by examination of certain parameters *in vivo*. Furthermore, these crude indices of injury-repair appear to have a relationship, or at least they can be correlated, with the subsequent appearance of tumors in and near the irradiated tissue volumes. It appears from some of these data that the quality of irradiation, that is, whether it is low or high LET, may be the predominant determinant on the shape and nature of the response curve, be it the net injury repair curve of tissues during the course of irradiation or the subsequent relative risk pattern for tumor development in experiments in which the doses have been graded.

Obviously, we have not reached a state in which the study of the best cancer mechanisms can be performed in experimental animals. Instead, we can attempt to collectively integrate bits and pieces derived from a series of studies. Of interest are some of the common threads seen in experiments in our own and other laboratories concerning the shape of the dose-response curve for tumor induction. To the extent that the shape of these curves is informative and suggestive of possible mechanisms of effect, we may be able to develop certain hypotheses. Hypotheses derived from an assessment of earlier data are not tenable in the light of our recent studies; indirect reasoning suggests other hypotheses might be more appropriate.

One of the more interesting inferences derived from animal studies relates to the balance between local cellular destruction following internal emitter dose absorption and possible subsequent tumor induction at these local sites.

It appears that, regarding the effects of internal emitters, the injury and the neoplasm are usually in the same general location. Abscopal effect is usually seen only in certain tumors involved with endocrine feedback, such as hypophyseal tumors following ablation of the thyroid. An attractive hypothesis, which we believe illuminates the sequence of initiation and promotion resulting in tumors, concerns the possible role of local tissue destruction as an extrinsic factor in the subsequent development of neoplasms. Much has been written about this role, and the general consensus seems to be that such local tissue destruction is not usually manifested until the radiation dose has reached a certain practical threshold value, and that this value is usually one that can be detected by careful histologic examination of irradiated tissue for pathologic change. At exceedingly high doses, the destruction can be so complete that the degree of cell sterilization and killing results in few remaining intact cells, and they possess limited replication potential; possibly this means an actual diminution of the tumor risk. The high dosage domain is sometimes jokingly referred to as "incandescent" radiation biology or the "biological Cherenkov reaction." Thus, in a practical sense, one is confined to the range of exposures or doses that results in a less than complete expression of neoplasia, that is, the range at which the percentage or incidence rate is below 100% and the minimal rates are at least sufficiently high as to eliminate the perpetual discussion of the significance of differences between small numbers. In a practical sense, we are talking about incidences in excess of 10% of the "spontaneous" level.

Although we suffer from a great paucity of information on this complex subject, there is no dearth of hypotheses. Two of the most commonly emphasized ones are the somatic mutation and radiation activation of a virus hypotheses (Kaplan, 1956). Both of them were well reviewed by van Bekkum (1974) and Upton (1974) at the Vth International Congress of Radiation Research in Seattle. At that meeting, van Bekkum further postulated that transformation occurs following the uptake of small pieces of DNA, which function as genes involved in proliferation of normal cells. He suggests that, if such genes are incorporated at the wrong sites in the DNA, that is, sites sufficiently distant from the appropriate repressor genes, they may release the cell from normal inhibition, thus leading to uncontrolled proliferation. He suggests further that the incorporation of transformed genes might occur during normal DNA synthesis, but the chance for such a mishap during repair of DNA following radiation damage would be substantially increased. He further proposes that the antigenic properties of such transformed cells would be expected to differ among the various tumors, since the process of DNA damage and repair by DNA fragments could vary considerably. It has been shown that genetic information can be introduced into cells to induce neoplastic transformation. Nucleic acid from oncogenic viruses is known to be integrated into the DNA of the host cell. Furthermore, with the discovery of reverse transcriptase (Temin and Mizutani, 1970; Baltimore, 1970), we know that tumor viral information can be integrated into the host genome. Of related interest is the oncogenic theory of Huebner and Todaro (1969), in which they propose that RNA or DNA oncogenic viruses transform cells that may not manifest neoplasia until appropriate manipulation occurs (e.g., by physical or chemical means).

Many authors have proposed that radiation-induced cancer may result from depressed immunocompetence (Kaplan, 1971; Cottier, 1974). Another interesting proposal is that cancer results from a radiation- and/or chemical-induced change in protein, RNA, or the cytoplasmic membranes, which results in a permanent change in expression (Pitot and Heidelberger, 1963; Boutwell, 1974; Pitot, 1974). Other hypotheses relate to cellular disorganization or damage and hormonal imbalance and/or stimulation. Numerous hypotheses reflect the complexity of the process and our abysmal ignorance regarding it. In view of this conclusion, we are moved to propose yet another cause of cancer under the heading, "Does No. 2 Cause Cancer?" Appropriately, this title appeared in Mad Magazine in December, 1967.

> No. 2 will probably deny that his cars bring on Cancer. He has that right.
> But Hertz has been busy the past few months digging up evidence to the contrary. We're not alarmists, but we think people should know that a recent survey shows that more doctors use Hertz than No. 2.
> Now why would a doctor pick one rent-a-car company over another? Obviously, because one is less dangerous to his health.
> And what's the worst health danger in the country today? Cancer, that's what!
> Just put two and two together, and one awful, horrible staggering fact emerges: No. 2 is a National Menace.
> No. 2 will probably not like this ad. He'll scream that he doesn't cause Cancer.
> Well, all Hertz had to say is: If No. 2 doesn't cause Cancer, let him prove it!

The reason we quote this is to remonstrate with you who are tempted to take yourself and your pet theory too seriously. We must keep our sense of humor and realize how little we know about this complex problem. We can only be humble about our knowledge and our hypotheses and at the same time be strident in our approach to our governing bodies and granting agencies, making certain they understand that we cannot obtain the much-needed information without increased research support. Also, we have the heavy responsibility to plan our studies well, to construct our hypotheses carefully, and to utilize them for designing experiments and not for hitting our friends and our opponents over the head.

In closing, we want to make a final point or two. We feel the greatest progress will be made if we conscientiously continue the type of exchange that characterizes this meeting among the many disciplines in which subcellular, cellular, tissue, and organ systems, and whole animals of varying species are studied; and if we listen to one another carefully. Most important in the final analysis is what happens in the heterogeneous whole animal and the whole human. We must continue to ask ourselves if what we are doing has relevance to the objective of understanding cancer in humans and animals. Unfortunately, however, understanding cancer doesn't cure it. We must develop effective means both to prevent and to control it. That is our most important challenge.

ACKNOWLEDGMENT

This work was supported by the United States Energy Research and Development Administration.

SUMMARY

Studies of heterogeneous populations of animals with long lives and humans, exposed to various radionuclides and particularly those related to the nuclear energy fuel cycle, are instructive for deriving inferences relative to a challenge posed by Dr. Alder in his introduction; i.e., How great a carcinogenic risk does this energy-related radiation pose? The characteristics and inferences of these studies include:

1. Dose-response curves for various radionuclides [with varying half-lives, qualities of radiation (LET), and metabolic characteristics] provide fascinating similarities regardless of the species studied or the tissues at risk.

2. Continuous exposure of the tissues at risk at rates that are low (<1 rads/hr, i.e., <0.01 rads/min) are emphasized instead of the more commonly utilized acute or fractionated external irradiation exposures.

3. Induction of neoplasms is confined chiefly to the irradiated tissues.

4. Over a relatively wide dose range, the response curve for tumor incidence is not linear.

5. Tumor appearance times are diminished with increasing dose rate.

6. Radiation doses sufficient to effect injury in target tissues may be quite carcinogenic; with no detectable injury, the tumor risk is minimal (and may even be absent).

7. Chronic radiation leads to chronic injury and repair, the consequences of which may be neoplasia.

8. The population restoration processes, which may be associated with carcinogenesis, appear to require a threshold or minimal injury, and the rates of such renewal may be related to cancer risk.

9. For a given cellular repopulation rate, there is an associated risk that may be independent of radiation quality (e.g., LET); the risk of tumor appearance may be highly correlated with the rate of cellular repopulation.

10. Within the tissues at risk, there are populations of pluripotential cells from which the neoplasms may arise. The repair and restoration phase may be more important than the initial injury. Such microenvironmental alterations might play a major role in the "promotional phase" of carcinogenesis.

11. Viruses may not be involved in all radiation-induced neoplasms.

12. Radiation-induced neoplasms may appear in the absence of any detectable changes in the immune system.

The elucidation of the mechanisms involved in carcinogenesis requires the further development of correlative studies involving molecular, cellular, tissue, organ, and animal studies and a continuing dialogue among the workers in the disciplines involved.

ACKNOWLEDGMENTS

We appreciate the helpfulness of Dr. Steven Book, Lynne Cuddy, Linda Hines, Glenn Horstman, Marion Lundquist, Dr. Dennis Mahlum, Dr. Harvey Ragan, Dr. Jean Starkey, and H. G. Wolf in the preparation of this manuscript.

REFERENCES

Albert, R. E., Burns, F. J., and Heimbach, R. D. (1967a): The effect of penetration depth of electron radiation on skin tumor formation in the rat. *Radiat. Res.*, 30:515–524.

Albert, R. E., Burns, F. J., and Heimbach, R. D. (1967b): The association between chronic radiation damage of the hair follicles and tumor formation in the rat. *Radiat. Res.*, 30:590–599.

Baltimore, D. (1970): RNA-dependent DNA polymerase in virions of RNA tumour viruses. *Nature*, 226:1209–1211.

Barendsen, G. W. (1968): Responses of cultured cells, tumors and normal tissues to radiations of different linear energy transfer. In: *Current Topics in Radiation Research*, edited by M. Ebert and A. Howard, pp. 293–356. North-Holland Publishing Co., Amsterdam.

Berenblum, I. (1941a): The cocarcinogenic action of croton resin. *Cancer Res.*, 1:44–48.

Berenblum, I. (1941b): Mechanism of carcinogenesis; Study of significance of cocarcinogenic action and related phenomena. *Cancer Res.*, 1:807–814.

Berenblum, I. (1954): A speculative review: The probable nature of promoting action and its significance in the understanding of the mechanism of carcinogenesis. *Cancer Res.*, 14:471–477.

Book, S. A., and Bustad, L. K. (1973): Effects of radioiodine and x-irradiation on beagle pups. In: *Annual Report, Radiobiology Laboratory*, UCD, 472–120, pp. 137–139. Davis, California.

Boutwell, R. K. (1974): The function and mechanism of promoters of carcinogenesis. *CRC Crit. Rev. Toxicol.*, 3:419–445.

Bustad, L. K. (1973): The problem and paradox that is cancer. In: *Radionuclide Carcinogenesis*, edited by C. L. Sanders, R. H. Busch, J. E. Ballou, and D. D. Mahlum, pp. 487–495. Proceedings of the Twelfth Annual Hanford Symposium at Richland, Washington, May 10–12, 1972.

Bustad, L. K., George, L. A., Jr., Marks, S., Warner, D. E., Barnes, C. M., Herde, K. E., and Kornberg, H. A. (1957): Biological effects of I-131 continuously administered to sheep. *Radiat. Res.*, 6:380–413.

Bustad, L. K., Goldman, M., Rosenblatt, L. S., Mays, C. W., Hetherington, N. W., Bair, W. J., McClellan, R. O., Richmond, C. R., and Rowland, R. E. (1971): Evaluation of long-term effects of exposure to internally deposited radionuclides. In: *Peaceful Uses of Atomic Energy*, Vol. 2, pp. 125–140. United Nations, New York, and IAEA, Vienna.

Bustad, L. K., Goldman, M., Rosenblatt, L. S., McKelvie, D. H., and Hertzendorf, I. I. (1969): Hematopoietic changes in beagles fed ^{90}Sr. In: *Delayed Effects of Bone-seeking Radionuclides*, edited by C. W. Mays, W. S. S. Jee, R. D. Lloyd, B. J. Stover,

J. H. Dougherty, and G. N. Taylor, pp. 279–291. University of Utah Press, Salt Lake City, Utah.

Bustad, L. K., McClellan, R. O., and Garner, R. J. (1965): The significance of radio-nuclide contamination in ruminants. In: *Physiology of Digestion in the Ruminant,* edited by R. W. Dougherty, pp. 131–146. Butterworths, Washington.

Cable, J. W., Horstman, V. G., Clarke, W. J., and Bustad, L. K. (1962): Effects of intradermal injections of plutonium in swine. *Health Phys.,* 8:629–634.

Casarett, G. W. (1973): Pathogenesis of radionuclide-induced tumors. In: *Radionuclide Carcinogenesis,* edited by C. L. Sanders, R. H. Busch, J. E. Ballou, and D. D. Mahlum, pp. 1–14. Proceedings of the Twelfth Annual Hanford Symposium at Richland, Washington, May 10–12, 1972.

Conard, R. A., Dobyns, B. M., and Sutow, W. W. (1970): Thyroid neoplasia as late effect of exposure to radioactive iodine in fallout. *JAMA,* 214:316–324.

Cottier, H. (1974): Immunological deficiency states and malignancy. In: *Interaction of Radiation and Host Immune Defense Mechanisms in Malignancy.* Conference, March 1974, Greenbrier, W. Va. BNL 50418, Brookhaven National Laboratory Report.

Dougherty, J. H., and Rosenblatt, L. S. (1969): Leukocyte depression in beagles injected with [226]Ra or [239]Pu. In: *Delayed Effects of Bone-seeking Radionuclides,* edited by C. W. Mays, W. S. S. Jee, R. D. Lloyd, B. J. Stover, J. H. Dougherty, and G. N. Taylor, pp. 457–470. University of Utah Press, Salt Lake City, Utah.

Evans, R. D. (1974): Radium in man. *Health Phys.,* 27:497–510.

Evans, R. D., Keane, A. T., Kolenkow, R. J., Neal, W. R., and Shanahan, M. M. (1969): Radiogenic tumors in the radium and mesothorium cases studied at M.I.T. In: *Delayed Effects of Bone-seeking Radionuclides,* edited by C. W. Mays, W. S. S. Jee, R. D. Lloyd, B. J. Stover, J. H. Dougherty, and G. N. Taylor, pp. 157–194. University of Utah Press, Salt Lake City, Utah.

Finkel, M. P., and Biskis, B. O. (1968): Experimental induction of osteosarcomas. *Prog. Exp. Tumor Res.,* 10:72–111.

Finney, D. J. (1952): *Probit Analysis,* 2nd ed. Cambridge University Press, Cambridge, England.

Garner, R. J. (1964): Comparative early and late effects of single and prolonged exposure to radioiodine in young and adults of various animal species—A review. In: *Biology of Radioiodine,* edited by L. K. Bustad. Pergamon Press, New York, pp. 253–259.

George, L. A., and Bustad, L. K. (1966): Comparative effects of beta irradiation of swine, sheep, and rabbit skin. In: *Swine in Biomedical Research,* edited by L. K. Bustad and R. O. McClellan, pp. 491–500. Pacific Northwest Laboratory, Richland, Washington.

Goldman, M., and Bustad, L. K. (1972): Proceedings synthesis. In: *Biomedical Implications of Radiostrontium Exposure,* edited by M. Goldman and L. K. Bustad, pp. 1–16. Proceedings of a symposium held at Davis, California, February 22–24, 1971.

Goldman, M., Della Rosa, R. J., and McKelvie, D. H. (1969): Metabolic, dosimetric, and pathological consequences in the skeletons of beagles fed [90]Sr. In: *Delayed Effects of Bone-seeking Radionuclides,* edited by C. W. Mays, W. S. S. Jee, R. D. Lloyd, B. J. Stover, J. H. Dougherty, and G. N. Taylor, pp. 61–67. University of Utah Press, Salt Lake City, Utah.

Goldman, M., and Rosenblatt, L. S. (1975): Some speculations in the role of radiation quality on "injury" and tumor risk from bone-seeking radionuclides, In: *Annual Report, Radiobiology Laboratory,* UCD, 472–122, pp. 165–167. Davis, California.

Goldman, M., Rosenblatt, L. S., Hetherington, N. W., and Finkel, M. P. (1973): Scaling dose, time, and incidence of radium-induced osteosarcomas of mice and dogs to man. In: *Radionuclide Carcinogenesis,* edited by C. L. Sanders, R. H. Busch, J. E. Ballou, and D. D. Mahlum, pp. 347–357. Proceedings of the Twelfth Annual Hanford Symposium at Richland, Washington, May 10–12, 1972.

Harrison, G. E. (1961): Calculation of the dose to the intestinal tract, thyroid and skeleton when mixed fission products are fed to a rabbit. In: *Progress in Nuclear Energy, Series* VI, Biol. Sci., Vol. 3, edited by J. F. Loutit and R. S. Russell, p. 60–68. Pergamon.

Henshaw, P. S., Snider, R. S., and Riley, E. F., Jr. (1951): Aberrant tissue developments of rats exposed to beta rays. Late effects of p^{32} beta rays. In: *Effects of Beta Radiation,* edited by R. E. Zirkle. McGraw-Hill, New York, pp. 227–228.

Hill, J. (1759): Cautions against the immoderate use of snuff. Founded on the known qualities of the Tobacco plant . . . and enforced by instances of persons who have perished . . . of diseases occasioned . . . by its use. London.

Huebner, R. J., and Todaro, G. J. (1969): Oncogenes of RNA viruses as determinants of cancer. *Proc. Natl. Acad. Sci. USA,* 64:1087–1094.

International Commission on Radiological Protection (1967): *A Review of the Radiosensitivity of the Tissues in Bone.* Publication 11. Pergamon Press, London.

Kaplan, H. S. (1957): *The Pathogenesis of Experimental Lymphoid Tumors in Mice,* p. 127. BEGG Proc. 2nd Canadian Cancer Research Conference, 1957. Academic Press, New York.

Kaplan, H. S. (1971): Role of immunologic disturbance in human oncogenesis: Some facts and fancies. *Br. J. Cancer,* 25:620–634.

Karagianes, M. T., Howard, E. B., and Palotay, J. L. (1968): Late effects of skin irradiation. In: *Pacific Northwest Laboratory Annual Report for 1967,* Vol. 1, edited by R. C. Thompson, P. Teal, and E. G. Swezea, pp. 10–11. Richland, Washington.

Leith, J. T., Welch, G. P., Schilling, W. A., and Tobias, C. A. (1973): Life-span measurements and skin tumorigenesis in mice following total-body helium-ion irradiation of the skin to different maximum penetration depths. In: *Radionuclide Carcinogenesis,* edited by C. L. Sanders, R. H. Busch, J. E. Ballou, and D. D. Mahlum, pp. 90–105. Proceedings of the Twelfth Annual Hanford Symposium at Richland, Washington, May 10–12, 1972.

Marks, S., and Bustad, L. K. (1963): Thyroid neoplasms in sheep fed radioiodine. *J. Natl. Cancer Inst.,* 30:661–673.

Marks, S., Seigneur, L. J., Hackett, P. L., Morrow, R. J., Horstman, V. G., and Bustad, L. K. (1962): Effects of the administration of single doses of I-131 to sheep of various ages. *Am. J. Vet. Res.,* 23:725–730.

Mays, C. W., Dougherty, T. F., Taylor, G. N., Lloyd, R. D., Stover, B. J., Jee, W. S. S., Christensen, W. R., Dougherty, J. H., and Atherton, D. R. (1969): Radiation-induced bone cancer in beagles. In: *Delayed Effects of Bone-Seeking Radionuclides,* edited by C. W. Mays, W. S. S. Jee, R. D. Lloyd, B. J. Stover, J. H. Dougherty, and G. N. Taylor, pp. 387–408. Salt Lake City, Utah.

McClellan, R. O. (1966): Use of swine in radionuclide toxicity studies. In: *Swine in Biomedical Research,* edited by L. K. Bustad and R. O. McClellan, pp. 447–462. Richland, Washington.

McClellan, R. O., and Bustad, L. K. (1964): Toxicity of significant radionuclides in large animals. *Ann. N.Y. Acad. Sci.,* 3:793–811.

McClellan, R. O., Clarke, W. J., Ragan, H. A., Wood, D. H., and Bustad, L. K. (1963): Comparative effects of I-131 and x-irradiation on sheep thyroids. *Health Phys.,* 9:1363–1368.

Nilsson, A. (1970): Pathologic effects of different doses of radiostrontium in mice. Dose effect relationship in ^{90}Sr-induced bone tumours. *Acta Radiol. [Ther.],* 9:155–176.

Nofal, M. M., Beierwaltes, W. H., and Patno, M. E. (1966): Treatment of hyperthyroidism with sodium iodide I-131: A 16-year experience. *JAMA,* 197:605–610.

Pitot, H. C. (1974): Neoplasia: A somatic mutation or a heritable change in cytoplasmic membranes? *J. Natl. Cancer Insti.,* 53:905–911.

Pitot, H. C., and Heidelberger, C. (1963): Metabolic regulatory circuits and carcinogenesis. *Cancer Res.,* 23:1694–1700.

Pott, P. (1775): Chirurgical observations relative to the cataract, the polypus of the nose, the cancer of the scrotum, the different kind of ruptures and the mortification of the toes and feet. London.

Rosenblatt, L. S., and Goldman, M. (1967): The use of probit analysis to estimate dose effects on postirradiation leukocyte depressions (a preliminary report). *Health Phys.,* 13:795–798.

Saenger, E. L., Seltzer, R. A., Sterling, T. D., and Kereiakes, J. G. (1963): Carcinogenic effects of I^{131} compared with x-irradiation—a review. *Health Phys.,* 9:1371.

Shifrine, M., Wolf, H. G., Taylor, N. J., Galligan, S. J., Wilson, F. D., Colgrove, G. S., and Bustad, L. K. (1973): Transplantation of radiation-induced canine myelomono-cytic leukemia. In: *Unifying Concepts of Leukemia,* edited by R. M. Dutcher and L. Chieco-Bianchi, pp. 158–169. Karger, Basel.

Temin, H. M., and Mizutani, S. (1970): RNA-dependent DNA polymerase in virions of Rous sarcoma virus. *Nature,* 226:1211–1213.

United Nations Scientific Committee on the Effects of Atomic Radiation (1972): *Ionizing Radiation: Levels and Effects,* Vol. 2, pp. 379–401.

Upton, A. C. (1974): *The Interplay of Viruses and Radiation in Carcinogenesis.* Fifth International Congress of Radiation Research, Seattle, Washington, July 14–19.

Van Bekkum, D. W. (1974): *Mechanisms of Radiation Carcinogenesis.* Fifth International Congress of Radiation Research, Seattle, Washington.

Van Cleave, C. D. (1968): *Late Somatic Effects of Ionizing Radiation.* Div. of Tech. Information, USAEC, Washington, D.C., pp. 117–120.

Walinder, G., Jonsson, C. J., and Sjöden, A. M. (1972): Dose rate dependence in the goitrogen stimulated mouse thyroid. *Acta Radiol. [Ther.],* 11:24–36.

Werner, S. C., editor (1971): *The Thyroid: A Fundamental and Clinical Text,* 3rd ed. Harper & Row, New York.

Williams, J. R., and Hansen, R. J. (1972): Radiographic changes in skeletons of beagles administered ^{90}Sr and [226]Ra. In: *Annual Report, Radiology Laboratory,* UCD 472–119, pp. 86–88. Davis, California.

Wolf, H. G., Taylor, N. J., Galligan, S. J., and Shiomoto, K. (1972): Karotypic alteration associated with radiation-induced and spontaneously occurring canine osteosarcomas. In: *Annual Report, Radiobiology Laboratory,* UCD 472–119, pp. 91–94. Davis, California.

Biology of Radiation Carcinogenesis, edited by
J. M. Yuhas, R. W. Tennant, and J. D. Regan.
Raven Press, New York © 1976.

Modifying Factors in Rat Mammary Gland Carcinogenesis

Claire J Shellabarger

Medical Department, Brookhaven National Laboratory, Upton, New York 11973

Mammary tumors often appear in large numbers in rats following exposure to ionizing radiation, administration of chemical carcinogens, modification of hormonal status, combinations of these manipulations, or often, simply, as the result of old age. Further, mammary tumor incidence, either experimental or spontaneous, depends strongly on the strain and sex of the rat chosen for study. Although an enormous literature exists on all of these topics, simple generalizations are not easily made, largely because few systematic comparison studies have been done, and partially because many papers fail to mention the strain of rat used, animal care conditions, statistics, or pathologic criteria. In attempting to deal with the topic of *modifications* of rat mammary gland carcinogenesis, I will emphasize reports that are both comparative in nature and contain sufficient detail of materials and methods so that the results can be evaluated. In some areas, to illustrate a particular point, only a few references will be cited, and an exhaustive literature search will not be attempted.

Before incidence statistics of rat mammary tumors can be understood, some consideration must be given to tumor pathology. Although mammary tumors may be first detected as subcutaneous nodules in mammary gland areas, anatomic location is not enough to be sure that the tumor is of mammary gland origin. Any lump or swelling in the region of the mammary gland should be examined to exclude salivary gland tumors, preputial gland tumors, epidermoid cysts, basal cell carcinomas, squamous cell carcinomas, lymph nodes, hibernomas, and lobular hyperplasia of the mammary gland. These exclusions then leave three types of mammary neoplasms, fibroepithelial, epithelial, and mesenchymal. The fibroepithelial neoplasms are clearly benign, and are given names ranging from adenoma through fibroma. In this report, the general term fibroadenoma will be used. Epithelial neoplasms of mammary gland origin are given names ranging from adenocarcinoma through anaplastic carcinoma, in this report I will use adenocarcinoma. Adenocarcinomas show some aspects of macroscopic, histologic, cytologic, and biologic malignancy. They do invade and metastasize, but only very rarely. The important point is that almost all mammary neoplasms are either fibroadenomas or adenocarcinomas and they can easily be diagnosed and separated with hemotoxylin and eosin sections. Sarcomas can be easily classi-

31

fied as sarcomas, however, verifying their origin is extremely difficult, at least for me, but fortunately so few sarcomas occur that they can usually be ignored. The classification of mammary neoplasms used here follows generally the very useful paper of Young and Hallowes (1973).

RAT STRAIN DIFFERENCES

The strain of rat chosen for study has important consequences in regard to both spontaneous and induced mammary neoplasia incidence. Some se-

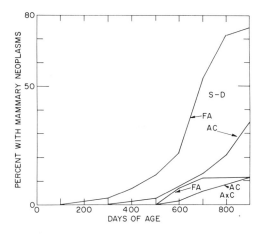

FIG. 1. Percent of rats "at-risk" (by life table technique) with mammary neoplasia in Sprague-Dawley (S-D) female rats and A × C female rats plotted against days of age: Mammary adenocarcinoma (AC), mammary fibroadenoma (FA).

lected illustrations of strain specificity follow. Females of the A × C strain have been reported to have "an essentially zero incidence of spontaneous breast cancer" (Segaloff and Maxfield, 1971) or "In 5329 normal adult and aged A × C rats necropsied at the Institute, the frequency of . . . mammary tumors was 1.8%" (Iglesias, 1974). In my own laboratory, we are following a small sample of A × C females, and they do have a reasonably low incidence of mammary neoplasia, especially compared to females of the Sprague-Dawley strain studied previously (Shellabarger et al., 1966). The difference in spontaneous incidence between the two strains (Fig. 1) holds for both mammary adenocarcinomas and mammary fibro-adenomas. No explanation has been put forward to account for this, or any other, particular strain difference. But, this one example of strain difference should suffice to illustrate that there are strain differences in regard to the spontaneous incidence of mammary neoplasia and to introduce the subject of rat strain differences in regard to the induction of mammary neoplasms.

INDUCED MAMMARY NEOPLASIA

The Lewis strain differs from the Sprague-Dawley strain in regard to incidence of mammary neoplasia in females following either whole-body X-irradiation or dimethylbenzanthracene (DMBA) administration (Table 1). Examination of these data, taken from a published paper (Shellabarger, 1972), shows clearly, in this direct comparison over a ten-month period, that

TABLE 1. *Mammary neoplasia in female rats of the Lewis or Sprague-Dawley strains*[a]

	Strain	
Treatment	Lewis	Sprague-Dawley
None		
start	22	44
end	21	40
rats with AC	0	1
total AC	0	1
rats with FA	0	2
total FA	0	2
DMBA[b]		
start	29	29
end	22	21
rats with AC	20	18
total AC	43	39
rats with FA	1	16
total FA	1	53
X-ray[b]		
start	40	40
end	38	36
rats with AC	3	10
total AC	4	11
rats with FA	3	23
total FA	4	39

[a] AC, mammary adenocarcinoma; FA, mammary fibroadenoma.

[b] DMBA administration: 13.3 mg/100 g body weight, or 350 r of 250 kVp total body X-irradiation on the 50th day of age; followed until autopsy 10 months later.

both the Lewis strain and the Sprague-Dawley strain show a high response to either DMBA or X-ray in regard to the incidence of mammary adenocarcinomas. Only the Sprague-Dawley strain, however, shows a large fibroadenoma response to either carcinogenic agent. Again, no explanation has been put forward to account for this strain difference. Less well studied is the strain difference between Long-Evans and Sprague-Dawley rats. It is clear, however, from the paper of Syndnor et al. (1962), and our own studies (Brown and Shellabarger, 1974) that in regard to mammary adenocarcinoma induction, the Long-Evans strain shows a smaller response than does the Sprague-Dawley strain to either X-irradiation or chemical carcinogens.

Again, although there is no clear known rationale for this strain difference, one experiment based on the *in vitro,* direct application of DMBA to mammary gland tissue was interpreted to mean that the strain difference was *not* at the level of carcinogen-tissue interaction (Brown and Shellabarger, 1974). The results of experiments cited above are all consistent with the thesis that strain sensitivity holds for both chemical carcinogens and for the physical carcinogen-ionizing radiation. That is to say, those strains that are relatively sensitive to DMBA are also apt to be sensitive to X-irradiation.

In addition to the differential susceptibility to chemical carcinogens shown by different strains, there are additional variables in regard to the mammary carcinogenic responses to chemical carcinogens and to radiation. There is probably a relationship between age at the time of carcinogen administration

TABLE 2. *Effect of age at time of 350 r exposure on mammary neoplasia in female Sprague-Dawley rats[a]*

	Days of age at time of 350 r exposure			
	24	42	84	225
start, number	29	30	30	30
end, number	28	27	24	25
rats with AC	2	10	12	12
total AC	2	13	12	12
rats with FA	15	19	19	19
total FA	19	33	35	35

[a] AC, mammary adenocarcinoma; FA, mammary fibroadenoma; X-rays were 250 kVp given as total body radiation on the days of age as indicated; all rats were studied 300 days. Three of thirty control rats, matched in age with those irradiated at 225 days exhibited a total of four FA.

and the amount of carcinogenic response. The mammary adenocarcinoma response to methylcholanthrene (MCA) in the female Sprague-Dawley rat appears to be at a maximum when the rats are about 50 to 65 days of age (Huggins et al., 1961). If the rats are younger or older at the time of MCA administration, a smaller mammary adenocarcinoma response occurs. Similarly, when total body X-irradiation was used as the carcinogenic agent, the juvenile Sprague-Dawley rat shows a smaller response than a younger, sexually mature rat (Shellabarger, 1974a). Whereas the MCA-treated rat shows a diminished response at ages older than 65 days of age, no loss of response to X-rays has been found in rats 225 days of age at the time of exposure to X-irradiation (Table 2). What has not yet been studied is the morphologic stage of development of the mammary gland at the time of the administration of the carcinogenic agents, the effect of age on the distribution of the chemical carcinogen, or the effects of the carcinogenic agents on ovarian and pituitary function. Perhaps one situation that is understandable is the following. In lactating rats, no mammary adenocarcinomas were produced by

MCA (Dao et al., 1960), whereas, in contrast, total body X-irradiation of the lactating rat (Shellabarger, 1974*b*) does produce mammary adenocarcinomas (Table 3). This lack of response to MCA in the lactating rat may well be due to a reduced carcinogenic stimulus to the mammary gland itself because the lactating gland rapidly eliminates the carcinogen via the milk. In the case of radiation, the dose to the mammary gland is little changed by the process of lactation. Even so, the factors responsible for the changing carcinogenic sensitivity of the mammary gland with age and with endocrine

TABLE 3. *Effect of lactation on mammary neoplasia response to 350 r of total body X-irradiation in Sprague-Dawley rats, strain 784*[a]

| | Treatment | | | |
| | X-rays | | Control | |
	Lactating	Virgin	Lactating	Virgin
Start, number	30	30	19	29
End, number	27	27	19	28
Rats with AC	11	11	0	0
Total AC	15	13	0	0
Rats with FA	6	5	0	1
Total FA	6	6	0	1

[a] AC, mammary adenocarcinoma; FA, mammary fibroadenoma; X-ray, 250 kVp, given on the fourth day of lactation, to virgin rats of the same age, or to non-irradiated rats of the same age; all rats were studied 300 days.

system maturation are neither understood nor thoroughly studied. This would appear, to me at least, a fruitful area of investigation.

RADIATION

Any of several types of low or high LET radiation produce mammary neoplasia in any of several strains of rats. There is general agreement that ionizing radiation acts by a scopal mechanism, that is, most of the mammary neoplasms following exposure are found in the irradiated volume of mammary gland tissue. There are two general types of evidence for the scopal mechanism. First, when Sprague-Dawley rats were partially shielded and exposed to X-rays (Bond et al., 1960), most of the mammary neoplasms were found in the irradiated mammary gland tissue (Fig. 2). A second approach was to remove mammary gland tissue, expose the tissue to X-irradiation *in vitro,* and then return the tissue to the rat from whence the tissue came (Shellabarger, 1971). When this was done, more mammary neoplasms were found in the irradiated tissue than in the nonirradiated tissue (Table 4).

Although there may be a sparing effect when low linear energy transfer (LET) radiation is spread out in time, over days or weeks, by lowering the dose rate (Shellabarger and Brown, 1972) or by fractionation and protrac-

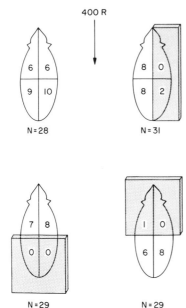

FIG. 2. Number of mammary neoplasms found in each quadrant of mammary tissue after 400 r of partial-body 250-kVp X-rays 11 months after exposure.

tion (Shellabarger et al., 1966), this has not been demonstrated unequivocally for mammary neoplasia in irradiated rats. Total body X-irradiation split into two equal doses separated by intervals up to 24 hr did not seem to diminish the mammary neoplastic response to 400 r of total body irradiation (Shellabarger, 1970) in Sprague-Dawley rats (Table 5) over a 315-day follow-up period. Also, split doses of 550 r plus 550 r of partial body irradiation, again with intervals up to 24 hr, did not diminish the mammary neoplastic response to 1100 r (Table 6) over a 300-day follow-up period. If repair or recovery does occur, it was not of sufficient magnitude to modify tumor incidence in these two experiments.

TABLE 4. Mammary neoplasia in transplants of tissue exposed in vitro to 800 r of 250 kVp X-rays or no irradiation[a]

Transplants	Irradiated	Sham-irradiated
No neoplasia	94	109
1 FA	11	1
2 FA	2	0
1 FA and 1 AC	1	0
1 AC	2	0
Total	110	110

[a] AC, mammary adenocarcinoma; FA, mammary fibroadenoma. Transplants were from 49- to 53-day-old female Sprague-Dawley rats; both the irradiated and non-irradiated mammary gland tissue were returned to the rat from whence they came. Transplants were recovered up to nine months after transplantation.

TABLE 5. Effect of split doses of 250 kVp X-ray, total body irradiation on mammary gland neoplasia in female Sprague-Dawley rats[a]

	Hours between 200 r + 200 r				No radiation
	0	2	6	24	
Start, number	24	24	24	24	15
End, number	22	23	21	23	15
Rats with AC	9	9	6	7	0
Total AC	10	12	7	9	0
Rats with FA	17	18	18	19	3
Total FA	37	27	43	32	4

[a] AC, mammary adenocarcinoma; FA, mammary fibroadenoma. The rats irradiated on their 55th day of age and followed 315 days.

High LET radiation seems to be more efficient, rad for rad, than low LET radiation, in inducing mammary neoplasia, provided that the comparisons are made at low doses and that the tumor observations are made relatively soon after exposure (Vogel, 1973; Shellabarger et al., 1973). Inspection of the plot of percent of rats with mammary neoplasia against dose, for neutrons or for X- or γ-rays suggests (Fig. 3) that neutrons have a reasonably high radiation biologic effectiveness (RBE), that the RBE is larger at low doses than at high doses, and that the shapes of the dose-response curves may be different for the two types of radiations. Rossi and Kellerer (1972), Kellerer and Rossi (1972), and Kellerer (*this volume*) have discussed the implications of these results in terms of mechanisms of action at the biophysical and cellular levels. But, from a biologic standpoint, it should be remembered that these results obtain only for one strain of rat, for overall mammary neoplasia, and for the temporal advancement of mammary neoplasia. Several laboratories have in progress experiments designed to study different strains of rats,

TABLE 6. Mammary neoplasia in irradiated volume after split doses of 250 kVp X-rays administered to the anterior one-half of female Sprague-Dawley rats[a]

	Hours between 550 r + 550 r			
	0	2	6	24
Start	35	35	35	35
End	33	34	33	33
Rats with AC	7	8	6	14
Total AC	8	8	7	16
Rats with FA	10	16	13	17
Total FA	13	24	15	22

[a] AC, mammary adenocarcinoma; FA, mammary fibroadenoma. The rats were exposed, with their posterior half shielded on their 60th day of age and studied 300 days. No neoplasia was found in 30 control rats.

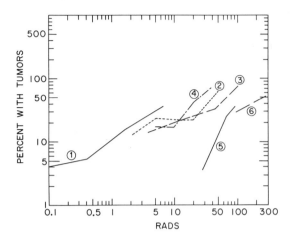

FIG. 3. Percent of rats with mammary neoplasia minus control values 11 months after exposure plotted against dose of radiation on log-log scales. Curve 1, 0.43-MeV neutrons, from Shellabarger et al. (1973). Curve 2, fission neutrons, from Vogel (1973). Curve 3, fission neutrons, from Shellabarger (*unpublished*). Curve 4, cyclotron (about 35 MeV) neutrons, from Montour (1975). Curve 5, 250-kVp X-ray, from Shellabarger et al. (1973). Curve 6, 250-kVp X-rays, from Shellabarger (*unpublished*). Curves 1 and 5 were done in one laboratory at the same time. Curves 3 and 6 were done in one laboratory at the same time.

with sample sizes large enough to look at both mammary adenocarcinomas and fibroadenomas, over the life-span of the rats, and at a wider range of doses in order to understand the RBE of neutrons.

COMBINATIONS OF CARCINOGENIC AGENTS

Because some chemical carcinogens seem to produce the same mammary neoplasms with about the same latent period as ionizing radiation produces, it seemed logical to study the interaction of chemical carcinogens and radiation on the induction of mammary neoplasia.

When MCA was given to Sprague-Dawley female rats with and without X-irradiation, or when the sequence reversed, and the incidence of mammary adenocarcinomas determined over a short period of time, the two agents appeared to act in an additive fashion (Shellabarger, 1967). Again, when MCA and fission neutrons were studied (Shellabarger and Straub, 1972), the interpretation was that the two agents were more nearly additive than inhibitory or synergistic. An additional observation is that what is close to the optimum dose of MCA seems to produce a larger mammary adenocarcinoma response than does a similar dose of radiation. In other words, the maximum response, in terms of percent of rats with one or more mammary adenocarcinomas produced by radiation seems to not exceed 20 to 30%, whereas it is not unusual to produce an almost 100% incidence with chemical carcinogens. In any event, if the additive result is accepted, it is then a usual step to continue to speculate and conclude that the two agents, one physical and one chemical, act at the same level of biologic organization. Proof of a common pathway for chemical and physical carcinogens has not yet been provided. Additional experiments are underway to learn, at lower doses of the two agents and over longer follow-up periods, if an additive result obtains for fibroadenoma induction also.

A long-standing concept in chemical carcinogenesis has been the idea of initiation and promotion. Recently, this concept has been extended to rat mammary carcinogenesis for the first time (Armuth and Berenblum, 1974). Armuth and Berenblum administered a relatively small amount of DMBA in a single dose and then administered phorbol twice a week for ten weeks. Their results can be easily interpreted as showing that DMBA acted as initiator and phorbol as a promotor. Despite the trouble that I have in reconciling the fact that DMBA itself can act as a "complete" carcinogen as well as appearing to serve as an initiator in the experiments of Armuth and Berenblum, we plan to test the effect of phorbol given after X-irradiation of rat mammary carcinogenesis.

VIRUSES

Any consideration of rat mammary gland carcinogenesis must include a consideration of viruses. Two recent reports are most pertinent. First, Ankerst et al. (1974) have reported that inoculation of adenovirus type 9 into seven newborn Wistar/Furth rats was followed by fibroadenoma development in all seven rats within 25 weeks, while none of their sisters (not inoculated or inoculated with adenovirus type 5) developed fibroadenomas. This report is of great interest, and I look forward to the results of attempts to confirm it. Second, Bogden et al (1974) reported that when R-35 mammary tumor virus, a C-type virus isolated from a transplantable rat mammary tumor, was inoculated into female, neonatal Sprague-Dawley rats, 10.6% of them developed mammary adenocarcinomas over a 20-month period, and only 1.6% of the controls developed adenocarcinomas during the same period. But, until survival rates are given for the two groups, the difference in tumor yield must be accepted with some reservations. Implantation of a 17, β-estradiol pellet in twenty virus-treated rats was followed by seven rats developing mammary adenocarcinomas within thirteen months, whereas no tumors were noted in twenty-one estrogen only–treated rats over the same period. Since the survival rates appear to be similar in this part of the experiment, a synergistic interaction between estrogen and virus may be postulated. Also, C-type virus was isolated from some of the tumors. At the very least, these two reports strongly suggest that viruses must be considered when discussing mammary carcinogenesis in the rat.

HORMONES

One of the most striking recent reports on the modification of rat mammary carcinogenesis was that of Segaloff and Maxfield (1971). Working with the A × C strain, they reported a synergistic interaction between X-irradiation and diethylstilbesterol (DES) on mammary adenocarcinoma formation. Since we have been able to reproduce their findings in A × C rats, using 0.43 MeV neutrons rather than X-rays, the findings with neutrons and DES will be described in these rats and contrasted with the findings in Sprague-Dawley strain. In both strains, a 20-mg cholesterol pellet containing 25% DES was implanted two days before 3.92 rad of neutrons. Even though the

TABLE 7. *Mammary neoplasia in A × C or Sprague-Dawley female rats given a DES pellet (5 mg diethylstilbestrol + 15 mg cholesterol), or DES and 3.92 rad of 0.43 MeV neutrons two days after DES, or neutrons only*[a]

	Neutrons (3.92 rad)		DES		Both	
	A × C	S-D	A × C	S-D	A × C	S-D
Start	23	34	23	34	23	34
End	22	32	0	16	0	16
Rats with AC	2	4	11	0	20	1
Total AC	2	6	48	0	300[b]	2
Rats with FA	1	14	0	0	0	0
Total FA	1	17	0	0	0	0

[a] AC, mammary adenocarcinoma; FA, mammary fibroadenoma. The rats studied 336 days after DES administration.
[b] Estimated.

experiment is not yet finished, the interim results are of interest (Table 7). It was clear to us that, 336 days after DES administration, DES had induced mammary adenocarcinomas in A × C rats but not in Sprague-Dawley rats. Radiation induced mammary fibroadenomas in Sprague-Dawley rats but not in A × C rats. Only in A × C rats did a synergistic interaction between estrogen and radiation occur and then only in regard to mammary adenocarcinomas. The A × C rats receiving both DES and neutron treatment developed mammary adenocarcinomas somewhat sooner than with either treatment alone, but what is more spectacular is that only the A × C rats receiving both treatments developed what Segaloff and Maxfield (1971) called "essentially" total carcinogenesis (Fig. 4). That is, so many adenocarcinomas were present that they were difficult to count. A possible clue as to the difference between strains may be the fact that only A × C rats developed pituitary tumors. These pituitary tumors where judged to be prolactin-secreting tumors. This has been proven to be true, since Dr. J. P. Stone has found, in a separate experiment, that prolactin blood levels are much higher in A × C rats with a DES pellet than in Sprague-Dawley rats with the same pellet, and because Dr. S. Holtzman has found, by immunofluorescent techniques, prolactin-secreting cells in these pituitary tumors. These results well illustrate the complexities of rat mammary gland carcinogenesis. There are strain differences in response to exogenous estrogen, in response to radiation, and in response to interactions of radiation and estrogen. These results suggest that prolactin may play a key role in the strain differences and the differences in response to radiation. It must also be mentioned that the results of this experiment are in full accord with the report of Yokoro and Furth

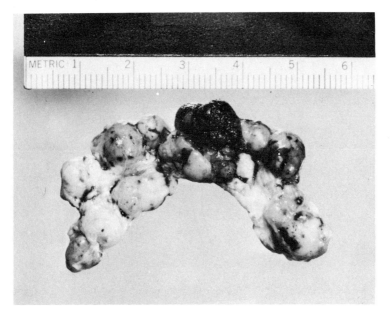

FIG. 4. A single quadrant of mammary gland tissue removed from an A X C female rat that received DES and neutron radiation, illustrating a multiple tumor response.

(1961), who reported a synergism between prolactin and radiation on mammary carcinogenesis some 15 years ago.

SUMMARY

1. The spontaneous incidence of mammary adenocarcinomas and mammary fibroadenomas is related to the strain of rat studied.

2. Strains of rats that are sensitive to chemical carcinogens in regard to induced mammary neoplasia tend to be the same strains of rats that are sensitive to radiation.

3. Following MCA and X-rays or MCA and neutron administration, induction of mammary adenocarcinomas is additive, when these agents were given together.

4. Lactating and older rats lose responsiveness to chemical carcinogens but do not lose responsiveness to radiation.

5. Radiation appears to act in a scopal fashion in the induction of mammary neoplasia, when studied over short periods of time.

6. Mammary neoplasia induction was not changed when low LET radiation was split into two equal fractions, when studied over short periods of time.

7. High LET radiation is more effective than low LET radiation in inducing mammary neoplasia, when studied over short periods of time.

8. One report suggests that DMBA can act as an initiator for the induction of mammary adenocarcinomas and that phorbol can act as a promotor.

9. Two reports were cited in which it is indicated that viruses may participate in mammary neoplasia induction.

10. Radiation and DES appear to act synergistically in the induction of mammary adenocarcinomas in one strain of rat but not in another strain.

ACKNOWLEDGMENT

Brookhaven National Laboratory is operated by Associated Universities, Inc., under contract to the U.S. Energy Research and Development Administration. Part of this research was done under contract Y01-CP-30213 with the Biological Models Segment of the Carcinogenesis Program of the National Cancer Institute.

REFERENCES

Ankerst, J., Jonsson, N., Kjellen, L., Norrby, E., and Sjorgren, H. O. (1974): Induction of mammary fibroadenomas in rats by adenovirus type 9. *Int. J. Cancer*, 13:286–290.

Armuth, V., and Berenblum, I. (1974): Promotion of mammary carcinogenesis and leukemogenic action by phorbol in virgin female Wistar rats. *Cancer Res.*, 34:2704–2707.

Bogden, A. E., Cobb, W. R., Ahmed, M., Alex, S., and Mason, M. M. (1974): Oncogenicity of the R-35 rat mammary tumor virus. *J. Natl. Cancer Insti.*, 1073–1077.

Bond, V. P., Shellabarger, C. J., Cronkite, E. P., and Fliedner, T. M. (1960): Studies on Radiation-induced mammary gland neoplasia in the rat. V. Induction by localized radiation. *Radiat. Res.*, 13:318–328.

Brown, R. D., and Shellabarger, C. J. (1974): Mammary neoplasia in Sprague-Dawley or Long-Evans rats after *in vitro* 7,12-dimethylbenzanthracene. *Cancer Res.*, 34:2594–2595.

Dao, T. L., Boch, F. G., and Greiner, M. J. (1960): Mammary carcinogenesis by 3-Methylcholanthrene. II. Inhibitory effect of pregnancy and lactation on tumor induction. *J. Natl. Cancer Inst.*, 25:991–1003.

Huggins, C., Grand, L. C., and Brillantes, F. P. (1961): Mammary cancer induced by a single feeding of polynuclear hydrocarbons, and its suppression. *Nature*, 189:204–207.

Iglesias, R. (1974): Secondary endocrine and mammary malignancies as main signs of hormonal syndromes produced by endocrine tumors. In: *Paraneoplastic Syndromes*, edited by T. C. Hall, Vol. 230. Annals of The New York Academy of Sciences, New York, pp. 500–507.

Kellerer, A. M., and Rossi, H. H. (1972): The theory of dual radiation action. *Curr. Top. Radiat. Res.*, 8:85–158.

Montour, J. L. (1975): Personal communication.

Rossi, H. H., and Kellerer, A. M. (1972): Radiation carcinogenesis at low doses. *Science*, 175:200–202.

Segaloff, A., and Maxfield, W. S. (1971): The synergism between radiation and estrogen in the production of mammary cancer in the rat. *Cancer Res.*, 31:166–168.

Shellabarger, C. J. (1967): Effect of 3-methylcholantrene and x-irradiation, given singly or combined on rat mammary carcinogenesis. *J. Natl. Cancer Inst.*, 38:73–77.

Shellabarger, C. J. (1970): Effect of short-term dose fractionation on mammary neoplasia incidence in the rat. In: *IV International Congress of Radiation Research*, p. 199 (Abstr.).

Shellabarger, C. J. (1971): Induction of mammary neoplasia after *in vitro* exposure to x-rays. *Proc. Soc. Exp. Biol. Med.*, 136:1103–1106.

Shellabarger, C. J. (1972): Mammary neoplastic response of Lewis and Sprague-Dawley female rats to 7,12-Dimethylbenzanthracene or x-ray. *Cancer Res.*, 32:883–885.

Shellabarger, C. J. (1974a): A comparison of rat mammary carcinogenesis following total-body irradiation at different ages. In: *Abstracts of Papers Presented at 5th International Congress of Radiation Research*, p. 103.

Shellabarger, C. J. (1974b): Mammary carcinogenesis in irradiated, lactating Sprague-Dawley female rats. In: *XI International Cancer Congress* (Abstr.), p. 634.

Shellabarger, C. J., Bond, V. P., Aponte, G. E., and Cronkite, E. P. (1966): Results of fractionation and protraction of total-body radiation on rat mammary gland neoplasia. *Cancer Res.*, 26 (1):509–513.

Shellabarger, C. J., and Brown, R. D. (1972): Rat mammary neoplasia following ^{60}Co irradiation at 0.03 R or 10 R per minute. *Radiat. Res.*, 51:493 (Abstr.).

Shellabarger, C. J., Brown, R. D., Rao, A. R., Shanley, J. P., Bond, V. P., Kellerer, A. M., Rossi, H. H., Goodman, L. J., and Mills, R. E. (1973): Rat mammary carcinogenesis following neutron or x-irradiation. In: *Biological Effects of Neutron Irradiation*, IAEA-SM-179/26, Vienna.

Shellabarger, C. J., and Straub, R. F. (1972): Effect of 3-methylcholanthrene and fission neutron irradiation, given singly or combined, on rat mammary carcinogenesis. *J. Natl. Cancer Inst.*, 48:185–187.

Syndnor, K. L., Butternandt, O., Brillantes, F. P., and Huggins, C. (1962): Race-strain factor related to hydrocarbon-induced mammary cancer. *J. Natl. Cancer Inst.*, 29:805–814.

Vogel, H. H., Jr. (1973): Neutron-induced mammary neoplasia. In: *Biological Effects of Neutron Irradiation*. IAEA-SM-179/32, Vienna.

Yokoro, K., and Furth, J. (1961): Relation of mammotropes to mammary tumors. V. Role of mammotropes in radiation carcinogenesis. *Proc. Soc. Exp. Biol. Med.*, 107:921–924.

Young, S., and Hallowes, R. C. (1973): Tumors of the mammary gland. In: *Pathology of Tumors in Laboratory Animals, Volume I- Tumors of The Rat, Part 1*, edited by V. S. Turusov, pp. 31–74. International Agency for Research on Cancer, Lyon, France.

Biology of Radiation Carcinogenesis, edited by
J. M. Yuhas, R. W. Tennant, and J. D. Regan.
Raven Press, New York © 1976.

The Feature in Common Among Persons at High Risk of Leukemia

Robert W. Miller

Epidemiology Branch, National Cancer Institute, Bethesda, Maryland 20014

THE FEATURE IN COMMON AMONG PERSONS AT HIGH RISK OF LEUKEMIA

Ionizing radiation was the first known human leukemogen. Certain heritable disorders were subsequently found to carry an increased risk of leukemia, e.g., the syndromes of Down, Bloom, and Fanconi [reviewed by Miller (1964, 1967) and by German (1972)]. In each syndrome, the old technique for staining chromosomes showed abnormality: long-lasting chromosomal breaks in Japanese survivors of the atomic bomb (Bloom, 1972), trisomy 21 due to an error in prezygotic chromosomal division in Down's syndrome (Lejeune et al., 1959), and chromosomal fragility in Bloom's and Fanconi's syndromes (German et al., 1965; Bloom et al., 1966). The known groups of persons at high risk of leukemia, then, had in common a cytogenetic abnormality, although it is not of a single type.

Relation to Leukemia in the General Population

What did this information based on rarities have to do with the usual course of leukemia? The only form of the neoplasm in the general population with a consistent chromosomal abnormality was chronic myelogenous leukemia (CML). In about 85% of cases, there appeared to be deletion of a long arm of a G-group chromosome—the so-called Philadelphia (Ph[1]) chromosome (Nowell and Hungerford, 1960), which is apparently clonal in origin (Barr and Fialkow, 1973; Moore et al., 1974; Gahrton et al., 1974). The Ph[1] chromosome has been described in CML among Japanese survivors of the atomic bomb (Kamada, 1969).

Recently, through the development of new staining techniques, it has become possible to identify chromosomes individually by their distinctive bands of light and dark areas, in contrast to the old method that grouped chromosomes that were morphologically similar with uniformly dark staining. Abnormalities previously invisible by the old techniques are now detectable by the new ones. Thus, it has been found that the cytogenetic abnormality in CML was not a deletion of chromosome 21, as originally thought, but a translocation from chromosome 22, usually to chromosome 9 (Caspersson et al., 1970; O'Riordan et al., 1971; Rowley, 1973).

Acute myelogenous leukemia (AML) was thought not to have a consistent chromosomal abnormality, but through the use of new staining procedures, is now reported to have 8/21 translocations or trisomy 9 in a substantial number of cases (Sakurai et al., 1974; Ford and Pittman, 1974; Rowley, 1975). There is some disagreement among the several groups as to the frequencies with which chromosomes 8, 9, and 21 are involved. The important point is that specific aberrations can now be seen where none was previously detectable.

From the original observations concerning rare mistakes in nature has come a generalization about leukemia: namely, myelogenous leukemia often, if not always, involves chromosomal abnormality, either inborn or acquired.

The Importance of Cell Type

Ionizing radiation induces CML or AML regardless of the age at exposure, but did not induce chronic lymphocytic leukemia (CLL) in the Japanese atomic-bomb survivors or in British men given radiotherapy for ankylosing spondylitis (Brill et al., 1962; Ishimaru et al., 1971a; Court Brown and Doll, 1965). Ionizing radiation has induced a few cases of acute lymphocytic leukemia (ALL), primarily among Japanese who were under 20 years of age at the time of exposure to the atomic bomb (Brill et al., 1962; Ichimaru et al., 1975).

There is thus something about age that affects susceptibility to radiogenic ALL, and about ethnicity that protects the Japanese against spontaneous CLL (Finch et al., 1969). There is something about the mechanism of cancer induction by radiation that does not evoke CLL even among the British, who are susceptible to it.

Chromosomal abnormalities have not been an important feature of CLL or of persons at high risk of lymphoma. Instead, these persons have in common cell-mediated immunodeficiency, either inborn—as in ataxia telangiectasia or the Wiskott-Aldrich syndrome, or acquired—as when immunosuppressive therapy is given for renal transplantation (Fraumeni and Miller, 1967; Kersey et al., 1973; Fraumeni et al., 1975; Hoover and Fraumeni, 1973).

Among persons at high risk of nonradiogenic leukemia, peculiarities in distribution by cell type have been observed. Acute monomyelogenous leukemia, which is rare in the general population, is the form of leukemia reported with Fanconi's anemia, after melphalan therapy for multiple myeloma, and among children in Ankara, Turkey, where 40% of all childhood leukemia is of this type (Dosik et al., 1970; Karchmer et al., 1974; Cavdar et al., 1971). In Bloom's syndrome, four cases of acute leukemia have been seen, and "classification . . . is difficult . . . but none . . . was lymphocytic" (German, 1974). In Down's syndrome, most leukemia is ALL, but the peak occurs at one year of age, instead of at four years as in the general population (Miller, 1970). There is also some excess of ALL in ataxia telangiectasia, an immunodeficiency disorder that predisposes primarily to lymphoma (Kersey et al., 1973). Hecht et al (1973) have presented evidence suggesting that D/D translocation in ataxia telangiectasia, and other conditions, can give rise to ALL. The differences in the types of leukemia according to the predisposing condition may well be related to differences in chromosomal anomalies characteristic of the high-risk group.

Are Some People Especially Susceptible to Radiogenic Leukemia?

Among Japanese atomic-bomb survivors, who were under ten years of age at the time of exposure, the risk of leukemia was about three times greater than when exposure occurred at older ages (Advisory Committee on the Biological Effects of Ionizing Radiation, 1972). The sex ratios (M/F) for radiation-exposed versus non-exposed persons with leukemia were similar, indicating no particular influence of sex.

The highest risk of radiogenic leukemia occurs among patients with polycythemia vera treated with X-ray and/or ^{32}P. One in six persons so treated developed leukemia within 12 years, as contrasted with one in sixty persons who were within 1,000 m of the hypocenter in Hiroshima (reviewed by Miller, 1967). Abnormalities of chromosomes 8 or 9 have been observed in polycythemia vera before radiotherapy (Rowley, 1975). These aberrations may enhance radiation leukemogenesis. A similar predisposition has been suggested as an explanation for the blast crisis (AML) that occurs terminally in patients with CML. In this instance, the chromosomal anomaly that typifies CML may increase the susceptibility to further (environmentally induced?) aberrations that lead to development of AML (Mastrangelo et al., 1967; Pedersen, 1973).

Recently, other interactions have been reported between ionizing radiation and inborn abnormalities:

1. Two children with ataxia telangiectasia developed lymphoma. Treatment with standard radiotherapy produced severe esophagitis in both, perhaps related to the chromosomal fragility sometimes seen in this genetically transmitted disorder (Gotoff et al., 1967; Morgan et al., 1968).

2. Several young children developed medulloblastoma as the earliest manifestation of the heritable disorder, multiple basal cell nevus syndrome. The brain tumors were treated with radiotherapy. Several years later, at the age when basal cell nevi typically appear in the syndrome, they were concentrated on the skin of the scalp in the field of radiotherapy (Meadows, unpub.).

3. There is a substantial frequency of orbital sarcomas in children after radiotherapy for retinoblastoma (Sagerman et al., 1969). It has recently been found that more than a dozen children with *bilateral* retinoblastoma, usually transmitted as an autosomal dominant trait, have developed osteo-

sarcoma of the femur, or less frequently, of the tibia. These second cancers were outside the radiation field or in children who received no therapy (Jensen and Miller, 1971; Kitchin and Ellsworth, 1974; Schimke et al., 1974). It appears that various tissues are at increased risk of neoplasia in children with heritable (as contrasted with sporadic) retinoblastoma, and their threshold for radiogenic cancer (of the orbit) may be lower than usual.

Rare mistakes of nature thus suggest an interaction between ionizing radiation and pre-existent genetic or cytogenetic abnormality. There is, of course, no reason to exclude the possibility that in man the effects of radiation, including leukemogenesis, may be enhanced by drugs, occupational or other environmental exposures, or certain infectious agents. With respect to leukemogenesis, interactions may be most likely with those agents that cause certain chromosomal abnormalities.

REFERENCES

Advisory Committee on the Biological Effects of Ionizing Radiation (1972): The effects on populations of exposure to low levels of ionizing radiation. National Academy of Sciences–National Research Council, Washington, D.C.

Barr, R. D., and Fialkow, P. J. (1973): Clonal origin of chronic myelocytic leukemia. *N. Engl. J. Med.,* 289:307–308.

Bloom, A. D. (1972): Induced chromosomal aberrations in man. In: *Advances in Human Genetics,* Vol. 3, edited by H. Harris and K. Hirschhorn, pp. 99–172. Plenum Press, New York.

Bloom, G. E., Warner, S., Gerald, P. S., and Diamond, L. K. (1966): Chromosome abnormalities in constitutional aplastic anemia. *N. Engl. J. Med.,* 274:8–14.

Brill, A. B., Tomonaga, M., and Heyssel, R. M. (1962): Leukemia in man following exposure to ionizing radiation: Summary of findings in Hiroshima and Nagasaki, and comparison with other human experience. *Ann. Intern. Med.,* 56:590–609.

Caspersson, T., Gahrton, G., Lindsten, J., and Zech, L. (1970): Identification of the Philadelphia chromosome as a number 22 by quinacrine mustard fluorescence analysis. *Exp. Cell Res.,* 63:238–240.

Cavdar, A. O., Arcasoy, A., Gozdasoglu, S., and Demirag, B. (1971): Chloroma-like ocular manifestations in Turkish children with acute myelomonocytic leukaemia. *Lancet,* 1:680–682.

Court Brown, W. M., and Doll, R. (1965): Mortality from cancer and other causes after radiotherapy for ankylosing spondylitis. *Br. Med. J.,* 2:1327–1332.

Dosik, H., Hsu, L. Y., Todaro, G. J., Lee, S. L., Hirschhorn, K., Selirio, E. S., and Alter, A. A. (1970): Leukemia in Fanconi's anemia: Cytogenetic and tumor virus susceptibility studies. *Blood,* 36:341–352.

Finch, S. C., Hoshino, T., Itoga, T., Ichimaru, M., and Ingram, R. H., Jr. (1969): Chronic lymphocytic leukemia in Hiroshima and Nagasaki, Japan. *Blood,* 33:79–86.

Ford, J. H., and Pittman, S. M. (1974): Duplication of 21 or 8/21 translocation in acute leukaemia. *Lancet,* 2:1458.

Fraumeni, J. F., Jr., and Miller, R. W. (1967): Epidemiology of human leukemia: Recent observations. *J. Natl. Cancer Inst.,* 38:593–605.

Fraumeni, J. F., Jr., Wertelecki, W., Blattner, W. A., Jensen, R. D., and Leventhal, B. G. (1975): Varied manifestations of a familial lymphoproliferative disorder. *Am. J. Med.,* 59:145–151.

Gahrton, G., Lindsten, J., and Zech, L. (1974): Clonal origin of the Philadelphia chromosome from either the paternal or maternal chromosome number 22. *Blood,* 43:837–840.

German, J. (1972): Genes which increase chromosomal instability in somatic cells and predispose to cancer. *Prog. Med. Genet.*, 8:61–101.

German, J. (1974): Bloom's syndrome. II. The prototype of human genetic disorders predisposing to chromosome instability and cancer. In: *Chromosomes and Cancer,* edited by J. German, pp. 601–617, John Wiley & Sons, New York.

German, J., Archibald, R., and Bloom, D. (1965): Chromosomal breakage in a rare and probably genetically determined syndrome of man. *Science*, 148:506–507.

Gotoff, S. P., Amirmokri, E., and Liebner, E. J. (1967): Ataxia telangiectasia. Neoplasia, untoward response to X-irradiation, and tuberous sclerosis. *Am. J. Dis. Child.*, 114:617–625.

Hecht, F., McCaw, B. K., and Koler, R. D. (1973): Ataxia-telangiectasia—clonal growth of translocation lymphocytes. *N. Engl. J. Med.*, 289:286–291.

Hoover, R., and Fraumeni, J. F., Jr. (1973): Risk of cancer in renal-transplant recipients. *Lancet*, 2:55–57.

Ichimaru, M., Ishimaru, T., Belsky, J. L., Tomiyasu, T., Tomonaga, M., Sadamori, N., Shimizu, N., Hoshino, T., and Okada, H. (In preparation): Leukemia in atomic-bomb radiation, Hiroshima and Nagasaki: October 1950–December 1971. Part 1. Dose-response relationship.

Ishimaru, T., Hoshino, T., Ichimaru, M., Okada, H., Tomiyasu, T., Tsuchimoto, T., and Yamamoto, T. (1971a): Leukemia in atomic bomb survivors, Hiroshima and Nagasaki, 1 October 1950–30 September 1966. *Radiat. Res.*, 45:216–233.

Jensen, R. D., and Miller, R. W. (1971): Retinoblastoma: Epidemiologic characteristics. *N. Engl. J. Med.*, 285:307–311.

Kamada, N. (1969): The effects of radiation on chromosomes of bone marrow cells. III. Cytogenetic studies on leukemia in atomic bomb survivors. *Acta Haem. Jap.*, 32:249–274.

Karchmer, R. K., Amare, M., Larsen, W. E., Mallouk, A. G., and Caldwell, G. G. (1974): Alkylating agents as leukemogens in multiple myeloma. *Cancer*, 33:1103–1107.

Kersey, J., Spector, B. D., and Good, R. A. (1973): Primary immunodeficiency diseases and cancer: The Immunodeficiency Cancer Registry. *Int. J. Cancer*, 12:333–347.

Kitchin, F. D., and Ellsworth, R. M. (1974): Pleiotropic effects of the gene for retinoblastoma. *J. Med. Genet.*, 11:244–246.

Lejeune, J., Gautier, M., and Turpin, R. (1959): Étude des chromosomes somatiques de neuf enfants mongoliens. *C. R. Acad. Sci.*, 248:1721–1722.

Mastrangelo, R., Zuelzer, W. W., and Thompson, R. I. (1967): The significance of the Ph[1] chromosome in acute myeloblastic leukemia: Serial cytogenetic studies in a critical case. *Pediatrics*, 40:834–841.

Meadows, A. T.: Unpublished observations.

Miller, R. W. (1964): Radiation, chromosomes and viruses in the etiology of leukemia. Evidence from epidemiologic research. *N. Engl. J. Med.*, 271:30–36.

Miller, R. W. (1967): Persons at exceptionally high risk of leukemia. *Cancer Res.*, 27 (Part 1):2420–2423.

Miller, R. W. (1970): Neoplasia and Down's syndrome. *Ann. NY Acad. Sci.*, 171:637–644.

Moore, M. A. S., Fitzgerald, M. G., and Carmichael, A. (1974): Evidence for the clonal origin of chronic myeloid leukemia from a sex chromosome mosaic: Clinical, cytogenetic and marrow culture studies. *Blood*, 43:15–22.

Morgan, J. L., Holcomb, T. M., and Morrissey, R. W. (1968): Radiation reaction in ataxia telangiectasia. *Am. J. Dis. Child.*, 116:557–558.

Nowell, P. C., and Hungerford, D. A. (1960): A minute chromosome in human chronic granulocytic leukemia. *Science*, 132:1497.

O'Riordan, M. L., Robinson, J. A., Buckton, K. E., and Evans, H. J. (1971): Distinguishing between the chromosomes involved in Down's syndrome (trisomy 21) and chronic myeloid leukaemia (Ph[1]) by fluorescence. *Nature*, 230:167–168.

Pedersen, B. (1973): The blastic crisis of chronic myeloid leukemia: Acute transformation of a preleukaemic condition? *Br. J. Haematol.*, 25:141–145.

Rowley, J. D. (1973): A new consistent chromosomal abnormality in chronic myelogenous leukaemia identified by quinacrine fluorescence and Giemsa staining. *Nature,* 243:290–293.

Rowley, J. D. (1975): Nonrandom chromosomal abnormalities in hematologic disorders of man. *Proc. Natl. Acad. Sci. USA,* 72:152–156.

Sagerman, R. H., Cassady, J. R., Tretter, P., and Ellsworth, R. M. (1969): Radiation-induced neoplasia following external beam therapy for children with retinoblastoma. *Am. J. Roentgenol. Radium Ther. Nucl. Med.,* 105:529–535.

Sakurai, M., Oshimura, M., Kakati, S., and Sandberg, A. A. (1974): 8–21 translocation and missing sex chromosomes in acute leukaemia. *Lancet,* 2:227–228.

Schimke, R. N., Lowman, J. T., and Cowan, G. A. B. (1974): Retinoblastoma and osteogenic sarcoma in siblings. *Cancer,* 34:2077–2079.

Biology of Radiation Carcinogenesis, edited by
J. M. Yuhas, R. W. Tennant, and J. D. Regan.
Raven Press, New York © 1976.

Dose-Response Curves and Their Modification by Specific Mechanisms

John M. Yuhas

Biology Division, Oak Ridge National Laboratory, Oak Ridge, Tennessee 37830

Many of the chapters contained in this volume demonstrate that certain biological mechanisms or processes are theoretically able to affect the yield of radiation-induced cancers *in vivo,* but there are opposing views regarding their actual importance. This stems, at least in part, from the fact that no two test systems used to assess the importance of a given mechanism are exactly alike, and different results are therefore to be expected. The point we wish to make here is that it is not necessary to compare different test systems in order to generate conflict, since it is possible to obtain diametrically opposed evaluations regarding the importance of a given mechanism merely by altering the region of the dose-response curve studied.

In specific terms, our proposal states that the relative importance of each biological mechanism will vary as a function of the total dose or dose rate, because these two variables affect not only the extent but also the nature of the injury induced in target and nontarget cells alike. In a sense, this proposal is not new, since it follows quite logically from a variety of predictions obtained in the study of dose-response curves (Rossi and Kellerer, 1972). What little originality exists stems from the combination of these predictions with biologically observable phenomena. If this proposal is valid, its value lies not only in resolving certain of the conflicts in the literature but also in providing a rational means of predicting the carcinogenic hazards associated with radiation exposure conditions that cannot be simulated in the laboratory.

A priori, there are a number of cases in which support for our proposal is self-evident: low radiation doses (<100 rads), which are at best marginally immunosuppressive (Celada and Carter, 1962) do not compromise the host's ability to cope with oncogenic virus or tumor cell antigens, whereas higher doses do (Yuhas et al., 1973); fractionation or protraction of a radiation dose can either increase or decrease the cancer yield, depending on the region of the dose-response curve studied (Nowell and Cole, 1965; Pazmino et al., 1975); and low doses of radiation can produce "negative injury" as evidenced by prolongation of the life-span of the exposed animal (Grahn

* These studies were supported by the Energy Research and Development Administration under contract with Union Carbide.

and Sacher, 1968). We concern ourselves here, not with these aspects, but with two, more subtle problems that have been the subject of debate in recent years: the dependence of recovery from radiation carcinogenic injury on dose size and the role of immunosuppression compared with target cell disturbances in radiation leukemogenesis.

RECOVERY FROM RADIATION CARCINOGENIC INJURY
AS A FUNCTION OF DOSE SIZE

The dose-response curves for low linear energy transfer (LET) induction of cancers are, at least theoretically (Kellerer, *this volume*), composed of three regions: the low dose region, in which tumor yield increases linearly with dose; the intermediate region, in which tumor yield increases as a greater than one power of the dose; and the high dose region, in which the cell-killing effects more than counterbalance the increased number of transformations and tumor yield declines progressively. The radiation doses that delimit these regions vary as a function of the tumor type in question (see below), but in most instances it is not possible to differentiate between the low and intermediate regions of the curve, i.e., the low dose region is small relative to the dose levels normally employed. We will use the terms low and linear interchangeably; this also holds true for the terms intermediate and curvilinear.

In the absence of a system that would allow differentiation of the low from the intermediate dose region, few of the questions relating to the role of dose size in radiation recovery from carcinogenic injury could be addressed. A number of test systems were studied in an attempt to develop one for this analysis, the most useful of which was the radiation induction of benign lung adenomas in the RF mouse (Yuhas and Walker, 1973). The unique features of this test system include negligible mortality between treatment and analysis; constant tumor yields between six and twelve months after treatment; and the development of multiple tumors in individual animals, thereby allowing use of "mean number of tumors per mouse" as the response end-point, as opposed to the more erratic incidence data (Yuhas and Walker, 1973).

In our pilot studies, the dose range of 750 to 3,000 rads of localized thoracic 250 kVp X-rays was studied (Yuhas and Walker, 1973). Two points were established in these experiments: that the dose-response curve between 750 and 1,500 rads was curvilinear, and that 1,500 rads was the upper limit of the intermediate dose region. In order to determine if the theoretically predicted linear component would be observed, we expanded these studies to include localized doses of as low as 250 rads. Figure 1 is a plot of the mean number of induced adenomas (treated mean minus control mean) per mouse observed 7 to 11 months after localized thoracic doses of 250 to 1,500 rads. Between 250 and 750 rads, the slope of the log-log plot of response on dose is not significantly different from 1, indicating that the induction of benign adenomas in this dose range is a simple linear function. At the higher doses (750 to 1,500 rads), the log-log slope of response on dose is significantly greater than 1 ($P < 0.01$), suggesting that an interaction between events is contributing to tumor yield. For comparison, we have included data on similar mice given graded doses of urethane (ethyl carbamate) instead of localized X-rays. The shape of the overall dose-response curve for this chemical carcinogen is essentially identical to that for the localized X-rays: 125 to 500 mg of urethane/kg body weight defines the linear portion of the dose-response curve, whereas higher doses are described by a curve with a log-log slope of greater than 1 ($P < 0.001$) (Fig. 1).

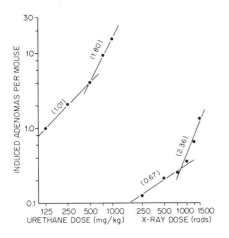

FIG. 1. Mean number of papillary lung adenomas per mouse induced by graded doses of urethane or localized X-rays. Induced values corrected for spontaneous control value (0.39 to 0.43 adenoma/mouse). Numbers on each of the curves represent the maximum likelihood estimates of the log-log slope.

The important point for the present discussion is not the specific doses that define the transition from a linear response to a curvilinear one, but rather the implications these two areas of the curve have for the process of recovery. For the case of the localized X-rays, at least, the linear relationship between dose and response (Fig. 1; 250 to 750 rads) indicates that a single ionizing event is responsible for tumor induction in this dose range. In the higher dose region, where the log-log slope is significantly greater than 1 (Fig. 1; 750 to 1,500 rads) an additional mechanism appears to be contributing to the yield of tumors, namely, the interaction of ionizations, each of which alone was unable to produce a tumor. A carcinogenic process that requires only a single ionization should be independent of the rate of carcinogen administration, whereas, if more than one ionization is required, a slow rate of administration might allow recovery of the initial injury before additional ionizations occur. In other words, there should be no recovery from total doses that fall on the linear portion of the dose-response curve, but there should be significant recovery from total doses that fall on

the curvilinear portion of the curve, when the doses are given over a prolonged period of time as opposed to acute X-irradiation.

In order to test this prediction of the dose-response curve (Fig. 1), we
chose the highest total X-ray doses that fell on the linear portion of the
dose-response curve (750 rads) and on the curvilinear portion of the same
curve (1,500 rads) and administered them either as a single dose or as two
equal doses separated by 24 hr. If no recovery occurred during the 24-hr
fractionation interval, then the tumor yield should be the same in the single
and split dose groups. If recovery from the first dose equaled 100%, then
the tumor yield in the split dose group should equal that of mice given only

TABLE 1. *Recovery from radiation carcinogenic injury to the
mouse lung as a function of dose size*

Exposure method[a]	Total radiation dose (rad)	Number of mice	Induced lung[b] adenomas (mean ± SE)	Recovery[c] (%)
Single dose	1,500	27	1.56 ± 0.21	—
Single dose	750	29	0.38 ± 0.09	—
Two fractions[d]	1,500	24	0.96 ± 0.19	51
Single dose	750	29	0.38 ± 0.09	—
Single dose	375	21	0.09 ± 0.04	—
Two fractions[d]	750	28	0.49 ± 0.06	−38

[a] Exposures given either as a single dose or as two equal fractions separated by 24 hr.

[b] Mean observed in the irradiated group minus the control mean of 0.39 adenoma/
mouse.

[c] 100% recovery equals a mean number of induced adenomas identical with that observed in mice given only one-half the total radiation dose, i.e., 750 and 375 rads, respectively.

[d] Two equal fractions given at a 24-hr interval.

one of the two fractions (i.e., one-half the total dose). The theoretical predictions of the dose-response curves were confirmed quite clearly, in that
highly significant recovery was observed in the group given the two fractions
that totaled a dose that fell on the curvilinear portion of the dose-response
curve, 1,500 rads (Table 1), whereas no recovery was apparent when a dose
that fell on the linear portion of the curve (750 rads) was fractionated
(Table 1).

Similar fractionation experiments were performed with urethane, since it
showed a single dose-response curve similar to that of localized X-rays
(Fig. 1). Table 2 summarizes the results of an experiment in which we fractionated urethane doses that fell either on the linear (500 mg/kg) or curvilinear (1,000 mg/kg) portions of the dose-response curve. Again, the same
pattern was observed (Table 2): significant recovery was observed when a
total dose within the curvilinear range was fractionated ($P < 0.02$), but no

recovery was apparent when a single dose on the linear portion of the curve was fractionated. Extension of the recovery interval from 24 to 96 hr (Table 2) failed to allow the demonstration of recovery in the low total dose group, and, in fact, apparent "negative recovery" was observed. It should be noted that urethane data similar to the data presented above (Fig. 1 and Table 2) have been published elsewhere (Shimkin et al., 1967; White et al., 1967), and extension of our analysis to it leads to essentially the same conclusions.

For the localized X-rays, we propose that the single events that are contributing to tumor yield in the linear range, and the single and multiple events that are contributing to tumor yield in the curvilinear range, are ioni-

TABLE 2. Recovery from urethane-induced carcinogenic injury to the mouse lung as a function of dose size

Injection method[a]	Total urethane dose (mg/kg)	Time between fractions (hr)	Number of mice	Induced lung[b] adenomas (mean ± SE)	Recovery[c] (%)
Single dose	1,000	—	31	16.64 ± 0.89	—
Single dose	500	—	36	4.12 ± 0.39	—
Two fractions[d]	1,000	24	32	8.73 ± 0.91	63
Single dose	500	—	36	4.12 ± 0.39	—
Single dose	250	—	35	2.13 ± 0.26	—
Two fractions[d]	500	24	31	3.97 ± 0.39	7
Two fractions[d]	500	48	31	4.56 ± 0.35	−22
Two fractions[d]	500	96	30	5.52 ± 0.39	−70

[a] Injections given either as a single dose or as two equal fractions separated by 24 to 96 hr.

[b] Mean observed in the treated group minus the control mean of 0.43 adenoma/mouse.

[c] 100% recovery equals a mean number of induced adenomas identical with that observed in mice given only one-half the total urethane dose, i.e., 500 and 250 mg/kg, respectively.

[d] Two equal fractions given at the specified intervals.

zations within the target cells of the irradiated lung. In brief, we propose that our results are compatible with the predictions of the dual action theory of radiation injury (Kellerer, this volume). The urethane data, although the kinetics are similar, need not be the product of identical or even similar processes. Urethane was administered systemically, and it is possible that the event interaction in the curvilinear portion of the dose-response curve (Fig. 1) reflects the development of significant immunosuppression (Malmgren et al., 1952) or prolonged retention time of the carcinogen (White, 1971), which does not occur in the low dose region.[1] Immunosuppression would appear to be an unlikely candidate for this additional event, since the adenomas are very weakly immunogenic, and mice treated with 1,000 mg/kg of urethane are no more or less resistant to transplants of this tumor

---

[1] The author acknowledges these suggestions by Professor N. Haran-Ghera and Professor J. Neyman, respectively.

(Yuhas, *unpublished observations*). Although unlikely, due to the time factors involved, a prolonged carcinogen retention time remains a possible interpretation.

Whether or not the event interaction involved in the two carcinogenic mechanisms is the same, it is interesting to note that recovery is dose dependent in both cases. However, at doses that are equally carcinogenic (e.g., a mean of one induced adenoma per mouse) one is well into the X-ray dose range in which recovery would occur (Fig. 1) but is still well within the "no recovery" dose range for urethane. Therefore, protraction of this X-ray dose would produce significantly fewer tumors, whereas protraction of the urethane dose would produce as many tumors as the same total dose given acutely. We suggest that information such as this may prove to be more valuable to those estimating comparative hazards than simple estimates of carcinogenic efficiency.

As a last point, it must be emphasized that the radiation doses that define the break between the linear, "no recovery" portion of the dose-response curve and the curvilinear portion are heavily dependent on the tumor being studied. As an example, in the ovarian tumor system, recovery is constant between doses of 49 and 392 rads (Yuhas, 1974a). In this highly radiosensitive system, we have been unable, as yet, to detect the linear portion of the dose-response curve. We concur, therefore, with the recommendations of the Aspen report (NRC/NAS, 1974), in which it was suggested that the definition of the low dose range is dependent on the test system employed and that for each system it is that region in which the effect is linearly proportional to dose.

ACUTE AND CHRONIC RADIATION EFFECTS ON RESISTANCE TO ONCOGENIC VIRUSES

For a number of years, it has been known that administration of 600 to 700 rads as four equal weekly fractions was far more leukemogenic than the administration of the same total dose acutely (Kaplan and Brown, 1952), at least in the C57BL mouse. This repeatedly observed phenomenon stands in contrast to what might be expected if significant recovery from immunosuppression occurred or if recovery from carcinogenic injury occurred in the fractionally exposed group. It has been suggested, therefore, that fractionation proves to be more leukemogenic because these exposures disturb the normal target cell kinetics, and thereby places more of them in a sensitive state (Kaplan, 1964). The exact nature of this disturbance is not clear, but recent evidence provided by Tennant (*this volume*) has demonstrated that actively dividing cells are more susceptible to radiation activation of endogenous leukemia viruses, and that chronic irradiation is more effective in this regard than is acute irradiation, even after cell survival is taken into account.

At the risk of overgeneralizing, we propose that radiation can increase the leukemia incidence either by inducing such a heavy viral burden that immune responsiveness is irrelevant, or by suppressing immune responsiveness such that even small viral burdens can prove to be significant. In addition to being a means of reconciling the opposing views in this argument, this proposal is consistent with established patterns—Those exposure regimens, such as fractionated or chronic exposures, which are highly leukemogenic in spite of their weak immunosuppressive capabilities, are highly efficient in activating endogenous leukemia viruses (Tennant, *this volume*); and, conversely, those exposure regimens, such as acute exposures, which are moderately leukemogenic in spite of their weak virus activation capabilities (see chapters by Tennant and Decleve, *this volume*), are strongly immunosuppressive (Yuhas et al., 1973). Consistency alone cannot prove or disprove a proposal, so we have initiated a series of experiments designed to test this proposal, and present below the results of our initial investigations.

For the host in these studies, we have used adult (4-month-old) BALB/c female mice), which are essentially insensitive to the induction of leukemia by either acute or chronic γ-rays over a wide range of doses and dose rates (Yuhas, unpub., 1974). Groups of these mice ($N = 16$) were exposed to 392 rads of ^{137}Cs γ-rays at dose rates of 41 rads/min (acute) or 28 rads/day (chronic). Following exposure, these mice, along with unirradiated controls, were allowed to recover through the age of 6-months, at which time all mice were given an intramuscular injection of 0.1 ml of the Moloney strain of the murine leukemia/sarcoma virus complex, henceforth referred to as MSV/MLV. Since our intent in these studies was to study the development of leukemia, we passaged our original low-leukemia line of this virus (Pazmino and Yuhas, 1973) through two *in vivo* passages, and thereby increased its leukemogenic potency (see below).

This experiment is still in progress, but the data obtained to date are more than sufficient to answer the question posed by these studies. It should be noted that unirradiated and irradiated (acute or chronic) mice demonstrated less than 7% mortality within the first 8 months of the experiment in the absence of MSV/MLV injection.

Figure 2 is a plot of the percent mortality versus time for the virus-injected control and irradiated mice. Control mice began to die between 90 and 100 days after virus injection, but this wave of deaths was completed by the 160th day after injection, with negligible further mortality through the 230th day. Radiation exposure of the mice prior to the virus injection altered the mortality pattern, but the direction of its alteration depended on the manner in which the 392 rads was applied (Fig. 2). Mice given 392 rads at 28 rads/day (Fig. 2; chronic) began to die between days 70 and 80 of the experiment, and all had died by the 160th day post-virus injection. Conversely, mice given 392 rads in a matter of minutes (Fig. 2; acute) did not start to die until the 110- to 120-day interval, and then only gradually, but significant mortality was observed between days 160 and 230 of the experiment. The apparent explanation for these anomalous patterns can be seen in the analysis of the causes of death in these mice. Typical MSV/MLV induced leukemias occurred exclusively within the first 160 days after virus injection, whereas none of the sarcomas that developed occurred before the 140th day after injection. This latter observation confirms our earlier estimates on the rate of development of sarcomas under similar conditions (Yuhas, 1974*b*). Table 3 summarizes the probabilities of dying of leukemia during the early period (through day 160) and of dying of a sarcoma during the later period (day 140 through 230) for each of the experimental groups. Relative to unirradiated mice, chronic irradiation increased the prob-

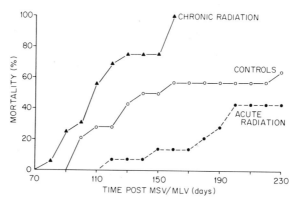

FIG. 2. Percent mortality as a function of time in BALB/c mice given MSV/MLV at the age of six months. Time zero on the plot coincides with the time of virus injection. Controls received no irradiated prior to the virus; the chronic radiation group received 392 rads of γ-rays at a rate of 28 rads/day, starting at the age of 4 months (exposure time = 14 days); and acute radiation group received 392 rads of γ-rays at 41 rads/min at the age of 4 months.

ability of developing leukemia, and acute irradiation suppressed it, and both of these alterations are statistically significant (Table 2). No valid estimate of the probability of dying with a sarcoma is available for the chronically irradiated group, but acute irradiation increased the risk of sarcoma relative to unirradiated mice. At the time of writing (day 230 of the experiment), the difference in risk of dying with sarcoma between the control and acutely irradiated group was not statistically significant ($P < 0.10$). It should be remembered, however, that almost all of these mice will eventually develop an injection site sarcoma (Yuhas, 1974*b*), with the acutely irradiated group demonstrating a much faster rate of development (see above, and Yuhas, 1974*b*). In support of our prediction regarding the eventual fate of the control and acutely irradiated mice still alive at day 230 of the experiment stands the observation that none of the control mice possessed palpable injection-site tumors on day 230 (0/6), whereas almost all of the acutely irradiated mice did (7/9). We conclude, therefore, that exposure of mice to chronic γ-rays prior to a large virus challenge sensitizes them to the development of leukemia, whereas acute preexposure makes them resistant to leukemia but sensitive to sarcoma induction.

Our proposal was that immunosuppression would only be important in the development of radiation induced leukemia if the viral burden were low but that disturbances in the target cell kinetics could more than counterbalance any lack of immunosuppression either by providing a source of sensitive cells in which the virus can accomplish transformation or by placing the target cells in a sensitive stage for activation of endogenous viruses (Tennant, *this volume*). The data presented above have provided only a partial

TABLE 3. *Deaths attributable to leukemia and sarcoma in control and preirradiated mice given MSV/MLV,[a] through the first 230 days of the experiment*

Preirradiation	Leukemia deaths[b]	Sarcoma deaths[c]
Controls	9/16	1/7[h]
Chronically exposed[d]	16/16[f]	—
Acutely exposed[e]	2/16[g]	5/14[i]

[a] MSV/MLV given intramuscularly at the age of 6 months; this equals day zero of the experiment.

[b] Cause of death, disseminated leukemia; no sarcomas detected, except in one on the two acutely exposed mice.

[c] Deaths due to local and metastatic sarcoma deposits.

[d] Given 392 rads at 28 rads/day starting at four months.

[e] Given 392 rads at 41 rads/min at the age of four months.

[f] Significantly greater than respective value in controls ($P < 0.005$) and in acutely exposed ($P < 0.0005$).

[g] Significantly smaller than respective value in controls ($P < 0.01$) and chronically exposed ($P < 0.0005$).

[h] None of the six mice surviving to 230 days possessed palpable sarcomas.

[i] Seven of the nine mice surviving to 230 days had palpable sarcomas.

test of this proposal, in that we have standardized the amount of virus present (by adding it exogenously) and determined the role of chronic versus acute exposure in altering sensitivity to the virus. Quite clearly, one cannot argue that immunosuppression is responsible for the radiation induced alterations in sensitivity to the exogenous virus. What appears more likely is that chronic irradiation enhances the sensitivity of the target population either quantitatively (more cells at risk) or qualitatively (more rapid cycle times), whereas acute irradiation depletes or at least reduces the size of the target population. We are at present testing these points directly. Preliminary results suggest that the chronic, radiation induced sensitization to leukemia declines as the time between completion of exposure and virus injection increases. Conversely, the acute irradiation effect does not alter appreciably as the interval between the two is increased. These observations are consistent with our proposal.

An interesting point observed in these studies is that although acute ir-radiation elevates resistance to the leukemogenic effect of MSV/MLV, it apparently sensitizes to the sarcomagenic effects of the same (Table 3). Undoubtedly, this is related to the fact that the target and effector cells in virus induced leukemia are one and the same, whereas in sarcomagenesis, they are quite distinct. Therefore, in the development of sarcomas, depletion of the lymphoid tissue can only serve to reduce host resistance to the devel-opment of tumors from muscle cells.

We are currently testing the second aspect of our proposal, i.e., that im-munosuppression can prove to be important in radiation leukemogenesis when the viral burden is low. The results are preliminary and thus do not warrant discussion, but they are not inconsistent with the argument that the immune system is able to cope with only limited tumor burdens (or viral burdens), and that their importance is restricted to a very limited range of experimental conditions (Klein, 1971).

SUMMARY

In the data presented above, we have demonstrated that at least three types of mechanisms can contribute to the yield of radiation induced can-cers, but that the relative contribution of each depends heavily on the ex-posure conditions and on the tumor type in question. A continued consid-eration of the mechanisms involved relative to the dose-response curves observed would appear to be the most fruitful approach to the study of the biology of radiation carcinogenesis.

ACKNOWLEDGMENTS

The author is indebted to Dr. Nelson Pazmino for his dedicated collabora-tion in these experiments, and to Miss Anita Walker and Mrs. Mildred Hayes for their invaluable assistance.

REFERENCES

Celada, F., and Carter, R. R. (1962): The radiosensitive nature of homograft-rejecting and agglutinin-forming capacities of isolated spleen cells. *J. Immunol.,* 89:161–169.
Grahn, D., and Sacher, G. (1968): Fractionation and protraction factors and the late effects of radiation in small mammals. In: *Dose Rate in Mammalian Radiation Biol-ogy,* edited by D. G. Brown, R. G. Cragle, and T. R. Noonan, pp. 2.1–2.27. USAEC, Division of Technical Information, CONF-680410.
Kaplan, H. S., and Brown, M. B. (1952): A quantitative dose response study of lymphoid tumor development in irradiated C57 black mice. *J. Natl. Cancer Inst.,* 13:185–208.
Kaplan, H. S. (1964): The role of radiation in experimental leukemogenesis. *National Cancer Inst. Monograph,* 14:207–220.
Klein, G. (1971): Immunologic studies on a human tumor: Dilemmas of the experi-mentalist. In: *Immunologic Parameters of Host-Tumor Relationships,* edited by D. W. Weiss, pp. 111–131. Academic Press, New York.

Malmgren, R. A., Bennison, E. B., and McKinley, T. W. (1952): Reduced antibody titers in mice treated with carcinogenic and cancer chemotherapeutic drugs. *Proc. Soc. Expt. Biol. Med.,* 79:484–488.

Nowell, P. C., and Cole, L. J. (1965): Hepatomas in mice: Incidence increased after gamma irradiation at low dose rates. *Science,* 148:96–97.

NRC/NAS (1974): Research needs for estimating the biological hazards of low doses of ionizing radiation. *Reports of an Ad Hoc Panel of the Committee on Nuclear Science,* 54 pp. National Academy of Sciences/National Research Council, Washington, D.C.

Pazmino, N. H., and Yuhas, J. M. (1973): Senescent loss of resistance to murine sarcoma virus (Moloney) in the mouse. *Cancer Res.,* 33:2668–2673.

Rossi, H. H., and Kellerer, A. M. (1972): Radiation carcinogenesis at low doses. *Science,* 175:200–202.

Shimkin, M. B., Wieder, R., and Marzi, D. (1967): Lung tumors in mice receiving different schedules of urethane. In: *Proceedings of the Fifth Berkeley Symposium on Mathematical Statistics and Probability.* Vol. IV, edited by L. M. LeCam and J. Neyman, pp. 707–720. University of California Press, Berkeley.

White, M. (1971): Studies on the mechanism of induction of pulmonary adenomas in mice. In: *Proceedings of the Sixth Berkeley Symposium on Mathematical Statistics and Probability.* Vol. IV, edited by L. M. LeCam, J. Neyman, and E. L. Scott, pp. 287–298. University of California Press, Berkeley.

White, M., Grendon, A., and Jones, H. B. (1967): Effects of urethane dose and time pattern on tumor formation. In: *Proceedings of the Fifth Berkeley Symposium on Mathematical Statistics and Probability.* Vol. IV., edited by L. M. LeCam and J. Neyman, University of California Press, Berkeley, pp. 721–734.

Yuhas, J. M. (1974a): Recovery from radiation carcinogenic injury to the mouse ovary. *Radiat. Res.,* 60:321–332.

Yuhas, J. M. (1974b): Discussion of paper by Zimmerman et al. In: *Interaction of Radiation and Host Immune Defense Mechanisms in Malignancy,* edited by V. P. Bond, Brookhaven National Laboratory, Upton, New York BNL-50418, pp. 73–74.

Pazmino, N. H., Ullrich, R. L., and Yuhas, J. M. (1975): Split dose recovery from radiation carcinogenic injury to the mouse lung. (Submitted to *Radiation Research.*)

Yuhas, J. M., Tennant, R. W., Hanna, M. G., and Clapp, N. K. (1973): Radiation-induced immunosuppression: Demonstration of its role in radiation leukemogenesis in the intact RF mouse. In: *Radionuclide Carcinogenesis,* edited by C. L. Saunders, R. H. Busch, J. E. Ballou, and D. D. Mahlum, pp. 312–321. USAEC, Washington, D.C.

Yuhas, J. M., and Walker, A. E. (1973): Exposure response curve for radiation induced lung tumors in the mouse. *Radiat. Res.,* 54:261–273.

Biology of Radiation Carcinogenesis, edited by
J. M. Yuhas, R. W. Tennant, and J. D. Regan.
Raven Press, New York © 1976.

Molecular Mechanisms in Radiation Carcinogenesis

R. B. Setlow

Biology Department, Brookhaven National Laboratory, Upton, New York 11973

A practical motivation behind molecular studies of radiation carcinogenesis is the desire to develop theories that permit us to extrapolate from cellular and animal models to man. The best example of this extrapolation—but one that is still incomplete—is that of skin cancer.

There are three reasons for the emphasis on skin cancer:

1. Skin cancer is the most common of all cancer among Caucasians (1) and there is a large amount of epidemiologic data for it (2). A better understanding of the many factors involved in its incidence could lead to improved data collection schemes.

2. There is persuasive biophysical, biochemical, and genetic evidence (2,3), some of which is discussed in this volume, that a causal relation exists between sunlight-induced photochemical damage to DNA and skin cancer in man. Since we know the wavelengths of UV radiation that affect DNA (3), we are on firm theoretical ground when we estimate the effective biological radiances in sunlight.

3. Some chemicals that result from man's activities (such as NO_x from supersonic transports and Freon (used as a propellant for sprays) tend to decrease the amount of ozone in the stratosphere and, hence, increase the biologically effective radiances at the Earth's surface (2).

The quantitative evaluation of the increase in the incidence rate of skin cancer for a decrease of ozone is a simplified model for most environmental carcinogens. Therefore, it is important to show explicitly the limitations in making such calculations and why better models, theories, and data are needed.

TABLE 1. *Some variables in sunlight-induced skin cancer*

I:	UV irradiance averaged over the year	
T:	Time of day at which exposure begins	Life
t:	Time duration per exposure	style
n:	Number of exposures per year	
A:	Age	Sampling
G:	Genetic background	factors
O:	Occupation	
E:	Other environmental factors (wind, visible light, temperature. . . .)	

There are many variables involved in the induction of skin cancer in man. Some of these are enumerated in Table 1.

The probability P of developing cancer at a particular time is a function of these variables [Eq. (1)]:

$$P = f(I,T,t,n,A,G,O,E, . . .) \tag{1}$$

and the quantitative evaluation of the risk to man of a decrease in ozone is represented by Eq. (2).

$$\frac{\partial P}{\partial O_3} = \frac{\partial f}{\partial I} \frac{\partial I}{\partial O_3} \tag{2}$$

Since we have good estimates of the change in irradiance with the change in ozone concentration (2), the evaluation of the environmental hazard depends upon a determination of $\partial f/\partial I$.

Approach I

There are two simple-minded approaches to the evaluation of $\partial f/\partial I$. The first is to use epidemiological data relating skin cancer to latitude (skin cancer increases with decreasing latitude). In formal terms, the change of P with latitude may depend upon many factors as shown in Eq. (3).

$$\begin{aligned}
\frac{\partial P}{\partial L} = &\frac{\partial f}{\partial I} \cdot \frac{\partial I}{\partial L} \\
&+ \frac{\partial f}{\partial T} \frac{\partial T}{\partial L} + \frac{\partial f}{\partial t} \frac{\partial t}{\partial L} + \frac{\partial f}{\partial n} \frac{\partial n}{\partial L} \quad \text{Life style factors} \\
&+ \frac{\partial f}{\partial A} \frac{\partial A}{\partial L} + \frac{\partial f}{\partial G} \frac{\partial G}{\partial L} + \frac{\partial f}{\partial O} \frac{\partial O}{\partial L} \quad \text{Sampling factors} \\
&+ \frac{\partial f}{\partial E} \frac{\partial E}{\partial L}
\end{aligned} \tag{3}$$

We know that, in addition to I, some of the factors under the headings life style and sampling are important in skin cancer and do depend upon latitude. Unfortunately, we do not know how. Therefore, we make the assumption that all these factors add up to zero and hence

$$\frac{\partial P}{\partial L} = \frac{\partial f}{\partial I} \cdot \frac{\partial I}{\partial L} \quad \text{or} \quad \frac{\partial f}{\partial I} = \frac{\partial P/\partial I}{\partial L/\partial L} \tag{4}$$

The results of this approach are given in a recent report (2). They indicate, for example, that a 10% reduction in ozone would result in an approximate 30% increase in skin cancer among Caucasians.

Approach II

A completely different way of looking at the problem assumes that the important factor in skin cancer is the total dose D accumulated up to the time skin cancer is detected.

$$D = kIA \tag{5}$$

where k depends on life style and includes variables T, t, and n in Table 1. The potentially important role of aging, for example, as a result of a less effective immune system, is ignored, and hence

$$P = f(D, G, O, E \ldots) \tag{6}$$

This formulation may be used at a particular latitude if one assumes that life style factors are independent of time. It is apparent from Eq. (5) that a 10% increase in ultraviolet irradiance, I, is equivalent to a 10% increase in the age, A, at which skin cancer is scored.

There is some theoretical basis for Eqs. (5) and (6). Blum (4) has shown that the induction of skin cancer in mice by repetitive exposures to UV depends upon the dose per fraction and the square of the total number of fractions delivered before the cancer is detected. At low intensities, however, the reciprocity law is not obeyed (perhaps because there is appreciable repair of damage before the carcinogenic changes become fixed in the genome), and incidence depends upon $I^2 t(nA)^2$, that is, on the square of the terms of Eq. (5). The use of approach II and age-specific incidence rates (1) indicates that a 10% decrease in ozone would result in a roughly 100% increase in the incidence of nonmelanoma skin cancer.

CONCLUSION

Although the two approaches outlined above give results that differ by a factor of three, I consider the agreement is good in view of the completely different assumptions involved and the crude averages used in data analysis. In the field of radiation carcinogenesis, we have gone much further than just the simple statement as to whether an agent is good or bad. We can make quantitative predictions. It is clear that for quantitative evaluation of hazardous environmental agents we need more than just extensive epidemiologic data. We need useful cellular and animal models as well as good molecular theories.

REFERENCES

1. Blum, H. F. (1974): Uncertainty of growth of cell populations in cancer. *J. Theoret. Biol.*, 46:143–166.
2. *Environmental Impact of Stratospheric Flight* (1975): National Academy of Sciences, Washington, D.C.
3. Scotto, J., Kopf, A. W., and Urbach, F. (1974): Nonmelanoma skin cancer among whites in four areas of the U.S. *Cancer Res.*, 34:1333–1338.
4. Setlow, R. B. (1974): The wavelengths in sunlight effective in producing skin cancer: A theoretical analysis. *Proc. Natl. Acad. Sci. USA*, 71:3363–3366.

Biology of Radiation Carcinogenesis, edited by
J. M. Yuhas, R. W. Tennant, and J. D. Regan.
Raven Press, New York © 1976.

Radiation-Induced Strand Breaks in the DNA of Mammalian Cells

M. G. Ormerod

Chester Beatty Research Institute, Institute of Cancer Research, Royal Cancer Hospital, Clifton Avenue, Sutton, Surrey, SM2 5PX England

The justification for including this topic in a meeting on radiation carcinogenesis is the hypothesis that radiation can induce cancer by means of a chemical change in the DNA of a cell. I think that it is fair to say that no one has yet established a direct link between a specific chemical change and a biological end-point (e.g., mutation, cell death) in a mammalian cell. Equally, if a mutation does lead to neoplastic growth, we have no idea what that mutation is nor do we know the biochemical product of such a mutation.

One of the many effects of ionizing radiation on DNA is to introduce breaks either in one strand of the double helix (single-strand breaks) or into both strands in close proximity (double-strand breaks). Because of the length of a molecule of DNA such breaks are relatively easy to detect.

Long molecules of DNA are susceptible to hydrodynamic shear. This effect hampered early workers until McGrath and Williams (1966) developed a method for determining the molecular weight of bacterial DNA that avoided handling solutions of DNA. Cells were lysed on top of a gradient of sucrose under conditions that deproteinized the nucleic acid; the molecular weight of the released DNA was measured by subsequent sedimentation through the solution of sucrose. Lett, Caldwell, Dean, and Alexander (1967) demonstrated that this technique could be used with mammalian cells, and since then, there have been many studies on the induction and restitution of strand breaks in the DNA of cells. This technique is probably of most value when used in parallel with measurements of other properties of the DNA and the cell—an example can be found in the study of the response of cells to photochemical damage (for a recent review, see Cleaver, 1974c). In the case of ionizing radiation, we know little about other chemical changes in DNA irradiated in a cell. We also do not have much information about the nature of the end-groups left after the introduction of a strand break. It is hoped that the development of improved techniques (Mattern, Hariharan, Dunlap, and Cerutti, 1973; Hariharan and Cerutti,

* This work was supported by grants to the Chester Beatty Research Institute, Institute of Cancer Research; Royal Cancer Hospital by the Cancer Research Campaign and the Medical Research Council.

1972; Coquerelle, Bopp, Kessler, and Hagen, 1973) will rectify this situation. Meanwhile, it should be realized that the wealth of literature reflects not the importance of the strand break but rather the ease with which it can be measured.

I have restricted this review to the observation of strand breaks in the DNA of mammalian cells after exposure to ionizing radiation. Most of the review deals with experiments that involve the sedimentation of DNA through a gradient of sucrose. I have assumed that the reader has some knowledge of the techniques involved. These techniques have been discussed in an earlier article, which also reviews the literature through 1971 (Ormerod, 1973).

This chapter illustrates various points with data obtained in my laboratory. In most cases, similar data have been published by other workers. I have used our own data because they are to hand and I am not thereby making any claim to originality.

ANALYSIS OF THE DATA

Correctly analyzed, the data obtained from use of a preparative ultra-centrifuge should yield not only the average molecular weight of the DNA but also its molecular weight distribution. Carefully isolated, the molecules of DNA from a bacteriophage are monodisperse, that is, they are all of the same molecular weight. Molecules of DNA from a cell usually have a poly-disperse distribution—a range of molecular weights is present. Ionizing radiation introduces strand breaks into DNA at random. The resulting molecular weight distribution is random and if the logarithm of the number of molecules of a given molecular weight is plotted against molecular weight, a linear plot results. The slope of this line equals $1/M_n$ where M_n is the number average molecular weight. If the molecules of DNA are radioactively labeled along most of their length, this can be realized experimentally by plotting $C/M \, \Delta \, M$ against M, where C is the radioactivity in a fraction the average molecular weight of which is M and which covers a range of molecular weights ΔM (Lehmann and Ormerod, 1970a). M_n can be read from this plot, which also confirms that the molecular weight distribution is indeed random. The method is simple to use and is superior to the calculation of molecular weight by summation because in a summation an error in one or two fractions can unduly influence the result. It has been used successfully by several workers (Dean, Ormerod, Serianni, and Alexander, 1969; Donlon and Norman, 1971; Palcic and Skarsgard, 1972a; Matsudaira and Furuno, 1972). Examples of this type of analysis are given later.

Alternatively, a computer can be used to simulate random strand breakage and the resulting sedimentation profile can be calculated and then compared to the experimental data (Lett and Sun, 1970; Gillespie, Gislason, Dugle, and Chapman, 1972; Ehmann and Lett, 1973). This method has the advantage that it can be applied to non-random distributions; for example, it can be used to estimate a molecular weight resulting from the introduction of a small number of breaks in a molecule of initially monodisperse distribution (Litwin, Shahn, and Kozinski, 1969). A random distribution will result only after the introduction of at least five breaks for every initial molecule (Charlesby, 1954).

If the ends of long molecules are labeled, then the label will have an apparent distribution of lower average molecular weight than that derived from fully labeled molecules (Lehmann and Ormerod, 1969). This condition is realized when growing cells are pulse-labeled with a radioactive precursor of DNA (Lehmann and Ormerod, 1970a), and the effect can be used to calculate the replication rate of the nucleic acid. The observation of a peak of radioactivity from pulse-labeled DNA sedimenting more slowly than fully labeled DNA should not be taken as evidence for the existence of an intermediate involved in replication. Great care must be taken in the analysis of data from pulse-labeled cells. For an example of pulse-labeling in the case of UV-irradiated cells, see Lehmann (1972).

DOUBLE-STRAND BREAKS

A double-strand break requires two single-strand breaks, one in each strand of the double helix, in sufficiently close proximity (probably between 2 and 20 nucleotides) (Freifelder and Trumbo, 1969). The single-strand breaks can either be a result of two independent events or a single event. The double breaks are usually detected by measuring the reduction in molecular weight of native DNA.

When murine lymphoma cells (L5178Y) were lysed in a variety of detergents on top of a gradient of sucrose, the DNA released was in a fast-sedimenting complex, which also contained lipid (Ormerod and Lehmann, 1971a). The density of this complex in a solution of sucrose and cesium chloride was approximately 1.4 as opposed to about 1.7 for free DNA. It was postulated that DNA is attached to the nuclear membrane by detergent-stable bonds spaced at on average interval of about 2×10^9 daltons (Ormerod and Lehmann, 1971a).

Radiation of the cells prior to lysis releases the DNA from this complex (Lehmann and Ormerod, 1970b; Corry and Cole, 1973), presumably by the introduction of breaks that release the DNA from the attached lipid. Using L5178Y cells, we found that 80% of the DNA was released by a dose of 30 krad, which yielded material of a number average molecular weight of 10^9 daltons (Ormerod and Lehmann, 1971a). Corry and Cole (1973) found that 5 krad was sufficient to release the DNA from Chinese hamster ovary cells. In these cells, this dose of radiation yielded DNA of molecular weight of about 2×10^9 daltons.

The DNA released from the lipid-DNA complex by radiation behaved upon centrifugation as freely sedimenting molecules. That is, no contamination by RNA, lipid, or protein could be detected by double-labeling; within experimental error, all the DNA was recovered from the gradient; the measured molecular weight was independent of the ionic strength of the gradient in the range 0.1 to 2; the molecular weight distribution was random, and the number of breaks produced was a linear function of radiation dose (Lehmann and Ormerod, 1970*b;* Ormerod, 1973). The last two criteria were fulfilled only when the speed of centrifugation was kept below 10^4 rpm. At higher rotor speeds, sharper, more slowly sedimenting profiles were obtained, due to an anomaly associated with DNA of high molecular weights (Zimm, 1974); it is discussed fully later.

From our data, we estimated that one double-strand break was introduced into the DNA of a murine lymphoma cell (L5178Y) per krad per 3×10^{10} daltons. This is equivalent to an energy absorption of 2900 eV per break (Lehmann and Ormerod, 1970*b*). Corry and Cole (1973) estimated that 1,250 eV was required per double-strand break in Chinese hamster ovary cells. In both cases, the plot of the reciprocal of number average molecular weight (M_n) against dose of radiation was linear, and it was concluded that the double-strand break is a single-hit event [a two-hit event would require that a plot of $1/M_n$ against $(dose)^2$ should be linear]. Metaphase chromosomes from Chinese hamster cells require only 600 eV/break; this increases to 4,000 eV/break in the presence of 0.05 M cystamine (Corry and Cole, 1968).

In rat thymocytes, irradiated in air, Coquerelle et al. (1973) estimated an efficiency for double-strand break production of 1,900 eV/break. The cells were irradiated in the dose range 0 to 6 Mrad, which is more than ten times the radiation doses used by Lehmann and Ormerod (1970*b*) and Corry and Cole (1973). It is possible that some of the breaks were formed by the close proximity of two single-strand breaks.

Lennartz, Coquerelle, and Hagen (1973) found that the electron volts required for each double-strand break decreased to 1,100 under oxygen and increased to 4,200 under nitrogen, an oxygen enhancement ratio of 3.8. This is the same ratio as was found for single-strand breaks in some experiments with rat thymocytes. The same criticism applies to this observation as was made above about that of Coquerelle et al. (1973).

Corry and Cole (1973) have demonstrated clearly that Chinese hamster ovary cells can rejoin at least some of the double-strand breaks introduced by up to 100 krad of ^{197}Cs γ-rays. The repair process was most efficient after doses of radiation of 50 krad or less. In constrast, the rejoining of double-strand breaks by L5178Y cells after 20 krad could not be detected (Lehmann and Ormerod, 1970*b*). Of course, this does not preclude the possibility that these cells might rejoin double-strand breaks after doses of radiation in the survival range (the survival curve has a shoulder of 100 rad and a D_{37} of 80 rads) (Lehmann, 1970).

It may be concluded that double-strand breaks are introduced into the DNA of mammalian cells as a single-hit event for every 1,000 to 3,000 eV of deposited energy. Repair of double breaks is possible.

SINGLE-STRAND BREAKS

The Release of Denatured DNA from a Mammalian Cell

Single-strand breaks are frequently detected by measuring a reduction in the molecular weight of denatured DNA. This is usually achieved by sedimenting the nucleic acid through gradients of alkaline (pH ~ 12) sucrose. The high pH denatures the DNA and helps to deproteinize it.

If untreated mammalian cells are lysed on top of such a gradient, DNA is released as a complex; it does not behave as a collection of freely sedimenting molecules (Lett et al., 1967; Elkind and Kamper, 1970; Elkind, 1971; McBurney, Graham, and Whitmore, 1972; Belli, Cooper, and Brown, 1972; Elkind and Chang-Liu, 1972a; Cleaver, 1974b). If the cells are lysed in alkali without a detergent, the complex may be associated with a material containing choline—probably lipid (Elkind, 1971; Elkind and Chang-Liu, 1972a). When cells were lysed in alkali and detergent, we could not detect any contaminating substance (Lehmann, 1970).

Any treatment that introduces strand breaks into the DNA releases DNA from the complex (for a fuller discussion, see Ormerod, 1973). It has been shown by many workers that long molecules of duplex DNA are not fully denatured in alkali (McBurney and Whitmore, 1972; Ahnstrom and Erixon, 1973; Simpson, Nagle, Bick, and Belli, 1973; Ahnstrom and Edvardsson, 1974; Cleaver, 1974a; Jolley and Ormerod, 1973; Rydberg, 1974). In particular, Ahnstrom and Erixon (1973), Cleaver (1974a), and Simpson et al. (1973) have fractionated DNA on gradients of alkaline sucrose and have shown that the "complexed" DNA is not fully denatured.

Introduction of single-strand breaks into the DNA allows the DNA to denature fully. This is usually achieved either by irradiating the cells to a dose of radiation between 700 and 1,000 rads (Elkind and Chang-Liu, 1972a; McBurney et al., 1972; Lehmann and Ormerod, 1971) or by allowing the DNA to degrade in alkali on top of the gradient (Lett, Klucis, and Sun, 1970; Elkind and Kamper, 1970). The resulting DNA, at speeds of centrifugation of 2×10^4 rpm or more, gives a sharp, nonrandom profile on the gradient (for example, see Lett and Sun, 1970; Elkind and Kamper, 1970; McBurney et al., 1971, 1972; Ormerod and Lehmann, 1971b; see also Fig. 7). This DNA has a sedimentation coefficient of 120 to 180 S. It is single stranded and seems to contain the largest piece of single-strand DNA obtainable by this technique. The DNA of larger size is not fully denatured (Ahnstrom and Erixon, 1973; Cleaver, 1974a).

It has been suggested that the DNA contained in this profile is monodisperse (i.e., all the same molecular weight) and that it represents a fundamental subunit in the organization of chromosomal DNA. It has also been postulated that the appearance of this profile is caused by anomalous sedimentation of long molecules and that much of the DNA therein is of higher molecular weight (McBurney and Whitmore, 1972; Ormerod and Lehmann, 1971b). I believe that the bulk of the experimental evidence favors the latter hypothesis, and for the rest of the discussion in this section, I will assume that the appearance of this type of DNA is indicative of the presence at random of about one single-strand break per 5×10^8 daltons of DNA and has no other significance. (This is approximately the number of strand breaks introduced by 1 krad of high-energy radiation, see below.)

This controversy is of importance in the discussion of the repair of strand breaks in DNA. It is proposed that two types of repair can be observed: first, the rejoining of random breaks to restitute the hypothetical subunits; this is followed by the reformation of the linkers between subunits (Elkind and Kamper, 1970; Elkind and Chang-Liu, 1972a; Lett, Sun, and Wheeler, 1972; Wheeler, Sheridan, Pautler, et al., 1973; Wheeler and Linn, 1974). If the subunit hypothesis holds, the reformation of the linkers could have special biological significance; on the other hand, if the so-called subunit reflects an anomaly of sedimentation, no second repair process is detected, and one is merely observing the rejoining of the last few single-strand breaks. Because of the importance of this topic, it is discussed in detail in a later section.

Doses of radiation of 5 krad or more release DNA with a random molecular weight distribution and a sedimentation coefficient that is independent of rotor speeds at present attainable ($< 5 \times 10^4$ rpm) (Elkind, 1971; McBurney et al., 1971; Ormerod and Stevens, 1971; Ormerod, 1973).

The Efficiency of Production of Single-Strand Breaks

Sedimentation in gradients of alkaline sucrose will reveal single-strand breaks introduced into the DNA of cells by radiation directly and indirectly (through attack by an endonulease) plus any alkali-labile bonds created by the radiation. If radiation is at 0°C (as is customary), endonuclease attack is unlikely (Palcic and Skarsgard, 1972b). Any postirradiation enzyme attack is probably obscured by a rapid rejoining of other strand breaks. Using DNA isolated conventionally from irradiated rat thymocytes, Lennartz et al. (1973) compared the number of single-strand breaks after denaturation by alkali with those revealed by heating in the presence of formaldehyde. They found that 28% of the breaks under oxygen and 50% of those formed by irradiation under nitrogen resulted from the production of alkali-labile bonds. Presumably, the remaining breaks were present as breaks in the DNA in the cell. Throughout the rest of this chapter, the term "single-strand break" will be used to include those breaks caused directly by radiation as well as those created by hydrolysis of radiation induced, alkali-labile bonds.

One single-strand break is produced in the DNA of a mammalian cell for every 30 to 100 eV of energy absorbed (see Table 1). It is not clear if the differences in efficiencies reflect a real variation between different types of cell or if they reflect differences in calibration (Wheeler, DeWitt, and Lett 1974). Certainly there has been no report from one laboratory of substantial differences in strand break production between one class of cell and another.

A careful study by Lett and Sun (1970) has shown that the number of strand breaks formed in the DNA of Chinese hamster ovary cells is independent of the position of the cells in the cell cycle.

TABLE 1. *The efficiency of production of single-strand breaks in the DNA of irradiated mammalian cells*

| Cell | eV/break | | References |
	Air or O_2	N_2	
Chinese hamster ovary	60		Lett and Sun (1970)
Murine lymphoma (L5178Y)	44	44	Omerod and Stevens (1971)
Human lymphocytes	55		Donlon and Norman (1971)
Murine L cells	72		McBurney et al. (1971)
Canine neurons	58		Wheeler and Lett (1972)
Ehrlich ascites nuclei	80		Matsudaira and Furano (1972)
Murine L-60	31	90	Palcic and Skarsgard (1972a)
Chinese hamster (V90)	29	77	Modig et al. (1974)
Chinese hamster (V9-379A)	83	284	Dugle et al. (1972)
Chinese hamster ovary	29	122	Roots and Smith (1974
Rat thymocytes	57	213	Lennartz et al. (1974)
Murine lymphoma (SL2)	44	44	—[a]
Rat fibrosarcoma (MC3)	~44	~90	—[a]

[a] This chapter.

In most mammalian cells three to four times more breaks are formed under nitrogen as compared to irradiation under air or oxygen (see Table 1). Although an oxygen effect on strand production in murine lymphoma cells (L5178Y) was originally reported from our laboratory (Lett et al., 1967), reanalysis of the data showed that this conclusion could not be drawn (Dean et al., 1969). Later data also demonstrated no effect (Ormerod and Stevens, 1971). We have now reexamined this problem. My colleague, Dr. P. Karran (*unpublished work*) found an oxygen effect of 1.3 using L5178Y cells (an effect only just outside the limit of experimental error). Using another murine lymphoma (SL2), I found no effect (see Fig. 1). In contrast, another experiment under identical conditions using a rat fibrosarcoma (MC3) gave an oxygen effect ratio (OER) of two (Fig. 2). It therefore seems that some cells show a much smaller oxygen effect than

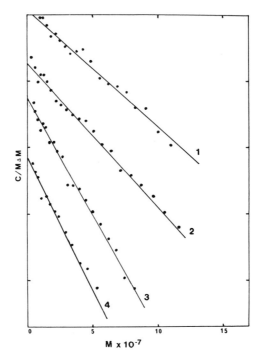

FIG. 1. Molecular weight plots from sedimentation profiles of DNA from murine lymphoma cells (SL2) irradiated at 0°C with 220-kVp X-rays, where C is the radioactivity in a fraction, M the molecular weight of that fraction, and $\triangle$ M the range of molecular weights covered by the fraction. The linear plot of C/M M against M demonstrates that the DNA had a random molecular weight distribution. The slope of the line equals $1/M_n$. Gradients: 5 to 20% sucrose, 0.1 M NaCl, 0.1 M NaOH, 5 mM EDTA. Cells lysed in 0.1 M NaOH, 0.02 M EDTA, 0.2% Sarkosyl. Centrifugation at 4.10^4 rpm for 1.5 hr. 1, Irradiated under air to 20 krad $M_n = 2.4 \times 10^7$; 2, irradiated under N_2 to 20 krad $M_n = 2.0 \times 10^7$; 3, irradiated under N_2 to 40 krad $M_n = 1.2 \times 10^7$; and 4, irradiated under air to 40 krad $M_n = 1.1 \times 10^7$.

others—possibly due to a lower level of intranuclear sulfhydryl compounds (see below).

Roots and Smith (1974) have studied the oxygen effect in some detail in Chinese hamster ovary cells. They found an OER ratio of about four. Preheating the cells to 70°C for 15 min sensitized the cells and reduced the OER to about two (13 eV/break under air, 29 eV/break under nitrogen). Addition of 5 mM cysteamine slightly protected heated cells irradiated in air, whereas for cells irradiated under nitrogen, the yield was reduced to that from unheated cells. Cysteamine had little effect on the yield of breaks in viable, unheated cells. They interpreted their results on the basis of the model suggested some years ago by Alexander and by Howard-Flanders, who proposed a competition for free radical sites between oxygen (fixation of damage) and sulfhydryl compounds (chemical repair of damage by hydrogen donation). (For example, see Ormerod and Alexander, 1963 and references cited therein.)

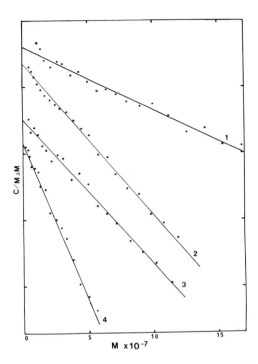

FIG. 2. Molecular weight plots from profiles of DNA from rat fibrosarcoma cells (MC3). Experimental details as in Fig. 1. 1, Irradiated under N_2 to 20 krad $M_n = 4.0 \times 10^7$; 2, irradiated under air to 20 krad $M_n = 1.9 \times 10^7$; 3, irradiated under N_2 to 40 krad $M_n = 2.0 \times 10^7$; and 4, irradiated under air to 40 krad $M_n = 0.95 \times 10^7$.

The MC3 cells and the SL2 cells used for Fig. 1 were gassed and irradiated under identical conditions.

In agreement with Roots and Smith (1974), Ormerod and Stevens (1971) found no effect of cysteamine or cystamine (up to 1 mM) on strand break production in L5178Y cells. Sawada and Okada (1970b) found that cysteamine protected their line of L5178Y cells at concentrations greater than 5 mM (a reduction factor of six at 50 mM), whereas cystamine had no effect. Roots and Okada (1972) obtained protection with cysteamine, cysteine, and mercaptoethanol, whereas Lohman et al. (1970) observed that concentrations of cysteamine of 4 mM or more protected the DNA of human T cells. One may conclude that a sufficiently high concentration of an added sulfhydryl compound can reduce the number of radiation-induced strand breaks. Smaller protective effects have also been observed using a range of alcohols (methanol, ethanol, t-butanol, ethylene glycol, and glycerol) (Lohmann et al., 1970; Roots and Okada, 1972).

The effects of oxygen on Chinese hamster cells can be mimicked by certain electron-affinic radiosensitizers (p-nitroacetophenone and three derivatives of nitrofuran) (Dugle, Chapman, Gillespie, Borsa, Webb, Meeker, and Reevers (1972). The dose-enhancement ratios for the production of strand breaks correlated closely with those for cell survival.

The incorporation of bromouracil into DNA in place of thymine sensitizes cells to the effects of radiation. The literature on the effect of bromouracil on the production and repair of strand breaks is somewhat contradictory. This may be due to different levels of incorporation. Lohmann et al. (1972) found that when less than 20% of the thymine bases were replaced, there was no increase in single-strand break production in human T cells. At higher levels of incorporation, the number of breaks was increased by about one and one-half. Sawada and Okada (1972) reported an increase of 2.4 in L5178Y cells at an unspecified level of incorporation, whereas Shipley and Elkind (1971) found no effect on Chinese hamster (V79) cells.

The Rejoining of Single-Strand Breaks

It has been reported by numerous authors that cells grown in tissue culture rapidly rejoin single-strand breaks. Sufficient data have been accumulated to permit the generalization that all cells growing in tissue culture can rejoin 90% or more of the single-strand breaks introduced by high energy radiation. About one-half of the breaks are rejoined during the first 10 to 20 min of a postirradiation incubation at 37°C, and about 90% of the breaks are rejoined within 60 min.

The rate of rejoining of single-strand breaks depends on temperature. The reaction is completely inhibited below 5°C (Sawada and Okada, 1970a; Ormerod and Stevens, 1971; Lee, Bennett, and Byfield, 1972). The rate of reaction is at a maximum at 40°C in human lymphocytes (Donlon and Norman, 1971) and 42°C in Chinese hamster (V79) cells (Ben-Hur and Elkind, 1974). In the temperature range 22 to 37°C, Donlon and Norman (1971) estimated an activation energy for the initial rejoining reaction of 19 kcal/mole.

The reaction is independent of the synthesis of RNA, DNA, or protein. This has been demonstrated using a variety of metabolic inhibitors: hydroxyurea (Sawada and Okada, 1970a; Kann, Kohn, and Lyles, 1974), thymidine (Sawada and Okada, 1970a; Ormerod and Stevens, 1971), 5-fluorodeoxyuridine (Tsuboi and Terasima, 1970), ouabain and mitomycin C (Sawada and Okada, 1970a), cytosine arabinoside (Lee et al., 1972; Karran, 1974), actinomycin D (Sawada and Okada, 1970; Tsuboi and Terasima, 1970; Ormerod and Stevens, 1971; Elkind, 1971; Elkind and Chang-Liu, 1972b; Kann et al., 1974), puromycin (Sawada and Okada, 1970a), and cycloheximide (Tsuboi and Terasima, 1970; Kann et al., 1974).

It has been claimed that actinomycin D prevents the rejoining of a small number of residual strand breaks (Lee et al., 1972; Elkind and Chang-Liu, 1972b). Since actinomycin D introduces a low level of strand breaks into DNA (Elkind and Chang-Liu, 1972b), it is possible that the wrong inference may have been drawn from the data. Cysteamine and cystamine also introduce strand breaks into the DNA of cells (Ormerod and Stevens, 1971), and the claim that they inhibit strand rejoining is probably untenable (Sawada and Okada, 1970).

Prolonged incubation of cells with metabolic inhibitors prior to irradiation and subsequent incubation in the presence of inhibitor blocks strand rejoining (Horikawa et al., 1972).

The reaction is blocked by 2,4-dinitrophenol, which uncouples oxidative phosphorylation at a sufficiently high dose of radiation (>15 krad) (Ormerod and Stevens, 1971) or with a brief preincubation of the drug (Moss, Dalrymple, Sanders, Wilkinson, and Nash, 1971; Palcic and Skarsgard, 1972b).

Rejoining is inhibited when the cells are incubated under anoxic conditions (Matsudaira, Nakagawa, and Hishizara, 1969; Matsudaira, Nakagawa, and Bannai, 1969; Modig et al., 1974).

Rejoining is also prevented by proflavine (Tsuboi and Terasima, 1970), quinacrine (Voiculetz, Smith, and Kaplan, 1974), and 2-chloroethylisocyanate (Kann et al., 1974). The first two of these compounds intercalate between adjacent base-pairs of the double helix. It is hypothesized that the third compound reacts directly with and inactivates the repair enzymes.

Matsudaira and Furuno (1972) have studied the rejoining of single-strand breaks in nuclei isolated from Ehrlich ascites cells. They observed maximal rejoining in the presence of adenosine triphosphate, nicotinamide adenine diphosphate, 3-phosphoglycerate, and a supernatant from the cytoplasm of unirradiated cells. The active factor in the supernatant was heat sensitive, but they did not attempt further identification.

Painter, Young, and Burki (1974) have found that Chinese hamster (V79) cells can only repair about one-half the breaks introduced by ^{125}I decay in the DNA (the isotope was introduced as [^{125}I]iododeoxyuridine). This failure is probably the reason for the extremely toxicity of ^{125}I in this situation.

Also of interest is the observation by Rainbow (1974) that breaks in an irradiated adenovirus are repaired following the infection of human cells.

In summary, in order to rejoin strand breaks, cells must undergo oxidative metabolism—probably to generate adenosine triphosphate. The enzymes involved are normally present in the nucleus and are not induced by radiation damage.

What is the function of these repair enzymes in an irradiated cell? Are they involved in replication or are they part of a system that constantly monitors DNA and repairs any defects that arise? The latter function would help maintain the information content of a cell during the lifetime of an animal. The two alternatives are not mutually exclusive. This question also raises the possibility that postmitotic cells may lack some repair enzymes and damage might accumulate in their DNA (Alexander, 1967). This could be a factor in aging.

These questions have stimulated investigation of the ability of nondividing cells to repair strand breaks. Since the DNA of these cells is not easily labeled with radioactive isotopes, the concentration of DNA from gradients of sucrose has been estimated using a sensitive fluorometric method (Kissane and Robins, 1958). In some experiments, cells were removed from the animal and irradiation and repair carried out *in vitro;* in others, irradiation and repair was *in vivo*.

In vitro experiments have shown that murine thymocytes and hepatocytes (Ono and Okada, 1974), rat thymocytes and splenic lymphocytes, and chicken peripheral blood lymphocytes (Karran and Ormerod, 1973) can all repair strand breaks. Rejoining has been demonstrated *in vivo* with murine thymocytes and hepatocytes (Ono and Okada, 1974), canine neurons (Wheeler and Lett, 1972), and retinal photoreceptor cells in rabbits (Wheeler et al., 1972; Wheeler et al., 1973). Actinomycin D did not block rejoining in rat thymocytes, indicating that the rejoining enzymes were normally present in these cells over 80% of which were not in cycle (Karran and Ormerod, 1973).

Karran and Ormerod (1973) found that cells prepared from the muscles of 1-day-old rats contained DNA of high molecular weight ($>10^9$ daltons) and could rejoin radiation-induced strand breaks. Cells from older animals (1 week or more) contained DNA of lower molecular weight and had lost their capacity for repair.

They also found that the DNA in the nucleus of newly formed chicken erythrocytes (unlike mammalian erythrocytes, avian erythrocytes retain their nucleus) was of high molecular weight, but the cells could not rejoin strand breaks. As the cells aged, *in vivo,* the molecular weight of the nuclear DNA decreased to about 2×10^8. This extreme example of a postmitotic cell lacks at least one class of repair enzymes and accumulates DNA damage *in vivo*.

Wheeler and Lett (1972) followed the rejoining of strand breaks *in vivo* in the DNA of internal granular layer neurons of the cerebellum of 7-week-old beagle pups. After a dose of 4.7 krad, breaks were rejoined during the following 2 hr. After about 5 hr, degradation was observed, and the DNA finally returned to its original molecular weight after about 2 days.

After doses of radiation less than 4.3 krad, the photoreceptor cells of rabbit retinas rejoined the strand breaks in their DNA (Wheeler et al., 1973). After doses greater than 4.3 krad, the initial process of rejoining was overtaken by a degradative reaction so that after about 10 hr, all the DNA was heavily degraded. At this critical dose of radiation, there was a sudden loss of the b-wave of the electroretinogram (Wheeler et al., 1972; Wheeler et al., 1973).

The overall picture that emerges is that cells undergoing division or cells that can be stimulated into division can repair radiation induced single-strand breaks. The necessary enzymes are a normal component of the nucleus. Fully differentiated cells may or may not lack one or more of the rejoining enzymes. Endonucleolytic attack on DNA in irradiated cells *in vivo* may be more important than was previously realized.

ALTERNATIVE METHODS FOR STUDYING REPAIR
OF SINGLE-STRAND BREAKS

Release of DNA from "Complex" on Gradients of Sucrose

Quantitative measurement on gradients of alkaline sucrose can only be made with freely sedimenting DNA and this restricts one to the use of DNA of molecular weight less than 5×10^8 daltons. If the DNA from unirradiated cells is sedimented without prolonged incubation in alkali, the DNA is in the form of a complex. Small doses of radiation release the DNA from this complex (for example, see Lett et al., 1967; Elkind, 1971; Ormerod, 1973, and references therein) and change its rate of sedimentation (Terasima and Tsuboi, 1969; McBurney et al., 1972; Belli et al., 1972). These changes can be used to follow the introduction and repair of single-strand breaks.

Alkaline Elution Analysis

Kohn and Grimek-Ewig (1973) have developed this novel method for the detection of single-strand breaks in mammalian cells. Cells were lysed with detergent on cellulose triacetate filters. The DNA bound to the filters. It was eluted off with 0.1 N NaOH–0.01 M trisodium ethylene diamine tetraacetate. Irradiation of the cells increased the rate of elution, and this effect could be used to detect the breaks introduced by as few as 200 rads.

Strand Separation in Alkali

DNA released from mammalian cells by lysis in alkali is not completely denatured unless some strand breaks are introduced (McBurney and Whitmore, 1972; Ahnstrom and Erixon, 1973; Simpson et al., 1973; Ahnstrom and Edvardsson, 1974; Cleaver, 1974a; Jolley and Ormerod, 1973, 1974; Rydberg, 1974). So that one may follow the introduction of strand breaks by radiation, the cells are lysed in a fixed molarity of alkali, incubated at a given temperature for a set time, the solution neutralized by the addition of acid, and the DNA sheared either by ultrasound or by vigorous mixing of the solution. The percentage of renatured DNA in the resulting solution is measured either by chromatography on hydroxyapatite (Ahnstrom and Erixon, 1973; Ahnstrom and Edvardsson, 1974; Rydberg, 1975) or by equilibrium sedimentation in a solution of cesium chloride (Jolley and Ormerod, 1973, 1974). The effect of a dose of radiation as low as 10 rad can be detected (Rydberg, 1975). An example of the results that can be obtained is shown in Figs. 3 and 4.

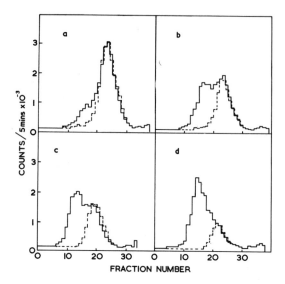

FIG. 3. DNA from irradiated murine lymphoma cells (L5178Y) banded isopycnically on neutral cesium chloride. The cells were lysed in 2% Na dodecyl sulfate, 0.02 M EDTA, 0.07 M NaOH, and neutralized with HCl after 30 min at 4°C. Cesium chloride solution was added, and the solution passed through a 21-gauge needle to sheer the DNA. The dotted profiles delineate the profile from native DNA (obtained by adding native [¹⁴C]DNA). Denatured DNA bands at a higher density (lower fraction number). No irradiation (a), 0.5 krad (b), 1.0 krad (c), 2.0 krad (d). Taken with permission from Jolley (1974).

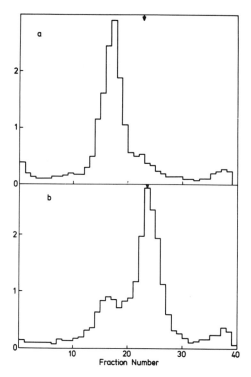

FIG. 4. The repair of single-strand breaks in the DNA of a murine lymphoma cell (L5178Y) demonstrated by a change in the renaturation of the DNA. Radiation dose, 2 krad. Experimental details as in Fig. 3. a: Cells lysed immediately after irradiation; b: cells lysed after 1 hr at 37°C. The arrow marks the position of native DNA. Note that in (a) little DNA has renatured; in (b) most of the DNA has renatured. Taken with permission from Jolley (1974).

ANOMALOUS SEDIMENTATION OF DNA OF HIGH MOLECULAR WEIGHT

Native DNA

Some years ago we observed that native DNA from a murine lymphoma cell (L5178Y) of molecular weight greater than 10^8 daltons sedimented anomalously at rotor speeds of 2×10^4 rpm or more (Lehmann and Ormerod, 1970b). At rotor speeds of 10^4 rpm or less, DNA from cells irradiated with at least 30 krad of X-rays yielded random profiles on the gradient of sucrose. At high speeds, much sharper nonrandom profiles were obtained, and the DNA in them had a lower sedimentation coefficient than that measured at low speeds. Similar effects were observed using DNA from the bacterium *Micrococcus radiodurans* (Burrell, Feldschreiber, and Dean, 1971).

Recently the inverse relationship between rotor speed and sedimentation velocity has been well documented, using DNA isolated from a variety of bacteria (Kavenoff, 1972; Levin and Hutchinson, 1973; Chia and Schumaker, 1974; Rubenstein and Leighton, 1974) and also from yeast (Petes and Fangman, 1972). Zimm (1974) has supplied the theoretical analysis of this effect. The complicated expression he derives predicts that at a given centrifuge speed, the sedimentation coefficient will have a maximum at a particular molecular weight and will be lower at higher molecular weights. In other words, in centrifugal fields, DNA of a given molecular weight can sediment faster than material of a higher molecular weight. This prediction has been confirmed experimentally (Chia and Schumaker, 1974).

Zimm and Schumaker (1975) have extended the theory to calculate the practical consequences of these effects. Of particular interest is the application to a collection of molecules the molecular weight distribution of which is random. They predict that at low rotor speeds the DNA would give the usual bell-shaped profile on the gradient, but at higher speeds, the profile would sharpen dramatically and have a much lower sedimentation coefficient. This is the behavior observed experimentally with mammalian DNA of molecular weight greater than 10^8 daltons (Lehmann and Ormerod, 1970b). Figure 5 shows the speed effect on DNA from a murine lymphoma irradiated with X-rays to a dose of 50 krad (Mn $\sim 5 \times 10^8$ daltons). The change from a "random" profile to a sharp, slower profile is dramatic. Figures 6 and 7 show profiles from cells irradiated to different doses. The rotor speed was 4×10^4 rpm. At the highest radiation dose (250 krad; $M_n \sim 10^8$), there is a bell-shaped profile typical of that obtained from DNA with a random molecular weight distribution. At lower doses (for example, 80 krad, $M_n \sim 3 \times 10^8$) a sharp profile is obtained, which is indistinguishable from that obtained from monodisperse DNA (such as phage DNA). At an even lower radiation dose (10 krad), much of the DNA is now sedimenting behind the sharp leading edge as predicted by Zimm and Schumaker (1975). [It should be noted that after a dose of 10 krad over one-half the DNA sedimented to the bottom of the centrifuge tube in the form of a complex;

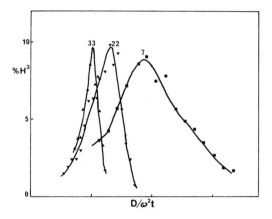

FIG. 5. Speed dependence of the sedimentation profile of native DNA from a murine lymphoma cell (SL2) irradiated at 0°C to a dose of 50 krad. The number on each profile is the rotor speed in 10^3 rpm. The entity $D/\omega^2 t$, where D is the distance sedimented, ω the rotor speed, and t the time of centrifugation (arbitrary units), is proportional to the sedimentation coefficient. DNA was labeled with [³H]thymidine. Gradients: 5 to 20% sucrose, 2 M NaCl, 0.01 M Na citrate, 1 mM EDTA, pH 8.9. Cells lysed in 0.2% sarkosyl, 0.08% Na deoxycholate, 2 M NaCl, 0.01 M Na citrate, and 0.02 M Na₄-EDTA. Beckman SW 50.1 rotor.

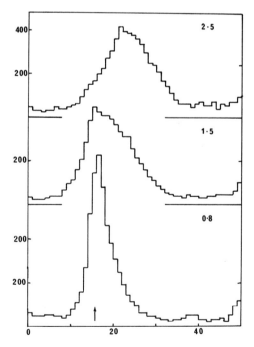

FIG. 6. Sedimentation profiles of native DNA from a murine lymphoma cell (L5178Y). The number by each profile is the dose of radiation ($\times 10^{-5}$ rad); the arrow is at the position equivalent to a molecular weight of 3×10^8 daltons. Gradients and lysing solution are similar to those in Fig. 5. Rotor speed, 4×10^4 rpm; centrifugation time, 1.5 hr; Beckman SW 50 rotor. This is an unpublished experiment by Dr. A. R. Lehmann run in this laboratory in 1968 (used by permission).

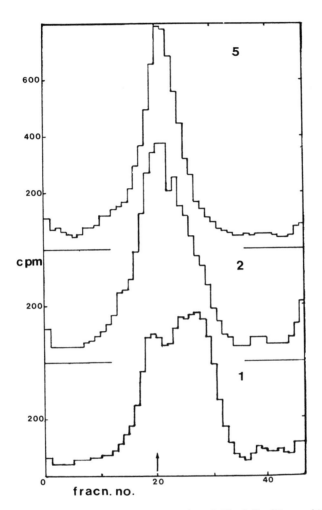

FIG. 7. Other sedimentation profiles from the experiment shown in Fig. 4. Conditions and key are similar except centrifugation time is 1.25 hr, and the numbers are the dose of radiation ($\times 10^{-4}$ rad).

see Ormerod and Lehmann (1971a). The profile is shown because of its close similarity to the theoretical profiles.]

The appearance of the profiles in Fig. 3 closely parallel the appearance of profiles expected from a monodisperse sample of DNA containing a few random breaks [for example, see Fig. 7 in Ormerod and Lehmann (1971) or Fig. 1 in Ehmann and Lett (1973)]. If the data at doses of radiation below 80 krad and the data obtained at lower rotor speeds were not available, it might be assumed, with some justification, that a dose of 50 to 80 krad released molecules of DNA about 3×10^8 daltons in size. The artifact introduced by high speed sedimentation can be curiously misleading.

Denatured DNA

Similar results can be obtained with denatured DNA sedimenting through alkaline gradients. The effects are not so dramatic for two reasons: (a) approximately one break for every 4×10^8 daltons has to be introduced into the DNA before it denatures fully (see discussion above) and (b) theoretically, longer molecules of denatured DNA are needed in order to observe a change in sedimentation coefficient with speed (Zimm and Schumaker, 1975). Several workers have reported the effects of rotor speed on the sedimentation of denatured DNA (Elkind, 1971; McBurney et al., 1971; Ormerod and Lehmann, 1971b; Palcic and Skarsgard, 1972a; Wheeler et al., 1974). Some of these results can be criticized, and not everybody accepts the fact that these effects are due to a sedimentation anomaly; this is discussed below.

An example of the effect of rotor speed on the sedimentation of denatured DNA is shown in Fig. 8. The changes in the high-speed sedimentation profiles caused by low doses of radiation to a murine lymphoma cell are shown in Fig. 9. Almost identical data have been published by Elkind and Kamper (1970), who used Chinese hamster cells, and McBurney et al. (1971, 1972), who used murine L-cells. If Fig. 7 is compared with Fig. 3, it can be seen that the profiles obtained from native and denatured DNA are almost identical. The behavior of denatured DNA also mirrors the behavior predicted theoretically by Zimm and Schumaker (1975).

Sharp, nonrandom profiles similar to those shown in the figures can be

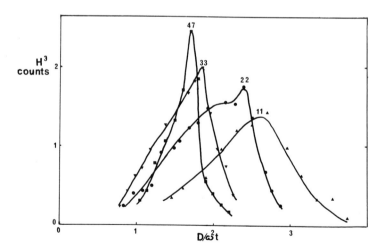

FIG. 8. Speed dependence of the sedimentation profile of denatured DNA from a murine lymphoma cell (SL2) irradiated at 0 °C to a dose of 2 krad. The number on each profile is the rotor speed in 10^3 rpm. Gradients and lysing solution as in Fig. 1. Beckman SW 50.1 rotor. The abscissa is proportional to the sedimentation coefficient. The ordinate is in arbitrary units, which have been selected for each profile to demonstrate best the change in the peak position.

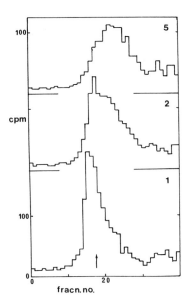

FIG. 9. Sedimentation profiles of denatured DNA from murine lymphoma cells (L5178Y) irradiated at 0°C. The number by each profile is the dose $\times$ 10^{-3} rads. The arrow is at a position of 2.10^8 daltons. Rotor speed, 4×10^4 rpm; centrifugation time, 40 min; Beckman SW 50 rotor. Gradients, 5 to 20% sucrose, 0.9 M NaCl adjusted to pH 12 with NaOH. Cells were lysed in a solution similar to that used for Fig. 1.

obtained with DNA from unirradiated cells by allowing it to degrade on top of the sucrose gradient in alkali (Lett et al., 1970; Elkind and Kamper, 1970). This process is accelerated by light (Elkind, 1971) and is fast in DNA containing bromouracil (Shipley and Elkind, 1971).

It has been postulated that the DNA responsible for sharp, nonrandom profiles is monodisperse and represents a special structural subunit of the chromosomal DNA (Lett et al., 1970; Elkind and Kamper, 1970). This subunit has been assigned a sedimentation coefficient of 165S and a molecular weight of 5.5×10^8 daltons (Lett et al., 1970; Wheeler et al., 1974). It is hypothesized that, in the intact chromosomal DNA, these subunits are joined by alkali-labile, radiation-sensitive markers (Lett and Sun, 1970; Lett, Sun, and Wheeler, 1972).

It has also been claimed that there is evidence for a second subunit with a sedimentation coefficient of either 150S (Lett and Sun, 1970) or 208S (Lett et al., 1970). Since these claims have not been supported by more recent evidence, I will not discuss them further. In the light of Cleaver's demonstration (1974a) that molecules of DNA on alkaline gradients with sedimentation coefficients greater than 165S are not fully denatured, the claim that multiples of the basic 165S subunit can be observed (Lett et al.,

1970; Wheeler and Lett, 1972; Wheeler et al., 1973) needs critical reexamination.

If this subunit is indeed a real entity, and the sharp profiles do represent monodisperse DNA and have nothing to do with a rotor speed effect, why do the profiles change shape at slower rotor speeds? Two possibilities come to mind: (1) degradation of the DNA occurs in alkali during the extended centrifugation time, and (2) large molecules of DNA are more susceptible to convective disturbance at slow rotor speeds.

If the low-speed sedimentation profiles of Elkind (1971) and McBurney et al. (1971) are inspected, it can be seen that the peaks of the broad profiles have about the same sedimentation coefficient as the narrow, high-speed profiles. This is not as predicted theoretically—the peak should have moved to a position of higher molecular weight. This does suggest that further alkaline degradation of the DNA has occurred. Despite this, the profiles still show an appreciable amount of DNA with a higher sedimentation coefficient at the slower speed.

The suggestion that large molecules may be more susceptible to convective disturbance is difficult to prove or disprove. I would not want to claim with any degree of certainty that such effects played no part in determining the shape of the profiles shown in Fig. 8.

The nature of the molecules linking the hypothesized subunits is of some interest. Its alkaline lability presents no problem—many such bonds are known. The precise way in which this linker is cleaved by radiation is unusual. It has been suggested that the linkage sites are in exposed positions susceptible to the indirect action of radiation (Lett and Sun, 1970; Lett et al., 1972). Even so, if a linker were equivalent in size to one hundred nucleotides it would still have a radiation sensitivity ten thousand times greater than the chromosomal DNA. It would seem that the linker contains thymidine since incorporation of bromouridine into DNA accelerates the production of "subunits" in alkali (Elkind and Shipley, 1971). The linker also appears to have a remarkably higher sensitivity to the combined action of alkali and light from standard fluorescent tubes (Elkind, 1971). I am suggesting that, on the basis of published experimental data, if the 165S structural subunits exist, their linkers must have some unusual chemical properties.

In conclusion, it is generally agreed that (1) denatured DNA of sedimentation coefficient 120 to 165S with an apparent monodisperse molecular weight distribution can be obtained from mammalian cells, and (2) at slower speeds of centrifugation, broader sedimentation profiles are obtained. The debate is about the interpretation of the data. I feel that the close parallel between the data obtained with native and denatured DNA and the close parallel between the experimental data and the theoretical calculations indicates that the sharp profile arises from a sedimentation anomaly. If this is accepted, then there is no longer evidence for the existence of a special structural subunit of fixed molecular length. The data on the production of this subunit can be reinterpreted as a demonstration of the random introduction of one single-strand break for about every 4×10^8 daltons of DNA. Similarly the observation of the linking-up of the subunits is just the observation of the repair of the last few strand breaks.

I do not question the existence of organizational subunits within the DNA molecule; replication would be impossible without some such unit. I do question the hypothesis that these organizational units are joined by alkali-labile, radiosensitive linkers and that they have been observed using gradients of alkaline sucrose.

CONCLUDING REMARKS

It has been known for many years that mammalian cells could recover from some of the effects of ionizing radiation [for example, see Elkind and Sutton (1960)]. The observation that single-strand breaks were rejoined was probably the first direct evidence for a mechanism for repair at the chemical level (Lett et al., 1967). The widespread existence of the necessary enzymes and the efficiency of the repair reaction in a variety of different cells indicate that the majority of the single-strand breaks introduced by radiation are not in themselves lethal. The same statement about double-strand breaks is possibly true, but more experimental evidence is needed.

When the unfortunate controversy over the interpretation of the so-called "subunit" profiles has been settled and more data on the formation and repair of double-strand breaks have been collected, there would seem to be little purpose to any further study of strand breaks in the DNA of cells on its own. The future of this powerful technique will be in its use as a tool in conjunction with other methods.

As far as radiation biology is concerned, the future must lie in obtaining a more detailed knowledge of the radiation chemistry of DNA in the cell. The chemical nature of the strand breaks is not known; they are probably heterogeneous, and the rejoining of the strand breaks probably reflects several different reactions. One hopes that the type of investigation being carried out in Professor Hagen's laboratory will give a lead (Coquerelle et al., 1973). Professor Cerutti and co-workers have recently shown that some mammalian cells can excise certain radiation products of thymine from their DNA (Mattern et al., 1973; Cerutti, 1974). When scientists are finally in a position to carry out conjointly analysis of end-groups, base products, and strand breaks, we will start to obtain a clearer picture of the chemical changes in cellular DNA caused by ionizing radiation. A study of cells defective in one or more repair mechanisms [such as those from patients with xerodema pigmentosum (Cleaver, 1968)] might indicate which types of damage are important in determining cell survival. By this time, some relationship between damage and repair of DNA and radiation carcinogenesis might have been established. We would still be a long way from determining the exact nature of this link, if it exists.

ACKNOWLEDGMENTS

I thank my colleagues, past and present, for all the help they have given me—Drs. C. J. Dean, G. M. Jolley, P. Karran, and A. R. Lehmann.

REFERENCES

Ahnstrom, G., and Edvardsson, K.-A. (1974): Radiation-induced single-strand breaks in DNA determined by rate of alkaline strand separation and hydroxylapatite chromatography: an alternative to velocity sedimentation. *Int. J. Radiat. Biol.*, 26:493–497.

Ahnstrom, G., and Erixon, K. (1973): Radiation induced strand breakage in DNA from mammalian cells. Strand separation in alkaline solution. *Int. J. Radiat. Biol.*, 23:285–289.

Alexander, P. (1967): The role of DNA lesions in the processes leading to ageing in mice. *Symp. Soc. Exp. Biol.*, 21:29–50.

Belli, J. A., Cooper, S., and Brown, J. A. (1972): Sedimentation properties of mammalian-cell DNA: Evidence that non-specific molecular aggregation does not occur during cell lysis. *Int. J. Radiat. Biol.*, 21:603–606.

Ben-Hur, E., and Elkind, M. M. (1974): Thermally enhanced radio-response of cultured Chinese hamster cells: Damage and repair of single-stranded DNA and a DNA complex. *Radiat. Res.*, 59:484–495.

Burrell, A. D., Feldschreiber, P., and Dean, C. J. (1971): DNA-membrane association and the repair of double breaks in X-irradiated *Micrococcus radiodurans*. *Biochim. Biophys. Acta*, 247:38–53.

Cerutti, P. A. (1974): Effects of ionizing radiation on mammalian cells. *Naturwissenschaften*, 61:51–59.

Charlesby, A. (1954): Molecular weight changes in the degradation of long-chain polymers. *Proc. R. Soc. (Lond.)*, A224:120–128.

Chia, D., and Schumaker, V. N. (1974): A rotor speed dependent crossover in sedimentation velocities of DNA's of different sizes. *Biochem. Biophys. Res. Commun.*, 56:241–246.

Cleaver, J. E. (1968): Defective repair replication of DNA in *xeroderma pigmentosum*. *Nature*, 218:652–656.

Cleaver, J. E. (1974a): Conformation of DNA in alkaline sucrose: The subunit hypothesis in mammalian cells. *Biochem. Biophys. Res. Commun.*, 59:92–99.

Cleaver, J. E. (1974b): Sedimentation of DNA from human fibroblasts irradiated with ultraviolet light: Possible detection of excision breaks in normal and repair-deficient xeroderma pigmentosum cells. *Radiat. Res.*, 57:207–227.

Cleaver, J. E. (1974c): Repair processes for photochemical damage in mammalian cells. In: *Advances in Radiation Biology*, Vol. 4, edited by J. T. Lett, H. Adler, and M. Zelle. Academic Press, New York.

Coquerelle, T., Bopp, A., Kessler, B., and Hagen, U. (1973): Strand breaks and 5' end-groups of DNA of irradiated thymocytes. *Int. J. Radiat. Biol.*, 24:397–404.

Corry, P. M., and Cole, A. (1968): Radiation-induced double-strand scission of the DNA of mammalian metaphase chromosomes. *Radiat. Res.*, 36:528–543.

Corry, P. M., and Cole, A. (1973): Double strand rejoining in mammalian DNA. *Nature [New Biol.]*, 245:100–101.

Dean, C. J., Ormerod, M. G., Serianni, R. W., and Alexander, P. (1969): DNA strand breakage in cells irradiated with x-rays. *Nature*, 222:1042–1044.

Donlon, T., and Norman, A. (1971): Kinetics of rejoining of single-strand breaks induced by ionizing radiation in DNA of human lymphocytes. *Mutat. Res.*, 13:97–107.

Dugle, D. I., Chapman, J. D., Gillespie, C. J., Borsa, J., Webb, R. G., Meeker, B. E., and Reuvers, A. P. (1972): Radiation-induced strand breakage in mammalian cell DNA. I. Enhancement of single-strand breaks by chemical radiosensitizers. *Int. J. Radiat. Biol.*, 22:545–555.

Ehmann, U. K., and Lett, J. T. (1973): Review and evaluation of molecular weight calculations from the sedimentation profiles of irradiated DNA. *Radiat. Res.*, 54:152–162.

Elkind, M. M. (1971): Sedimentation of DNA released from Chinese hamster cells. *Biophys. J.*, 11:502–520.

Elkind, M. M., and Chang-Liu, C.-M. (1972a): Repair of a DNA complex from X-irradiated Chinese hamster cells. *Int. J. Radiat. Biol.*, 22:75–90.

Elkind, M. M., and Chang-Liu, C.-M. (1972b): Actinomycin D inhibition of repair of a DNA complex from Chinese hamster cells. *Int. J. Radiat. Biol.*, 22:313–324.

Elkind, M. M., and Kamper, C. (1970): Two forms of repair of DNA in mammalian cells following irradiation. *Biophys. J.*, 10:237–245.

Elkind, M. M., and Sutton, H. (1960): Radiation response of mammalian cells grown in culture. 1. Repair of x-ray damage in surviving Chinese hamster cells. *Radiat. Res.*, 13:556–593.

Freifelder, D., and Trumbo, B. (1969): Matching of single-strand breaks to form double-strand breaks in DNA. *Biopolymers*, 7:681–693.

Gillespie, C. J., Gislason, G. S., Dugle, D. L., and Chapman, J. D. (1972): Random break analysis of DNA sedimentation profiles. *Radiat. Res.*, 51:272–279.

Hariharan, P. V., and Cerutti, P. A. (1972): Formation and repair of gamma ray induced thymine damage in *Micrococcus radiodurans. J. Mol. Biol.*, 66:65–81.

Horikawa, M., Fukuhara, M., Suzuki, F., Nikaido, O., and Sugahara, T. (1972): Comparative studies on induction and rejoining of DNA single-strand breaks by radiation and chemical carcinogen in mammalian cells *in vitro. Expt. Cell Res.*, 70:349–359.

Jolley, G. M. (1974): The use of high energy radiation in the study of normal, crosslinked and newly replicated DNA from a mammalian cell. Ph.D. Thesis, University of London.

Jolley, G. M., and Ormerod, M. G. (1973): An improved method for measuring crosslinks in the DNA of mammalian cells: the effect of nitrogen mustard. *Biochim. Biophys. Acta*, 308:242–252.

Jolley, G. M., and Ormerod, M. G. (1974): The incomplete separation of complementory strands of high molecular weight DNA in alkali. *Biochim. Biophys. Acta*, 353:200–214.

Kann, H. E., Jr., Kohn, K. W., and Lyles, J. M. (1974): Inhibition of DNA repair by the 1, 3-Bis (2-Chloroethyl)-1 Nitrosourea breakdown product, 2-Chloroethyl Isocyanate. *Cancer Res.*, 34:398–402.

Karran, P. (1973): The repair of methyl methane sulphonate induced lesions in the DNA of a murine lymphoma cell. *Chem. Biol. Interact.*, 7:389–398.

Karran, P., and Ormerod, M. G. (1973): Is the ability to repair damage to DNA related to the proliferative capacity of a cell? The rejoining of x-ray produced strand breaks. *Biochim. Biophys. Acta*, 299:54–64.

Kavenoff, R. (1972): Characterization of the *Bacillus subtilis* W23 genome by sedimentation. *J. Mol. Biol.*, 72:801–806.

Kissane, J. M., and Robins, E. (1958): The fluorometric measurement of deoxyribonucleic acid in animal tissues with special reference to the central nervous system. *J. Biol. Chem.*, 233:184–188.

Kohn, K. W., and Grimek-Ewig, R. A. (1973): Alkaline elution analysis, a new approach to the study of DNA single-strand interruptions in cells. *Cancer Res.*, 33:1849–1853.

Lee, Y. C., Bennett, L. R., and Byfield, J. E. (1972): Inhibition of repair of DNA single strand breaks in mouse leukaemia cells by Actinomycin D. *Biochem. Biophys. Res. Commun.*, 49:758–765.

Lehmann, A. R. (1970): X-ray induced breaks in the DNA of a mammalian cell and its application to DNA replication. Ph.D. Thesis, University of London.

Lehmann, A. R. (1972): Postreplication repair of DNA in ultraviolet-irradiated mammalian cells. *J. Mol. Biol.,* 66:319–337.

Lehmann, A. R., and Ormerod, M. G. (1969): Artefact in the measurement of the molecular weight of pulse-labelled DNA. *Nature,* 221:1053–1056.

Lehmann, A. R., and Ormerod, M. G. (1970*a*). The replication of DNA in murine lymphoma cells (L5178Y). I. Rate of replication. *Biochim. Biophys. Acta,* 204:128–143.

Lehmann, A. R., and Ormerod, M. G. (1970*b*): Double strand breaks in the DNA of the mammalian cell after x-irradiation. *Biochim. Biophys. Acta,* 217:268–277.

Lehmann, A. R., and Ormerod, M. G. (1971): The replication of DNA in murine lymphoma cells (L5178Y). II. Size of replicating units. *Biochim. Biophys. Acta,* 272:191–201.

Lennartz, M., Coquerelle, T., and Hagen, U. (1973): Effect of oxygen on DNA strand breaks in irradiated thymocytes. *Int. J. Radiat. Biol.,* 24:621–625.

Lett, J. T., Caldwell, I., Dean, C. J., and Alexander, P. (1967): Rejoining of x-ray induced breaks in the DNA of leukaemia cells. *Nature,* 214:790–792.

Lett, J. T., Klucis, E. S., and Sun, C. (1970): On the size of the DNA in the mammalian chromosome. *Biophys. J.,* 10:277–292.

Lett, J. T., and Sun, C. (1970): The production of strand breaks in mammalian DNA by x-rays: At different stages in the cell cycle. *Radiat. Res.,* 44:771–787.

Lett, J. T., Sun, C., and Wheeler, K. T. (1972): Restoration of the DNA structure in x-irradiated eucaryotic cells: *in vitro* and *in vivo. Johns Hopkins Med. J.* (Suppl. 1): 147–158.

Levin, D., and Hutchinson, F. (1973): Neutral sucrose sedimentation of very large DNA from *Bacillus subtilis.* I. Effect of random double-strand breaks and centrifuge speed on sedimentation. *J. Mol. Biol.,* 75:455–478.

Litwin, S., Shahn, E., and Kozinski, A. W. (1969): Interpretation of sucrose gradient sedimentation pattern of deoxyribonucleic acid fragments resulting from random breaks. *J. Virol.,* 4:24–30.

Lohman, P. H. M., Bootsma, D., and Hey, A. H. (1972): The influence of 5-Bromodeoxyuridine on the induction of breaks in the deoxyribonucleic acid of cultivated human cells by x-irradiation and ultraviolet light. *Radiat. Res.,* 52:627–641.

Lohman, P. H. M., Vos, O., Van Sluis, C. A., and Cohen, J. A. (1970): Chemical protection against breaks induced in DNA of human and bacterial cells by x-irradiation. *Biochim. Biophys. Acta,* 224:339–352.

McBurney, M. W., Graham, F. L., and Whitmore, G. F. (1971): Anomalous sedimentation of high molecular weight denatured mammalian DNA. *Biochem. Biophys. Res. Commun.,* 44:171–177.

McBurney, M. W., Graham, F. L., and Whitmore, G. F. (1972): Sedimentation analysis of DNA from irradiated and unirradiated L-cells. *Biophys. J.,* 12:369–383.

McBurney, M. W., and Whitmore, G. F. (1972): Molecular weight analysis of mammalian DNA. *Biochem. Biophys. Res. Commun.,* 46:898–904.

McGrath, R. A., and Williams, R. W. (1966): Reconstruction *in vivo* of irradiated *Escherichia coli* deoxyribonucleic acid; the rejoining of broken pieces. *Nature,* 212: 534–535.

Matsudaira, H., and Furuno, I. (1972): The rejoining of x-ray-induced DNA strand breaks in nuclei isolated from Ehrlich ascites tumor cells. *Biochim. Biophys. Acta,* 272:202–211.

Matsudaira, H., Nakagawa, C., and Bannai, S. (1969): Rejoining of x-ray-induced breaks in the DNA of Ehrlich ascites-tumour cells *in vitro. Int. J. Radiat. Biol.,* 15: 575–581.

Matsudaira, H., Nakagawa, C., and Hishizawa, T. (1969): Rejoining of x-ray-induced breaks in the DNA of Ehrlich ascites tumour cells *in vivo. Int. J. Radiat. Biol.,* 15: 95–100.

Mattern, M. R., Hariharan, P. V., Dunlap, B. E., and Cerutti, P. P. (1973): DNA degradation and excision repair in γ-irradiated Chinese hamster ovary cells. *Nature,* 245:230–232.

Modig, H. G., Edgren, M., and Revesz, L. (1974): Dual effect of oxygen on the induction and repair of single-strand breaks in the DNA of x-irradiated mammalian cells. *Int. J. Radiat. Biol.,* 26:341–353.

Moss, A. J., Dalrymple, G. V., Sanders, J. L., Wilkinson, K. P., and Nash, J. C. (1971): Dinitrophenol inhibits the rejoining of radiation-induced DNA breaks by L cells. *Biophys. J.,* 11:158–173.

Ono, T., and Okada, S. (1974): Estimation *in vivo* of DNA strand breaks and their rejoining in thymus and liver of mouse. *Int. J. Radiat. Biol.,* 25:291–301.

Ormerod, M. G. (1973): The measurement of radiation-induced strand breaks in the DNA of mammalian cells. In: *Physico-chemical Properties of Nucleic Acids,* edited by J. Duchesma, Vol. 3, pp. 139–159. Academic Press, New York.

Ormerod, M. G., and Alexander, P. (1963): On the mechanism of radiation protection by cysteamine: An investigation by means of electron spin resonance. *Radiat. Res.,* 18:475–509.

Ormerod, M. G., and Lehmann, A. R. (1971a): The release of high molecular weight DNA from a mammalian cell (L5178Y). Attachment of the DNA to the nuclear membrane. *Biochim. Biophys. Acta,* 228:331–343.

Ormerod, M. G., and Lehmann, A. R. (1971b): Artefacts arising from the sedimentation of high molecular weight DNA on sucrose gradients. *Biochim. Biophys. Acta,* 247:369–372.

Ormerod, M. G., and Stevens, U. (1971): The rejoining of X-ray induced strand breaks in the DNA of a murine lymphoma cell (L5178Y). *Biochim. Biophys. Acta,* 232: 72–82.

Painter, R. B., Young, B. R., and Burki, H. J. (1974): Non-repairable strand breaks induced by ^{125}I incorporated into mammalian DNA. *Proc. Natl. Acad. Sci. USA,* 71: 4836–4838.

Palcic, B., and Skarsgard, L. D. (1972a): The effect of oxygen on DNA single-strand breaks produced by ionizing radiation in mammalian cells. *Int. J. Radiat. Biol.,* 21: 417–433.

Palcic, B., and Skarsgard, L. D. (1972b): DNA single-strand breaks produced in mammalian cells by ionizing radiation after treatment with 2, 4-dinitrophenol. *Int. J. Radiat. Biol.,* 21:535–544.

Petes, T. D., and Fangman, W. L. (1972): Sedimentation properties of yeast chromosomal DNA. *Proc. Natl. Acad. Sci. USA,* 69:1188–1191.

Rainbow, A. J. (1974): Repair of radiation-induced DNA breaks in human adenovirus. *Radiat. Res.,* 60:155–164.

Roots, R., and Okada, S. (1972): Protection of DNA molecules of cultured mammalian cells from radiation-induced single-strand scissions by various alcohols and SH compounds. *Int. J. Radiat. Biol.,* 21:329–342.

Roots, R., and Smith, K. C. (1974): On the nature of the oxygen effect on x-ray-induced DNA single-strand breaks in mammalian cells. *Int. J. Radiat. Biol.,* 26:467–480.

Rubenstein, I., and Leighton, S. B. (1974): The influence of rotor speed on the sedimentation behaviour in sucrose gradients of high molecular weight DNAs. *Biophys. Chem.,* I:292–299.

Rydberg, B. (1975): The rate of strand separation of alkali of DNA of irradiated mammalian cells. *Radiat. Res.,* 61:274–287.

Sawada, S., and Okada, S. (1970a): Rejoining of single-strand breaks of DNA in cultured mammalian cells. *Radiat. Res.,* 41:145–162.

Sawada, S., and Okada, S. (1970b): Cysteamine, Cystamine and single-strand breaks of DNA in cultured mammalian cells. 44:116–132.

Sawada, S., and Okada, S. (1972): Effects of BUdR-labelling on radiation-induced DNA breakage and subsequent rejoining in cultured mammalian cells. *Int. J. Radiat. Biol.,* 21:599–602.

Shipley, W. U., and Elkind, M. M. (1971): DNA damage and repair following irradiation: The effect of 5-Bromodeoxyuridine in cultured Chinese hamster cells. *Radiat. Res.,* 48:86–94.

Simpson, J. R., Nagle, W. A., Bick, M. D., and Belli, J. A. (1973): Molecular nature of mammalian cell DNA in alkaline sucrose gradients. *Proc. Natl. Acad. Sci. USA,* 70: 3660–3664.

Terasima, T., and Tsuboi, A. (1969): Mammalian cell DNA isolated with minimal shearing. A sensitive system for detecting strand breaks by radiation. *Biochim. Biophys. Acta,* 174:309–314.

Tsuboi, A., and Terasima, T. (1970): Rejoining of single breaks of DNA induced by x-rays in mammalian cells: effects of metabolic inhibitors. *Mol. Gen. Genet.,* 108: 118–128.

Voiculetz, N., Smith, K. C., and Kaplan, H. S. (1974): Effect of Quinacrine on survival and DNA repair in X-irradiated Chinese hamster cells. *Cancer Res.,* 34:1038–1044.

Wheeler, K. T., DeWitt, J., and Lett, J. T. (1974): A marker for mammalian DNA sedimentation. *Radiat. Res.,* 57:365–378.

Wheeler, K. T., and Lett, J. T. (1972): Formation and rejoining of DNA strand breaks in irradiated neurons: *In vivo. Radiat. Res.,* 52:59–67.

Wheeler, K. T., and Linn, J. D. (1974): Differential sensitivity of DNA strand-break rejoining mechanisms to split doses of x-rays. *Int. J. Radiat. Biol.,* 26:411–420.

Wheeler, K. T., Pautler, E. L., and Lett, J. T. (1972): Irradiation of photoreceptor cells *in vivo* DNA repair and retinal function. *Expt. Cell Res.,* 74:281–284.

Wheeler, K. T., Sheridan, R. E., Pautler, E. L., and Lett, J. T. (1973): *In vivo* restitution of the DNA structure in gamma irradiated rabbit retinas. *Radiat. Res.,* 53:414–427.

Zimm, B. H. (1974): Anomalies in sedimentation. IV. Decrease in sedimentation coefficients of chains at high fields. *Biophys. Chem.,* 1:279–291.

Zimm, B. H., and Schumaker, V. N. with an appendix by C. B. Zimm. (1975): Anomalies in sedimentation. V. Chains at high fields, practical consequences. (Submitted to *Biophysical Chemistry.*)

Biology of Radiation Carcinogenesis, edited by
J. M. Yuhas, R. W. Tennant, and J. D. Regan.
Raven Press, New York © 1976.

Gamma-Ray Excision Repair in Normal and Diseased Human Cells

Peter A. Cerutti and Joyce F. Remsen

Department of Biochemistry, University of Florida, College of Medicine, Gainesville, Florida 32601

Ionizing radiation damages both the phosphodiester backbone and the heterocyclic bases of DNA *in situ* in the living cell. The major reactions of the bases involve the addition of radicals formed by water radiolysis, most importantly hydroxyl radicals, to the aromatic ring systems (see, for example, Alexander and Lett, 1968; Johansen and Howard-Flanders, 1965; Roots and Okada, 1972; Blok and Loman, 1973; Roti Roti and Cerutti, 1974). Radical addition results in ring saturation and may in secondary reactions lead to ring-fragmentation and ring-elimination. In the case of thymidine irradiated under aerobic conditions, hydroxyl radicals preferentially add to the 5,6-double bond and subsequent addition of oxygen and hydrogen leads to the formation of products of the hydroxy-hydroperoxy-dihydrothymine type (Ekert and Monier, 1959; Cadet and Téoule, 1972). Part of the saturated rings are spontaneously released from the DNA backbone under formation of "clean" apyrimidinic sites (i.e., unsubstituted deoxyribose residues) or sugar residues carrying a small fragment originating from the heterocyclic moiety (Dunlap and Cerutti, 1975). Unsubstituted deoxyribose residues in DNA are also formed in secondary reactions following purine alkylation (see, for example, Strauss et al., 1975) or heat treatment or even "spontaneously" at 37°C (Lindahl and Nyberg, 1972). The similarity of the biological effects of ionizing radiation and certain alkylating agents ("radiomimetic drugs") (see, for example, Regan and Setlow, 1974; Verly, 1974; Strauss, 1974) may, therefore, find an explanation in the formation of unsubstituted deoxyribose residues—apyrimidinic or apurinic sites—by both classes of DNA-damaging agents. A second type of radiation-chemical reaction undergone by thymine *in situ* in the cell involves the removal of a hydrogen atom from the methyl substituent under formation of a 5-methylene-uracil radical and a molecule of water (Roti Roti and Cerutti, 1974; Swinehart and Cerutti, 1975). These reactive radicals may revert back to thymine by picking up a hydrogen atom, they may react to 5-hydroxymethyl or 5-hydroperoxymethyl-thymine (Latarjet et al., 1963) by radical recombination reactions, or they may conceivably represent reactive inter-

---

* This work was supported by a grant from the National Institutes of Health and a contract from the USAEC.

mediates in the formation of DNA-DNA or DNA-protein cross-links. Deoxy-cytidine in DNA probably undergoes radical addition reactions to the 5,6-double bond similar to those of thymidine, but the resulting products are expected to be less stable and to undergo rapid secondary reactions (Alexander and Lett, 1968; Hahn et al., 1973). Exposure of cells to ionizing radiation also leads to the destruction of the purine bases in DNA. *In vitro* irradiation of the free purine bases leads to ring saturation and subsequent fragmentation by the addition of hydroxyl radicals to the central 4,5-double bond (Weiss, 1964), but addition to carbon-8 under formation of 6-amino-8-hydroxy-7,8-dihydro-purine has also been observed (Van Hemmen, 1971). It is not known, however, if these reactions occur in DNA.

From physicobiochemical studies of the effects of saturated pyrimidine bases on the structure of ribopolynucleotide model compounds (Cerutti et al., 1966; Swinehart et al., 1972) it is expected that radiation products of the 5,6-dihydroxy-dihydrothymine type distort the native conformation of DNA. In our recently proposed structural classification of DNA base-damage, pyrimidine ring saturation products fall into Class II, i.e., "monofunctional lesions causing minor helix distortion" (Cerutti, 1974a, Cerutti, 1975). Ring-saturated pyrimidine residues are expected to affect the functional properties of DNA. Uridine-photohydrates, 6-hydroxy-5,6-dihydrouridine were shown to be responsible for the ultraviolet inactivation of the single-stranded RNA phage R17 (Remsen et al., 1970) and to miscode as cytidine in an *in vitro* translation system (Remsen and Cerutti, 1972). Uridine photohydrates are structurally closely related to the major thymine products formed in DNA by ionizing radiation.

Radiation products of the 5,6-dihydroxy-dihydrothymine type (t') are efficiently removed from the DNA during postirradiation incubation of bacterial (Hariharan and Cerutti, 1974a,b,c) and mammalian cells. In this chapter we describe the t'-excision system contained in normal human cells, in human carcinoma HeLa S-3 cells, and in skin fibroblasts from xeroderma pigmentosum (XP) and Fanconi's anemia (FA) patients. The latter diseases are characterized among other symptoms by a genetically increased susceptibility for the development of cancer.

EFFICIENCY OF FORMATION OF γ-RAY-INDUCED THYMINE DAMAGE IN MAMMALIAN CELLS

Products of the 5,6-dihydroxy-dihydrothymine type (t') are formed under aerobic conditions in human diploid lung fibroblasts WI-38 with an efficiency of 0.5×10^{-3} t'/krad/10^6 daltons of DNA (Cerutti, 1974b). The t'-content of acid-precipitable DNA was determined by the alkali-acid degradation assay (Hariharan and Cerutti, 1974a) immediately following irradiation at 0°C. A similar value of 0.32×10^{-3}[^{3}H]H_2O/krad/10^6 daltons of DNA was determined for the formation of [^{3}H]H_2O from thymine-methyl[^{3}H] in Chi-

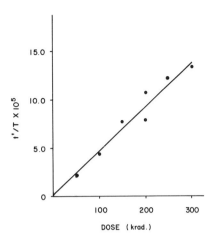

FIG. 1. Formation of γ-ray-induced thymine damage of the 5,6-dihydroxydihydrothymine type (t') in the DNA of human lung fibroblasts WI-38. The WI-38 cells were grown in monolayers, labeled with thymidine-methyl [³H] and exposed to ¹³⁷Cs γ-rays under protective, aerobic conditions at 0°C essentially as described for chinese hamster ovary cells by Mattern et al. (1973). The acid-precipitable DNA was immediately analyzed without postirradiation incubation for t', according to Hariharan and Cerutti (1974a). The data are presented as t'/T, i.e., the amount of radioactivity obtained from the 5% trichloroacetic acid-precipitable material by the alkali-acid degradation assay divided by the total radioactivity contained in each sample. The values for unirradiated controls have been subtracted. The data have not been extrapolated to total thymine ring destruction (from Mattern et al., 1975).

nese hamster ovary cells (CHO) (Roti Roti and Cerutti, 1974). The latter reaction is a measure of the radiation chemical reactivity of the thymine-methyl group. As shown in Fig. 1 and in Roti Roti and Cerutti (1974), linear dose-response curves were obtained for t' and [³H]H₂O formation. The efficiency of single-strand breakage in CHO-cells has been estimated at 1.92×10^{-3} breaks/krad/10^6 daltons DNA (Lett and Sun, 1970). Because additional damage not measurable by our assays undoubtedly occurs from thymine and the other DNA bases, it follows that base damage and strand breakage are produced with comparable efficiency in mammalian cells. It should be noted that single-strand breaks and t'-type products may not be completely unrelated. Products of the t'-type are alkali sensitive and may in part represent alkali-labile bonds (Achey et al., 1971; Kessler et al., 1971) under the conditions of alkaline sucrose gradient centrifugation.

EXCISION OF DAMAGED THYMINE FROM THE DNA OF MAMMALIAN CELLS EXPOSED TO HIGH DOSES OF γ-RAYS

The rapid, selective removal of t' from acid-precipitable DNA was demonstrated during postirradiation incubation of thymine-methyl[³H]-labeled WI-38, simian virus 40 (SV40) transformed WI-38 (line 2RA from L. Hayflick), and CHO-cells, which had received 250 krads of ¹³⁷Cs γ-rays. The high dose was necessary because of the limited sensitivity of the alkali-acid degradation assay, which at best allows the determination of one t'-type product in 20,000 undamaged thymine residues. Approximately 80% of t' had disappeared from the DNA within a 15-min incubation at 37°C in all three cell lines. Acid solubilization of total thymine label was determined as a measure of radiation-induced DNA degradation. The maximal level of

DNA degradation was reached after 20 to 30 min of incubation and reached approximately 1% for WI-38, 9% for CHO, and 15% for 2RA. For WI-38 cells, where DNA degradation was very low, it follows that the gap size, i.e., the number of undamaged residues released per t′, must be small. This result is in agreement with the determination of a small patch size of one to three nucleotides for γ-ray repair in human cells estimated by a different experimental approach (Painter and Young, 1972; Setlow and Regan, 1973). It is interesting to note that SV40 transformation of WI-38 leads to increased radiation-induced DNA degradation; however, the significance of this observation is not clear (Mattern et al., 1975).

EXCISION OF DAMAGED THYMINE FROM γ-IRRADIATED EXOGENOUS DNA BY WHOLE CELL SONICATES AND NUCLEAR PREPARATIONS OF HeLa S-3 CELLS

The properties of the t′-excision repair system of human cells were studied using whole cell sonicates and purified nuclear preparations of HeLa S-3 cells and γ-irradiated bacteriophage DNA as exogenous substrate. The most important advantage of this experimental design lies in the use of a chemically and physically well-defined DNA substrate and of unirradiated cellular preparations. Cell sonicates and intact or sonicated nuclei prepared under hypertonic conditions in the presence of 0.3% Triton X-100 by a modification of the procedure of Berkowitz et al. (1969) had similar capabilities to remove t′ selectively from γ-irradiated λ- or PM-2 DNA. The disappearance of t′ from acid-precipitable bacteriophage DNA was determined by the alkali-acid degradation assay (Hariharan and Cerutti, 1974a). It follows that all the repair enzymes necessary for t′ removal are still contained in hypertonic–0.3% Triton X-100 nuclei, which are essentially free of cytoplasmic contamination but have also lost part of the nuclear content. The excision kinetics were nonlinear, and excision remained incomplete even after prolonged incubation. The highest degree of completeness of the reaction, approximately 50% of t′ removed within 40 min of incubation at 37°C, was obtained at the lowest initial t′ concentration of 0.3×10^{-6} μmoles t′/sample. Unspecific degradation of the exogenous DNA substrate was only 2 to 3% within 60 min incubation. The t′-excision process is therefore highly selective. Ring-damaged thymine t′ was also removed by whole cell sonicates from the DNA of γ-irradiated, sonicated thymine-methyl [³H]-labeled HeLa nuclei, i.e., from chromatin rather than naked bacteriophage DNA.

Average rates of product excision by nuclear sonicates from irradiated λ-DNA were determined as a function of substrate (t′) concentration. A Lineweaver-Burk plot of the data is shown in Fig. 2 and is characterized by a $V_{\mathrm{max\ apparent}}$ of 3.16×10^{-6} μmoles of t′ removed in 40 min by 5×10^{6} nuclear equivalents and a $K_{\mathrm{max\ apparent}}$ of 5.7×10^{-6} μmoles.

The t′-excision capacity of preparations from human skin fibroblasts and

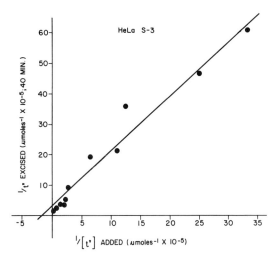

FIG. 2. Capacity of sonicated, hypertonic-0.3% Triton X-100, HeLa S-3 nuclei for the excision of γ-ray-damaged thymine (t') as a function of substrate concentration. The amount t' removed from acid-precipitable γ-irradiated bacteriophage λ-DNA within 40 min incubation at 37°C by 5 × 10⁶ nuclear equivalents was measured by the alkali-acid degradation assay (Hariharan and Cerutti, 1974a) as a function of the initial t' concentration, which varied from 0.3 to 90 × 10⁻⁶ μmoles t'/sample. Each sample also contained ATP and an ATP-generating system, bovine serum albumin, dithiothreitol, and the four deoxynucleoside triphosphates. The data are presented according to Lineweaver and Burk. The curve was calculated by the least-square-fit method. A correlation coefficient of 0.985 was obtained; $V_{max\ apparent}$ is 3.16 × 10⁻⁶ μmoles t' in 40 min by 5 × 10⁶ nuclear equivalents and $K_{max\ apparent}$ 5.7 × 10⁻⁶ μmoles.

young, medium-aged, but not senescent lung fibroblasts WI-38 (Mattern and Cerutti, 1975) was similar to that described above for HeLa S-3 cells, whereas preparations from mouse embryo 3T3 cells were only approximately one-half as active.

γ-RAY EXCISION REPAIR CAPACITY OF NUCLEAR PREPARATIONS FROM XERODERMA PIGMENTOSUM AND FANCONI'S ANEMIA SKIN FIBROBLASTS

There are a number of rare autosomal recessive diseases in humans that are characterized by an increased frequency for the development of leukemia and other forms of cancer (e.g., FA, Bloom's syndrome, Louis-Bar syndrome, XP). A higher than normal frequency of chromosomal aberrations has been detected in part of these diseases (see, for example, German, 1972). For the case of XP and FA (see below and Poon et al., 1974), a DNA repair deficiency has been demonstrated. The defects in these diseases have not been defined in precise molecular terms, however. It has been speculated that a causal relationship may exist between unrepaired DNA damage and malignant transformation and chromosomal aberration.

A depression or complete absence of unscheduled synthesis was found in most XP cells following exposure to UV light but not to ionizing radiation. Mostly on the basis of this observation, it was concluded that the endonucleolytic incision step in prereplication repair of photodimers was deficient, but considerable doubt has recently arisen concerning this conclusion. Resealing of X-ray-induced single-strand breaks is normal in XP cells. An appraisal of the present status of xeroderma research can be found in the article by Robbins et al. (1974) and in this volume and a recent review by Cleaver (1974). We have compared the t'-excision repair capacity of sonicated hypotonic–0.3% Triton X-100 nuclei of normal and XP skin fibroblasts using the experimental design and conditions described in the preceding section for HeLa S-3 preparations. Average rates of t'-excision were measured as a function of the substrate concentration (0.3 to 4×10^{-6} μmoles t') for the normal skin fibroblast lines CRL 1121 and 1141 and for the XP lines CRL 1223, 1199, and 1166 (from ATCC) corresponding to the ultraviolet-complementation groups A, B, and C. All three XP lines have drastically decreased levels of ultraviolet-induced, unscheduled DNA synthesis. The capacity of nuclear preparations for the excision of γ-ray–damaged thymine was found to be normal for the three lines in our experiments, however.

A first indication that a deficiency in the repair of chromosomal damage may exist in FA comes from the detection of an increased efficiency of formation of chromosomal aberrations by ionizing radiation (Higurashi and Conen, 1971) and DNA cross-linking agents (Sasaki and Tonomura, 1973) in FA lymphocytes and skin fibroblasts. Enhanced sensitivity to cell killing was observed for mitomycin C but not for γ-rays and ethylmethane sulfonate (Finkelberg et al., 1974). A deficiency in the excision of photodimers was recently described for the FA skin fibroblast line CCL 122 from ATCC (Poon et al., 1974). Decreased rates for the resealing of γ-ray-induced DNA single-strand breaks were observed in some FA cells in preliminary experiments (J. Little, *personal communication*). It is interesting to note that some FA cell lines were transformed at an increased frequency by simian virus 40 (Miller and Todaro, 1969). We have compared the capacity for the excision from DNA of γ-ray-damaged thymine by nuclear preparations of three FA and two normal skin fibroblast lines. The average rate of t' excision was determined as a function of damage concentration (0.3–5 $\times$ 10^{-6} μmoles t') for sonicated crude nuclei and sonicated hypotonic Triton X-100 nuclei from normal skin fibroblasts CRL 1121 and 1141 and FA skin fibroblasts CCL 122 and CRL 1196 (from ATCC) and 1265T (from Dr. G. Todaro). As shown in Fig. 3 for purified sonicated nuclei preparations, the t'-excision capacity was found to be considerably lower for CCL 122 and slightly lower for CRL 1196 and 1265T relative to preparations derived from normal cells. Qualitatively, the same relative differences were found for the repair capacities of the corresponding crude nuclear preparations that are expected to retain most of the nuclear content during their preparation. It is con-

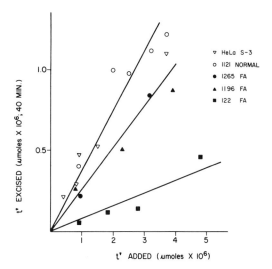

FIG. 3. Capacity of sonicated, hypotonic-0.3% Triton X-100 nuclei from normal human skin fibroblasts, HeLa S-3 cells, and Fanconi skin fibroblasts for the excision of γ-ray-damaged thymine (t') as a function of substrate concentration. The experimental conditions were as described in the legend to Fig. 2. HeLa S-3 (▽), CRL 1121 normal skin fibroblasts (○), CRL 1196 Fanconi's anemia skin fibroblasts (▲), 1265T Fanconi's anemia skin fibroblasts (●), CCL 122 Fanconi's anemia skin fibroblasts (■).

cluded that nuclear preparations from the Fanconi cell lines tested in our experiments possess a decreased capacity for the excision of γ-ray-damaged thymine. The molecular step(s) responsible for this repair deficiency have not yet been identified.

REFERENCES

Achey, P., Billen, D., and Beltranena, H. (1971): Single-strand breaks in gamma-irradiated φX174 DNA induced by exposure to alkali. *Int. J. Radiat. Biol.,* 20:501–504.

Alexander, P., and Lett, J. (1968): Effects of ionizing radiations on biological macro-molecules. In: *Comprehensive Biochemistry,* Vol. 27, edited by M. Florkin and E. Stotz, Elsevier, Amsterdam, pp. 267–356.

Berkowitz, D., Kakefuda, T., and Sporn, M. (1969): A simple and rapid method for the isolation of enzymatically active HeLa cell nuclei. *J. Cell. Biol.,* 42:851–855.

Blok, J., and Loman, H. (1973): The effects of γ-radiation in DNA. *Cur. Top. in Rad. Res.,* 9:165–245.

Cadet, J., and Téoule, R. (1972): Irradiation Gamma de la thymidine en solution aqueuse aéreé. *Tetrahedron Letters,* 31:3225–3228.

Cerutti, P. (1974*a*): Excision repair of DNA base damage. *Life Sci.,* 15:1567–1575.

Cerutti, P. (1974*b*): Effects of ionizing radiation on mammalian cells. *Naturwissenschaften,* 61:51–59.

Cerutti, P. (1975): Structural classification of DNA base damage. In: *Molecular Mechanisms for the Repair of DNA,* Part A. edited by P. C. Hanawalt and R. B. Setlow. Plenum Press, New York.

Cerutti, P., Miles, H. T., and Frazier, J. (1966): Interaction of partially reduced polyuridylic acid with polyadenylic acid. *Biochem. Biophys. Res. Commun.,* 22:466–742.

Cleaver, J. (1974): Repair processes for photochemical damage in mammalian cells. In: *Advances in Radiation Biology,* edited by J. Lett, H. Adler, and M. Zelle, Vol. 4, pp. 1–69. Academic Press, New York.

Dunlap, B., and Cerutti, P. (1975): Apyrimidinic sites in gamma-irradiated DNA. *FEBS Letters,* 51:188–190.

Ekert, B., and Monier, R. (1959): Structure of thymine hydroperoxide produced by X-irradiation. *Nature,* 184:58–59.

Finkelberg, R., Thompson, M., and Siminovitch, L. (1974): Survival after treatment with EMS, γ-rays and mitomycin C of skin-fibroblasts from patients with Fanconi's Anemia. *Am. J. Hum. Genet.,* 26:A30.

German, J. (1972): Genes which increase chromosomal instability in somatic cells and predispose to cancer. In: *Medical Genetics,* edited by A. Steinberg and A. Bearn, Vol. VIII, pp. 61–101. Grune & Stratton, New York.

Hahn, B. S., Wang, S. J., Flippen, J. L., and Karle, I. L. (1973): Radiation chemistry of nucleic acids. Isolation and characterization of 1-carbamylimidazolidone as product of cytosine, *J. Am. Chem. Soc.,* 95:2711–2712.

Hariharan, P. V., and Cerutti, P. A. (1974a): Excision of damaged thymine residues from gamma-irradiated polyd(A-T) by crude extracts of E. coli. *Proc. Natl. Acad. Sci. USA,* 71:3532–3536.

Hariharan, P. V., and Cerutti, P. A. (1974b): Excision of γ-ray damaged thymine by E. coli extracts is due to the 5′ → 3′ exonuclease associated with DNA polymerase I. *Biochem. Biophys. Res. Commun.,* 61:971–976.

Hariharan, P. V., and Cerutti, P. A. (1974c): The incision and strand rejoining step in the excision repair of 5,6-dihydroxy-dihydrothymine by crude E. coli extracts. *Biochem. Biophys. Res. Commun.,* 61:375–379.

Higurashi, M., and Conen, P. (1971): *In vitro* chromosomal radiosensitivity in Fanconi's Anemia. *Blood,* 38:336–342.

Johansen, I., and Howard-Flanders, P. (1965): Macromolecular repair and free radical scavenging in the protection of bacteria against X-rays. *Radiat. Res.* 24:184–200.

Kessler, E., Bopp, A., and Hagen, U. (1971): Radiation-induced single strand breaks in double-stranded circular DNA. *Int. J. Radiat. Biol.,* 20:75–78.

Latarjet, R., Ekert, B., and Demersman, P. (1963): Peroxidation of nucleic acids by radiation: Biological implications. *Radiat. Res. (Suppl.),* 3:247–256.

Lett, J., and Sun, C. (1970): The production of strand breaks in mammalian DNA by X-rays: At different stages in the cell cycle. *Radiat. Res.,* 44:771–787.

Lindahl, T., and Nyberg, B. (1972): Rate of depurination of native deoxyribonucleic acid. *Biochemistry,* 11:3610–3618.

Mattern, M., and Cerutti, P. (1975): Age-dependent excision repair of damaged thymine from γ-irradiated DNA by isolated nuclei from human fibroblasts. *Nature,* 254:450–452.

Mattern, M., Hariharan, P., and Cerutti, P. (1975): Selective excision of gamma-ray damaged thymine from the DNA of cultured mammalian cells. *Biochim. Biophys. Acta,* 395:48–55.

Mattern, M., Hariharan, P., Dunlap, B., and Cerutti, P. (1973): DNA degradation and excision repair in γ-irradiated Chinese hamster ovary cells. *Nature [New Biol.],* 245:230–232.

Miller, R. W., and Todaro, G. (1969): Viral transformation of cells from persons at high risk of cancer. *Lancet,* 81.

Painter, R., and Young, B. (1972): Repair replication in mammalian cells after X-irradiation. *Mutat. Res.,* 14:225–235.

Poon, P., O'Brien, R., and Parker, J. (1974): Defective DNA repair in Fanconi's Anemia. *Nature,* 250:223–225.

Regan, J., and Setlow, R. (1974): Two forms of repair in the DNA of human cells damaged by chemical carcinogens and mutagens. *Cancer Res.,* 34:3318–3325.

Remsen, J. F., and Cerutti, P. (1972): Ultraviolet inactivation and miscoding of irradiated R17-RNA in vitro. *Biochem. Biophys. Res. Commun.,* 48:430–436.

Remsen, J. F., Miller, N., and Cerutti, P. (1970): Photohydration of uridine in the RNA of coliphage R17, II. The relationship between ultraviolet inactivation and uridine photohydration. *Proc. Natl. Acad. Sci. USA*, 65:460–466.

Robbins, J., Kraemer, L., Lutzner, M., Festoff, B., and Coon, H. (1974): Xeroderma pigmentosum: An inherited disease with sun sensitivity, multiple cutaneous neoplasms and abnormal DNA repair. *Ann. Intern. Med.*, 80:221–248.

Roots, R., and Okada, S. (1972): Protection of DNA molecules of cultured mammalian cells from radiation-induced single-strand scissions by various alcohols and SH compounds. *Int. J. Radiat. Biol.*, 21:329–342.

Roti Roti, J., and Cerutti, P. (1974): Gamma-ray induced thymine damage in mammalian cells. *Int. J. Radiat. Biol.*, 25:413–417.

Sasaki, M., Tonomura, A. (1973): A high susceptibility of Fanconi's anemia to chromosome breakage by DNA cross-linking agents. *Cancer Res.*, 33:1829–1836.

Setlow, R., and Regan, J. (1973): The average size of the repaired regions in human DNA damaged by γ-rays. *Biophys. Soc. Abstr. FPM-G5,* 17th Annual Meeting of the Biophys. Society, Columbus, Ohio.

Strauss, B. (1974): Repair of DNA in mammalian cells. *Life Sci.*, 15:1685–1693.

Strauss, B., Scudiero, D., and Henderson, E. (1975): The nature of the alkylation lesions in mammalian cells. In: *Molecular Mechanisms for the Repair of DNA,* Part A. edited by P. C. Hanawalt and R. B. Setlow. Plenum Press, New York.

Swinehart, J., Bobst, A., and Cerutti, P. (1972): The effect of saturated pyrimidine bases on RNA conformation. *FEBS Lett.*, 21:56–58.

Swinehart, J., and Cerutti, P. A. (1975): Gamma-ray induced thymine damage in the DNA in coliphage φX174 and in *E. coli. Int. J. Radiat. Biol.*, 27:83.

Van Hemmen, J. J. (1971): 6-Amino-8-hydroxy-7,8-dihydropurine: Radiation product of adenine. *Nature [New Biol.]*, 231:79–80.

Verly, W. (1974): Monofunctional alkylating agents and apurinic sites in DNA. *Biochem. Pharmacol.*, 23:3–8.

Weiss, J. (1964): Chemical effects of ionizing radiations on nucleic acids and related compounds. In: *Progress in Nucleic Acid Research and Molecular Biology,* Vol. 3, pp. 103–142. Academic Press, New York.

Biology of Radiation Carcinogenesis, edited by
J. M. Yuhas, R. W. Tennant, and J. D. Regan.
Raven Press, New York © 1976.

Repair of Human DNA: Radiation and Chemical Damage in Normal and Xeroderma Pigmentosum Cells

James D. Regan and R. B. Setlow

Biology Division, Oak Ridge National Laboratory, Oak Ridge, Tennessee 37830 and Biology Department, Brookhaven National Laboratory, Upton, New York 11973

Recent reviews on DNA repair dealing with microorganisms and eukaryotic cells have appeared (Setlow and Setlow, 1972; Van Lancker, 1972; Cerutti, 1974). DNA repair in human cells has also been reviewed recently (Cleaver, 1974) as has the well-known genetically heterogeneous disease xeroderma pigmentosum (XP), involving defective DNA repair (Editorial, 1974). It is therefore, unnecessary for us to review the literature in these areas.

We present the experimental evidence we have gathered, using a particular assay for DNA repair in human cells—the photolysis of bromodeoxyuridine (BrdUrd) incorporated during repair. This assay characterizes the sequence of repair events that occur in human cells after radiation, both ultraviolet (UV) and ionizing, and permits an estimation of the size of the average repaired region after these physical insults to DNA (Regan, Setlow, and Ley, 1971; Regan, Setlow, Kaback, Howell, Klein, and Burgess, 1971). We will discuss chemical insults to DNA and attempt to liken the repair processes after chemical damages of various kinds to those repair processes that occur in human DNA after damage from physical agents (Regan and Setlow, 1974). We will also show results indicating that, under certain conditions, repair events resembling those seen after UV-irradiation can be observed in normal human cells after ionizing radiation. Furthermore the XP cells, defective in the repair of UV-induced DNA damage, show defective repair of these UV-like DNA lesions induced by ionizing radiation.

ULTRAVIOLET- AND IONIZING RADIATION DAMAGE AND REPAIR

Figure 1 is a diagrammatic representation of the BrdUrd photolysis method. The method has been described in detail in previous publications (Regan, Setlow, and Ley, 1971; Regan, Setlow, Kaback, Howell, Klein, and Burgess, 1971; Regan and Setlow, 1974).

Figure 2 shows typical sedimentation results obtained with normal human skin fibroblasts that have received as an insult 200 erg/mm^2 of 254-nm UV-irradiation. The 313-nm irradiation given subsequent to harvesting of

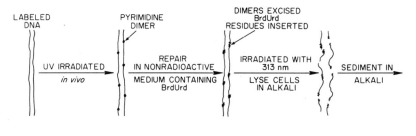

FIG. 1. Diagram of the BrdUrd photolysis assay for DNA repair.

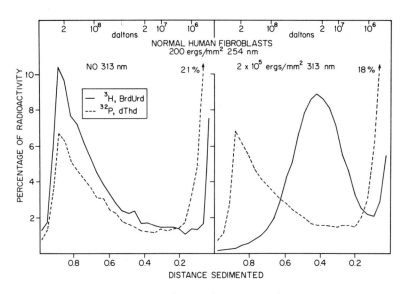

FIG. 2. Typical results of alkaline sucrose gradients analysis with normal human fibroblasts that received as insult 200 erg/mm² of 254-nm UV-irradiation 20 hr earlier. Note that the cells previously bulk-labeled with tritium have, post-insult, been incubated in BrdUrd whereas the control cells, previously bulk-labeled with ³²P, have, post-insult, been incubated in dThd. The left-hand panel shows the sedimentation profiles of the DNA from these cells that received no 313-nm irradiation and in the right-hand panel, DNA of cells that received 2 × 10⁵ erg/mm² of 313-nm irradiation.

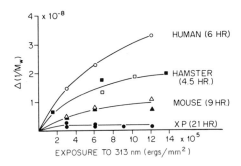

FIG. 3. Relationship of the change in the difference in the reciprocal of the weight-average molecular weight to the fluence of 313-nm radiation in various mammalian cells incubated at various times after the delivery of 200 erg/mm² of 254-nm UV-irradiation. Note that the human cells appear to exhibit the greatest sensitivity to 313-nm radiation, hamster cells less, mouse cells even less, and XP cells, even at extended times (21 hr after irradiation), are insensitive, in terms of molecular weight changes, to this irradiation. (Regan and Setlow, 1973.)

the cells causes a marked decrease in the molecular weight of the DNA of cells, which are incubated post-insult in BrdUrd. The magnitude of the shift observed is an indication of the amount of BrdUrd in the DNA and thus of the magnitude of repair. In Fig. 3 we see these kinds of data translated to represent the change in the reciprocal of the weight-average molecular weight $(\Delta 1/M_w)$, with increasing fluences of 313-nm radiation. Human cells at only 6 hr after the UV-irradiation appear to be extensively substituted with

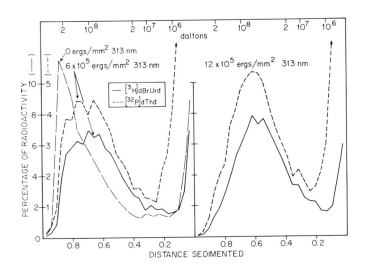

FIG. 4. Sedimentation profiles of the DNA of normal cells irradiated with 10 krad of ^{60}Co γ-rays and sedimented after 60 min through alkaline sucrose. In the left-hand panel are sedimentation profiles of cells that received either no or 6×10^5 erg/mm² of 313-nm radiation. In the right-hand panel are sedimentation profiles of DNA from cells that received 12×10^5 erg/mm² 313-nm radiation. (Regan and Setlow, 1974.)

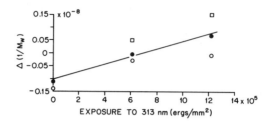

FIG. 5. Relationship of the change in the reciprocal of the molecular weight to the fluence of 313-nm radiation in normal human cells irradiated with 10 krad of ^{60}Co γ-rays and incubated for 60 min before assay on alkaline sucrose gradients. (Regan and Setlow, 1974.)

BrdUrd after 200 erg/mm^2 of 254-nm UV-irradiation. This figure also contains data from hamster, mouse, and XP cells. The human cells, in terms of the change in the reciprocal of the weight-average molecular weight, clearly are the best repairers among these species.

In Fig. 4, this assay is applied to normal human cells after 10 krad of ^{60}Co γ-rays. There is little or no difference in the shift induced by 313-nm radiation either in the BrdUrd- or the thymidine(dThd)-incubated controls. This indicates that the BrdUrd substitution is either zero or extremely low and suggests that the size of the repaired region is very small.

Figure 5 shows the relationship between $\Delta 1/M_w$ and the fluence of 313-nm radiation. The type of curve generated from these data is quite dif-

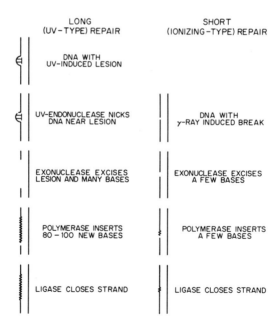

FIG. 6. Diagram of the two forms of prereplication repair in human cells. (Regan and Setlow, 1974.)

ferent from that seen in Fig. 3. It suggests a great insensitivity to the 313-nm radiation of the BrdUrd-substituted DNA. Moreover, we see no indication that this curve levels off at high fluences suggesting that, even at the highest fluences we can reach, we are not hitting all of the BrdUrd-substituted regions.

The preceding results (UV- versus ionizing radiation) indicate that we are observing two rather different repair systems (Fig. 6); the UV type or "long" repair and the ionizing type or "short" repair. The terms short and long have meaning both with regard to the patch size in the DNA and the time it takes to repair these lesions. Long repair takes 20 hr or more. Short repair takes 60 min. The typical patch size in long repair is about 100 nucleotides (200 erg/mm² of 254-nm UV) in agreement with estimates made in other ways (Cleaver, 1974). In short repair, the patch size is about three nucleotides (10 krad of ⁶⁰Co γ-rays). Our short patch size estimate of three nucleotides is in agreement with the findings of Painter and Young (1972) who used repair replication methods.

REPAIR OF CHEMICALLY INDUCED DAMAGE IN HUMAN DNA

Chemical damage to DNA both in normal and XP cells and repair has been studied by a number of workers (Cleaver, 1973; Stich and San, 1973; Stich, San, and Kawzoe, 1971, 1973; Stich, San, Miller, and Miller, 1972;

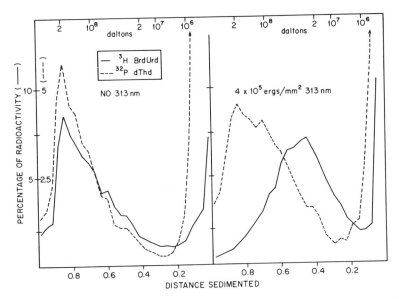

FIG. 7. Normal human fibroblasts. Alkaline sucrose gradient profiles of the DNA from cells insulted with 7 × 10⁻⁶ M N-acetoxyacetylaminofluorene and assayed after 20 hr. Note the similarity of these data to the data shown in Fig. 3 illustrating such gradients after UV-irradiation of human cells. (Setlow, Faulcon and Regan, 1976.)

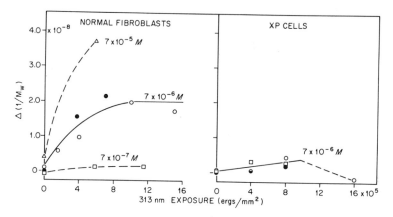

FIG. 8. Relationship of the difference in the reciprocal of the weight-average molecular weight to the fluence of 313-nm irradiation in normal and XP cells after treatment with N-acetoxyacetylaminofluorene. (Setlow, Faulcon, and Regan, 1976.)

see also review by Cleaver, 1974). We have applied the BrdUrd photolysis assay to the study of damage induced in human DNA by chemical carcinogens (Regan and Setlow, 1974). Figure 7 shows gradient results with N-acetoxy acetylamino fluorene (N-acetoxy AAF; kindly supplied by Dr. James A. Miller). The results with this carcinogen resembled quite closely results seen with UV-irradiation. Note, in Fig. 8, that the relationship of $\Delta 1/M_w$ to 313-nm fluence (at a dose of 7×10^{-6} M N-acetoxy AAF) is very similar to the results with 200 erg/mm^2 254-nm radiation shown in Fig. 3. Note also in the right-hand panel of Fig. 8 that XP cells are defective in

TABLE 1. *Classification of DNA-damaging agents according to the type of repair induced*

Treatment	Dose or conc.	Duration	Strand breaks/ 10^8 daltons after BrdUrd incubation and 10^6 erg/mm^2 of 313-nm radiation	BrdUrd nucleotides inserted/ lesion	Type of repair
UV (254 nm)	200 ergs/mm^2	24 s	10	25	Long[a]
^{60}Co γ-rays	10 krad	4 min	0.6	1	Short[b,c]
N-acetoxy AAF	7×10^{-6} M	60 min	4	~40	Long[a]
4-NQO	5×10^{-7} M	90 min	~2		Long and short
EMS	10^{-2} M	120 min	~1.0		Short[c]
MMS	5×10^{-5} M	5 min	~0.4		Short
Propane sultone	2×10^{-4} M	2 hr	~0.4		Short
ICR-170	10^{-6} M	1 hr	~1	~10	Long[a]

[a] Repair in normal cells 10-fold greater than in XP cells.
[b] Repair equal in normal and XP cells.
[c] See text for recent results.

repairing *N*-acetoxy AAF-induced lesions. Thus we would classify *N*-acetoxy AAF as an UV type or long repair-inducing agent. Similar experiments with other agents have resulted in the classification scheme summarized in Table 1.

ULTRAVIOLET-LIKE DAMAGE AND REPAIR AFTER IONIZING RADIATION (SETLOW, FAULCON, AND REGAN, 1976)

Figure 9 again shows the relationship between $\Delta 1/M_w$ and the fluence of 313-nm radiation in another series of BrdUrd photolysis experiments. In these experiments, the cells received 10 krad of ^{60}Co γ-rays in air and were

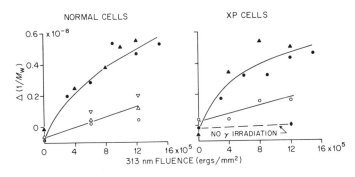

FIG. 9. Relationship of the difference in the reciprocal of the weight-average molecular weight to fluence of 313-nm irradiation in normal and XP cells at short and long times after γ-ray radiation (10 krad, air; incubation: 1.5 hr, open symbols; 20 hr, filled symbols). (Setlow, Faulcon, and Regan, 1976.)

then incubated for either 1.5 hr or 20 hr in the BrdUrd-containing medium. At 1.5 hr after irradiation, the same kind of relationship is seen in both normal and XP cell types as was previously shown in Fig. 5. But at long incubation times (20 hr), in the normal cells, there appears to be a definite tendency toward an UV type of pattern with a much increased sensitivity to 313 nm and a relatively curvilinear response to increasing fluences of 313 nm. In the right panel, the XP cells show greater variability but follow a pattern similar to that of normal cells.

In the next series of experiments, we changed the gas phase to nitrogen and increased the dose of ionizing radiation to 30 krad. Figure 10 shows the results with normal cells under anoxic conditions and incubated for 20 hr. In the left-hand panel are the two DNAs that received no 313-nm radiation. They appear to be sedimenting nearly identically. In the right-hand panel are the sedimentation profiles of DNA that received 12 × 10⁵ erg/mm² of 313-nm radiation at the conclusion of the experiment. The cells that have been incubated in BrdUrd subsequent to the 30 krad of ionizing radiation, delivered in an anoxic atmosphere, have a greater sensitivity to the 313-nm

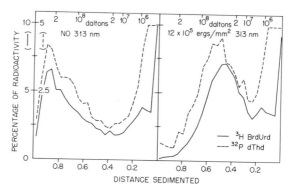

FIG. 10. Sedimentation profiles of the DNA from normal cells irradiated with 30 krad under nitrogen and incubated 20 hr, post-insult, either in BrdUrd-containing medium ([³H]bulk-labeled cells) or, for controls, dThd-incubated cells ([³²P]bulk-labeled cells). (Setlow, Faulcon, and Regan, 1976.)

radiation and show a lower molecular weight average than the cells labeled with ³²P and incubated in dThd. This result is reminiscent of a UV type effect.

In Fig. 11, a similar experiment on XP cells is shown. The two DNA receiving no 313-nm radiation had essentially the same sedimentation profiles, and the DNA receiving 12×10^5 erg/mm² 313-nm radiation before sedimentation showed only a very slight difference in the sedimentation profiles. There is much less of a difference than in Fig. 10. Figure 12 summarizes a number of experiments in terms of $\Delta 1/M_w$ as a function of fluence of 313-nm radiation. In the left-hand panel are results with normal cells assayed at 1.5 hr and 20 hr. Note the slowly rising, insensitive curve seen in normal cells incubated for 1.5 hr and the initial rapid rise and curvilinear relationship seen in normal cells incubated for 20 hr. The right panel shows

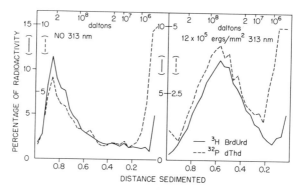

FIG. 11. Sedimentation profiles of the DNA of XP cells irradiated with 30 krad under nitrogen and incubated for 20 hr, post-insult, either in BrdUrd-containing medium ([³H]bulk-labeled cells) or in dThd-containing medium ([³²P]bulk-labeled cells). Conditions for this experiment were exactly the same as those in Fig. 10, except that XP cells rather than normal cells were used. (Setlow, Faulcon, and Regan, 1976.)

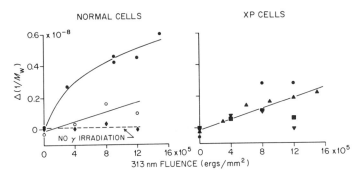

FIG. 12. Relationship of the difference in the reciprocal of the weight-average molecular weight of either normal cells or XP cells irradiated with 30 krad of ^{60}Co γ-rays under nitrogen and incubated either at long times or short times before assay (1.5, *open circles;* 20 hr, *closed symbols*). The different symbols refer to different experiments. (Setlow, Faulcon, and Regan, 1976.)

several experiments with XP cells incubated for 20 hr. They do not show this sensitivity to the 313-nm radiation. This result indicates that there are not extensive runs of BrdUrd inserted into these DNA, and suggests that in these cells, unlike the normal cells, UV-like lesions induced by ionizing radiation are poorly repaired just as in the case of UV-induced pyrimidine dimers in XP cells.

The results we have presented here, taken together with results of previous investigators (summarized by Setlow and Setlow, 1972) suggest that ionizing radiation induces some UV-like lesions in human DNA. These lesions are repaired in the usual prereplication repair mode in normal cells. In XP cells, it appears that these UV-like lesions are poorly repaired as are the UV-induced pyrimidine dimers.

The murine rodents (our models for ionizing radiation carcinogenesis) perform prereplication repair of pyrimidine dimers close to the level of human XP cells. What then is the role of these ionizing radiation-induced, UV-like lesions in murine rodent carcinogenesis? How might the difference between the ability of man and rodents to perform prereplication repair of ionizing radiation-induced, UV-like DNA lesions affect our evaluation of the quantitative aspects of radiation carcinogenesis as it is experimentally investigated in murine rodents and extrapolated to man?

RECENT RESULTS WITH AN "IONIZING-TYPE" CHEMICAL MUTAGEN

As indicated in Table 1, we have investigated a number of chemical carcinogens and constructed a classification of these agents according to the type of repair sequence they induce in the DNA. With our finding of UV-type repair, which occurred after ionizing radiation at long times in normal cells, and the reduced repair of this γ-ray induced damage in XP cells, we were encouraged to investigate further ethyl methanesulfonate (EMS), which we

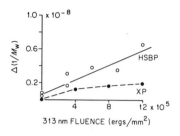

FIG. 13. Results of an analysis of normal and XP cells after treatment with 2×10^{-5} M ethyl methane sulfonate and a BrdUrd photolysis assay done at 20 hr, post-insult (10^{-2} M 2 hr, incubated 18–20 hr in BrdUrd + HO − urea and dThd + HO − urea, both at 313 n m). Conditions for these experiments were the same as in the experiments described in the preceding figures. Note that the XP cells under these conditions appear to display defective repair of lesions induced by this chemical agent when assayed at long times after the delivery of the original insult and normal cells appear to exhibit a UV-type repair response, in contrast to the result previously found at short times after treatment with this chemical agent. (*Unpublished experiments.*)

have classified as an ionizing-type agent because it results in similar repair patterns in normal and XP cells at short times after treatment. Figure 13 presents data relating $\Delta 1/M_w$ to increasing fluences of 313-nm radiation in normal and XP cells treated with EMS. These results are derived a long time, i.e., 18 to 20 hr, after treatment with EMS. In the normal cells, the data are typical of UV-induced lesions, and UV-type repair. Furthermore, in the XP cells we see evidence of reduced repair. This result indicates that EMS also has an UV-type capability in terms of DNA damage and repair along with its ionizing-type function.

It is not inconceivable that many DNA-damaging agents, such as ionizing radiation and certain chemical carcinogens, produce several types of changes in DNA. They may induce ionizing-type damage—the repair of which is rapid and is optimally observed at short times after treatment and at the same rate in normal and XP cells; additionally, they may also induce UV-type damage, the repair of which is observable only a long time after treatment and which appear to be rather differently repaired in normal and XP cells. Perhaps we should be prepared to expect that DNA-damaging agents may induce several types of damages and that these damages will be repaired according to the structural configurations of the damage they induce and the sites of enzymes, available and evolved, for dealing with such damage in human cells.

ACKNOWLEDGMENT

This research was jointly sponsored by the National Cancer Institute and the Energy Research and Development Administration under contract with the Union Carbide Corporation.

REFERENCES

Cerutti, P. (1974): Excision repair of DNA base damage. *Life Sci.,* 15:1567–1575.

Cleaver, J. D. (1973): DNA repair with purines and pyrimidines in radiation- and carcinogen-damaged normal and xeroderma pigmentosum human cells. *Cancer Res.,* 33:362–369.

Cleaver, J. E. (1974): Repair processes for photochemical damage in mammalian cells. In: *Advances in Radiation Biology,* Vol. 4, pp. 1–75, edited by J. T. Lett, H. Adler, and M. Zelle, Academic Press, New York.

Editorial (1974): Xeroderma pigmentosum—an inherited disease with sun sensitive multiple cutaneous neoplasms, and abnormal DNA repair. *Ann. Inter. Med.* 80:221–248.

Painter, R. B., and Young, B. R. (1972): Repair replication in mammalian cells after X-irradiation. *Mutat. Res.,* 14:225–235.

Regan, J. D., and Setlow, R. B. (1973): Repair of chemical damage to human DNA. In: *Chemical Mutagens,* Vol. 3, edited by A. Hollaender. Plenum, New York.

Regan, J. D., and Setlow, R. B. (1974): Two forms of repair in the DNA of human cells damaged by chemical carcinogens and mutagens. *Cancer Res.,* 34:3318–3325.

Regan, J. D., Setlow, R. B., and Ley, R. D. (1971): Normal and defective repair of damaged DNA in human cells: A sentitive assay utilizing the photolysis of bromodeoxyuridine. *Proc. Natl. Acad. Sci., USA,* 68:708–712.

Regan, J. D., Setlow, R. B., Kaback, M. M., Howell, R. R., Klein, E., and Burgess, G. (1971). Xeroderma pigmentosum: A rapid, sensitive method for prenatal diagnosis. *Science,* 174:147–150.

Setlow, R. B., and Setlow, J. K. (1972): Effects of radiation on polynucleotides. In: *Annual Review of Biophysics and Bioengineering,* Vol. 1, edited by M. F. Morales, pp. 293–345. Annual Reviews, Inc., Palo Alto, Calif.

Setlow, R. B., Faulcon, F. M., and Regan, J. D. (1976): Defective repair of gamma-ray-induced DNA damage in xeroderma pigmentosum cells. (In press.)

Stich, H. F., San, R. H. C., Miller, J. A., and Miller, E. C. (1972): Various levels of DNA repair synthesis in xeroderma pigmentosum cells exposed to the carcinogens, *N*-hydroxy and *N*-acetoxy-2-acetylaminofluorene. *Nature [New Biol.],* 238:9–10.

Stich, H. F., and San, R. H. C. (1973): DNA repair synthesis and survival of repair deficient human cells exposed to the K-region epoxide of benz(a)anthracene. *Proc. Soc. Exp. Biol. Med.,* 142:155–158.

Stich, H. F., San, R. H. C., and Kawzoe, Y. (1971): DNA repair synthesis in mammalian cells exposed to a series of oncogenic and non-oncogenic derivatives of 4-nitroquinoline-1-oxide. *Nature,* 416–419.

Stich, H. F., San, R. H. C., and Kawzoe, Y. (1973): Increased sensitivity of xeroderma pigmentosum cells to some chemical carcinogens and mutagens. *Mutat. Res.,* 17:127–137.

Van Lancker, J. L. (1974): Carcinogenesis and DNA repair. In: *Chemical carcinogenesis,* edited by P. O. P. Tso and J. A. DiPaolo, Part A, Dekker, New York.

Biology of Radiation Carcinogenesis, edited by
J. M. Yuhas, R. W. Tennant, and J. D. Regan.
Raven Press, New York © 1976.

Inherited DNA Repair Defects in *H. sapiens:* Their Relation to UV-Associated Processes in Xeroderma Pigmentosum

Jay H. Robbins, Kenneth H. Kraemer, and Alan D. Andrews

Dermatology Branch, National Cancer Institute, National Institutes of Health, Bethesda, Maryland 20014

Xeroderma pigmentosum (XP) is an autosomal recessive disease in which patients develop pigmentation abnormalities and numerous malignancies on areas of skin exposed to sunlight (Robbins, Kraemer, Lutzner, Festoff, and Coon, 1974). Some XP patients have neurological abnormalities in addition to their cutaneous pathology (De Sanctis and Cacchione, 1932; Robbins, Kraemer, Lutzner, Festoff, and Coon, 1974). Genetic defects in DNA repair have now been found in all studied XP patients. Here, we shall review and present studies relating the different inherited DNA repair defects of XP to several UV-associated processes.

MATERIALS AND METHODS

Peripheral blood lymphocytes were obtained from patients of the NIH series and prepared as described previously (Burk, Lutzner, Clarke, and Robbins, 1971). Fibroblasts were obtained from the American Type Culture Collection, Rockville, Maryland and cultured as described by Kraemer, Coon, Petinga, Barrett, Rahe, and Robbins (1975). The UV-induced thymidine incorporation was measured by autoradiography (Kraemer, Coon, Petinga, Barrett, Rahe, and Robbins, 1975) or by scintillation spectroscopy (Burk, Lutzner, Clarke, and Robbins, 1971). The radioactive thymidine ([3]HTdR; specific activity, 15–22 Ci/mmole) was used in a final concentration of 10 μCi/ml of culture fluid.

RESULTS

Excision Repair in XP

During excision repair of UV-damaged DNA in cultured cells, [3]HTdR in the culture medium is incorporated into newly synthesized segments which replace regions of DNA containing UV-induced pyrimidine dimers (Cleaver, 1968; Robbins, Kraemer, Lutzner, Festoff, and Coon, 1974). This rate of unscheduled DNA synthesis (UDS) can be determined autoradiographically

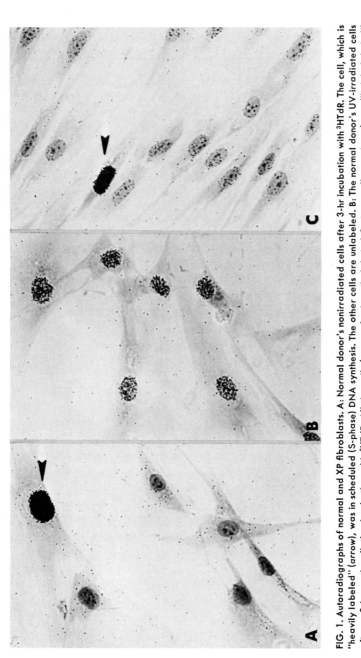

FIG. 1. Autoradiographs of normal and XP fibroblasts. A: Normal donor's nonirradiated cells after 3-hr incubation with ³HTdR. The cell, which is "heavily labeled" (arrow), was in scheduled (S-phase) DNA synthesis. The other cells are unlabeled. B: The normal donor's UV-irradiated cells after a 3-hr postirradiation incubation with ³HTdR. All the cells (except for heavily labeled S-phase cells not shown) are "lightly labeled" owing to the UV induced incorporation of ³HTdR during DNA repair synthesis. (C) Irradiated cells of strain XP2BE after a 3-hr postirradiation incubation with ³HTdR. All cells other than the heavily labeled cell in S-phase synthesis (arrow) are lightly labeled, owing to repair synthesis, but the amount of labeling and, therefore, of repair synthesis is considerably less than that of the normal donor's cells. Fibroblasts irradiated in saline with 300 erg/mm² of UV light from a General Electric germicidal lamp (No. G15T8), emitting predominantly 2,537 Å UV light. The cells were incubated for 3 hr with ³HTdR in a 37 °C air:CO_2 (95%:5%) incubator. Then they were washed with phosphate-buffered saline, fixed in a glutaraldehyde-cacodylate solution, and prepared for autoradiography (emulsion, NTB-3; exposed time, one week). (Acid hematoxylin; magnification, ×300.) (From Robbins, Kraemer, Lutzner, Festoff, and Coon, 1974.)

(Fig. 1). Cells from most XP patients are unable to perform a normal rate of excision repair of DNA containing these dimers as shown by the reduced ³HTdR incorporation of the XP cells of Fig. 1C.

This DNA excision repair defect is also demonstrable in XP patients' peripheral blood lymphocytes (Burk, Lutzner, Clarke, and Robbins, 1971; Robbins and Kraemer, 1972a,b). Figure 2 shows decreased UV-induced ³HTdR incorporation into the lymphocytes from patients XP1BE, XP2BE and XP3BE during each of the first 3 hr after irradiation. In contrast, the last frame in Fig. 2 shows a normal rate of incorporation into lymphocytes from patient XP4BE. Subsequent studies have shown that this patient's dermal fibroblasts (Burk, Yuspa, Lutzner, and Robbins, 1971), epidermal cells (Robbins, Levis, and Miller, 1972; Robbins and Burk, 1973), and basal cell carcinoma cells (Robbins, Kraemer, and Flaxman, 1975) also have normal rates of UV-induced ³HTdR incorporation. This patient has been designated an "XP variant" (Cleaver, 1972), and four other variant kindred have subsequently been found (Day, 1975; Lehmann, Kirk-Bell,

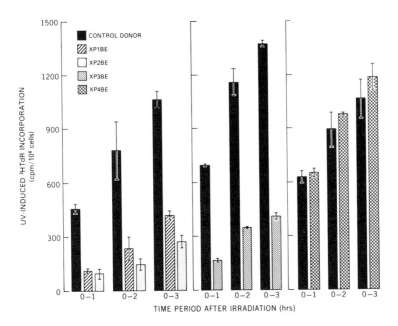

FIG. 2. Ultraviolet induced ³HTdR incorporation into 10^6 peripheral blood lymphocytes from normal control donors and from XP patients 1, 2, 3, and 4 of the NIH series. For each time period, the mean counts per minute (cpm) of duplicate unirradiated cultures of a person's cells were subtracted from the mean cpm of duplicate irradiated cultures of those cells, and the differences of the means so obtained are represented by the vertical columns (with the standard errors of the mean differences indicated). The preparation, irradiation (150 erg/mm²), and determination of ³HTdR uptake of the lymphocytes are described in detail by Burk et al. (1971a). Hydroxyurea, which has no effect on the UV induced ³HTdR incorporation of DNA repair, was added to a final concentration of 10^{-3} M immediately after irradiation to retard any S-phase DNA synthesis associated with normal preparation for mitosis occurring in a small percentage of the cells. (From Robbins and Burk, *unpublished data*.)

Arlett, Patterson, Lohman, De Weerd-Kastelein, and Bootsma, 1975). A variety of methods other than UDS have been utilized to measure DNA excision repair. These methods include assays of repair replication by equilibrium density gradient centrifugation (Cleaver, 1968) and by bromo-deoxyuridine photolysis (Regan, Setlow, and Ley, 1971), and assays of pyrimidine dimer removal by measuring loss of UV-endonuclease-susceptible sites in irradiated DNA (Patterson, Lohman, and Sluyter, 1973). Each of these methods has confirmed the UDS findings of normal DNA excision repair in the variants (Cleaver, 1972; Buhl, Setlow, and Regan, personal communication; Lehmann, Kirk-Bell, Arlett, Patterson, Lohman, De Weerd-Kastelein, and Bootsma, 1975) and defective repair in the cells of all other XP patients so tested.

Complementation Among Excision-Deficient XP Strains

De Weerd-Kastelein, Keijzer, and Bootsma (1972) were the first to dem-onstrate that when fibroblasts from certain pairs of excision-deficient XP patients are fused in culture, the nucleus of each strain in the resulting bi-nuclear heterokaryons is complemented, i.e., both nuclei in such cells ac-quire the capacity to perform UV-induced UDS at a normal rate. By such studies, these investigators found three complementation groups among their Rotterdam XP strains (De Weerd-Kastelein, Keijzer, and Bootsma, 1974). Similar studies at the NIH (Fig. 3) subsequently distinguished four com-plementation groups (designated A, B, C, and D) among the NIH strains (Kraemer, Coon, and Robbins, 1973; Robbins, Kraemer, Lutzner, Festoff, and Coon, 1974; Kraemer, Coon, Petinga, Rahe, and Robbins, 1975). The restored UV-induced UDS observed in the complemented nuclei of the XP heterokaryons was shown to represent DNA repair by virtue of its resistance to hydroxyurea (Kraemer, Coon, Petinga, Rahe, and Robbins, 1975) and by assays of repair replication (De Weerd-Kastelein, Kleijer, Sluyter, and Keijzer, 1973) and thymine dimer excision (Patterson, Lohman, Wester-veld, and Sluyter, 1974).

All the strains within a complementation group should fail to complement each other. This requirement was fulfilled for all the strains in groups con-taining more than one kindred (groups A, C, and D) tested at the NIH (Kraemer, Coon, Petinga, Rahe, and Robbins, 1975).

In collaborative studies by Rotterdam and NIH investigators, it has been determined that the third Rotterdam complementation group (De Weerd-Kastelein, Keijzer, and Bootsma, 1974) is different from all of the four NIH groups and has been designated group E. Thus, there are five currently known UDS complementation groups in XP (Bootsma, De Weerd-Kastelein, Kleijer, and Keijzer, 1975; Kraemer, De Weerd-Kastelein, Robbins, Petinga,

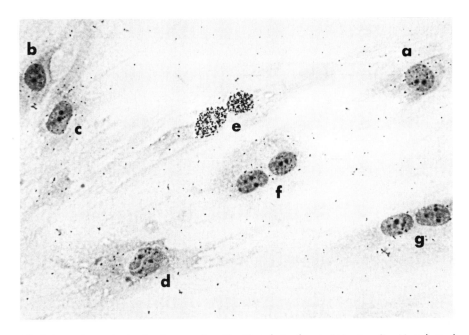

FIG. 3. Autoradiograph of unfused mononuclear fibroblasts (a to d) and of binuclear fibroblasts (e to g) in a Sendai virus-treated culture containing cells from patients 1 and 12, who are in different complementation groups. The cells were exposed to 300 erg/mm² of UV light and treated as described in the legend of Fig. 1. The binuclear cell with numerous grains over its nuclei (e) is a heterokaryon the nuclei of which have complemented each other, since both nuclei seem to have a normal or nearly normal amount of UV induced ³HTdR incorporation, compared with the incorporation in the normal cells in Fig. 1B. The other binuclear cells (f and g) are presumed homokaryons, and their nuclei have no more incorporation than the nuclei of the unfused mononuclear cells (a to d). (Acid hematoxylin; magnification, ×420.) (From Robbins, Kraemer, Lutzner, Festoff, and Coon, 1974.)

Barrett, and Bootsma, 1975). Each of the five complementation groups has a characteristic rate of UV-induced UDS (Table 1, Column II).

Experiments have been performed (Day, Kraemer, and Robbins, 1975) to determine whether the quantitatively normal levels of excision repair observed in heterokaryons formed from complementing XP strains represent a functionally normal repair, which restores full biological activity to UV-damaged DNA. These experiments were performed using the host-cell reactivation technique of Day (1974) in which the plaque-forming ability of UV-irradiated adenovirus 2 (a double-strand DNA virus) is assayed on fibroblast monolayers. Excision-deficient XP strains have a reduced ability to functionally repair the irradiated virus and thereby restore its plaque-forming ability (Day, 1974). With this technique, it has been shown (Day, Kraemer, and Robbins, 1975) that heterokaryons of complementing XP strains do indeed restore full biological activity to the irradiated virus.

TABLE 1. Characteristics of the different genetic forms of XP

XP mutation	I. Clinical manifestations[a]		II. UV-induced [3H]TdR incorporation[e] (% of normal rate)	III. Host cell reactivation[g] (% of normal)	IV. Post-UV colony-forming ability[i] (% of normal)	V. Post-aromatic amide carcinogen colony-forming ability[j] (% of normal)	VI. Repair of X-ray breaks[k]	VII. Post-replication repair
	Cutaneous	Neurologic						
Group A	+	+	<2	3.4–6.8	u	11–32	Proficient	Partly deficient[l]
Group B	+	?[c]	3–7	11	u	u	u	Partly deficient[m]
Group C	+	–[d]	10–20	11–35	25	43–56	Proficient	Partly deficient[l]
Group D	+[b]	+	25–50	3.5	15	u	u	Partly deficient[m]
Group E	+[b]	–[b]	>60[f]	47	u	u	Proficient	Proficient[m]
Variant	+	–	100	57–64[h]	56	59–83	Proficient	Markedly deficient[l]

+, present; –, absent; ?, unknown; u, untested

[a] Refs. 2, 17, From Bootsma, DeWeerd-Kastelein, Kleijer, and Keijzer, 1975), Kleijer, DeWeerd-Kastelein, Sluyter, Keijzer, DeWit, and Bootsma (1973), Kraemer, DeWeerd-Kastelein, Robbins, Petinga, Barrett, and Bootsma (1975), and Robbins, Kraemer, Lutzner, Festoff, and Coon (1974).

[b] From DeWeerd-Kastelein, Keijzer, and Bootsma (1974) and Kleijer, DeWeerd-Kastelein, Sluyter, Keijzer, DeWit, and Bootsma (1973).

[c] The neurological abnormalities of the one patient in this complementation group may be attributed entirely to her coincident Cockayne's syndrome Robbins, Kraemer, Lutzner, Festoff, and Coon (1974).

[d] The only patient in group C with any known neurological abnormality has a dull-normal IQ (Robbins, Kraemer, Lutzner, Festoff, and Coon, 1974) which is probably coincidental to her XP.

[e] From Kraemer, Coon, Petinga, Rahe, and Robbins (1975) and Robbins, Kraemer, Lutzner, Festoff, and Coon (1974).

[f] From Kraemer, DeWeerd-Kastelein, Robbins, Petinga, Barrett, and Bootsma (1975).

[g] Day (1974).

[h] Day (1975).

[i] The D_{37} of a strain (determined from the exponential portion of its curve in Fig. 4) was expressed as a percent of the average D_{37} of two normal strains (control donors L and P). Maher et al. (1975) have reported post-UV colony-forming ability for a strain from Group A, Group C and the variant class, which, if expressed as above, we calculate to be 17, 53, and 77% of normal, respectively. C. F. Arlett has also reported that XP variants have decreased colony-forming ability after UV-irradiation (cf. note added in proof, Lehmann et al., 1975).

[j] The values are calculated from data presented by Maher et al. (1975).

[k] From Kleijer, DeWeerd-Kastelein, Sluyter, Keijzer, DeWit, and Bootsma (1973).

[l] Lehmann, Kirk-Bell, Arlett, Patterson, Lohman, DeWeerd-Kastelein, and Bootsma (1975).

[m] Lehmann, personal communication.

XP Variants

Day (1974, 1975) has found that the five known XP variants all have from 57 to 64% of the normal level of host-cell reactivation of UV-irradiated adenovirus 2 (Table 1, Column III). Although Day's studies do not indicate what aspect of DNA repair may be defective in these XP variant strains, the findings of Lehmann et al. (1975) indicate that the variants are markedly defective in the rate at which they convert low molecular weight DNA synthesized in UV-irradiated cells into high molecular weight DNA. This process, which is also known as post-replication repair (Lehmann, 1974), is believed to involve the filling in of gaps created in daughter-strand DNA when S-phase synthesis is interrupted by UV-induced dimers on the parental template strand. The variants' post-replication repair defect is greatly intensified by caffeine, which has no effect on post-replication repair in normal human cells. Similar, but less severe impairment in post-replication repair and sensitivity to caffeine is present in strains from all the UDS complementation groups except group E (Lehmann, Kirk-Bell, Arlett, Patterson, Lohman, De Weerd-Kastelein, and Bootsma, 1975; Lehmann, *personal communication*) (Table 1, Column VII).

Post-UV Colony-Forming Ability

Kraemer, Barrett, and Robbins (1974) reported that some XP fibroblast strains had greater reductions in post-UV colony-forming ability than other XP strains. Furthermore, strains within a complementation group had similar levels of post-UV colony-forming ability. As shown in Fig. 4, strains XP6BE and XP7BE (representing different kindreds in complementation group D) have a similar post-UV colony-forming ability, which is less than that of strain XP2BE (group C). Preliminary experiments indicate that the colony-forming ability of strain XP12BE (group A) is similar to that of the group D strains, whereas that of XP11BE (group B) may be intermediate between that of the group D and C strains. Strain XP4RO (group C) appears to have a UV sensitivity similar to that of the group C strain shown in Fig. 4. Maher, Birch, Otto, and McCormick (1975) found that strains XP12BE and XP2BE had D_{37} values of 3 and 8 erg/mm^2, respectively, which are similar to the values of 5 and 9 erg/mm^2 for our group D and group C strains, respectively (cf. Fig. 4). C. F. Arlett (cf. note added in proof in Lehmann, Kirk-Bell, Arlett, Patterson, Lohman, De Weerd-Kastelein, and Bootsma, 1975) and Maher, Birch, Otto and McCormick (1975) have recently found that XP variants also have reduced post-UV colony-forming ability. We have confirmed their findings using variant strain XP4BE (Fig. 4), which has a post-UV colony-forming ability intermediate between that of the normal strain and strain XP2BE of group C (Fig. 4; Table 1, Column IV).

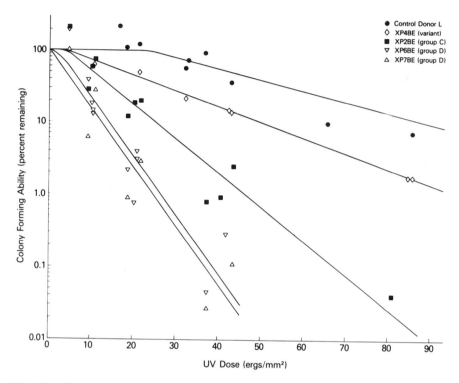

FIG. 4. Post-UV colony-forming ability of different XP fibroblast strains. Each point is calculated by dividing the mean colony-forming efficiency of replicate plates at a given UV dose by the mean colony-forming efficiency of the cells when unirradiated. The colony-forming efficiency per plate is the number of colonies per plate divided by the number of cells plated. For unirradiated cells, the colony-forming efficiency ranged from 0.013 to 0.27. Each line was determined by the method of least squares, utilizing points obtained from two to four experiments. Two points from Control Donor L at doses greater than 90 erg/mm² are not shown. The cells were irradiated in phosphate-buffered saline in log-phase growth in Petri dishes at fluxes of 0.5 to 2.2 erg/mm²/s. The cells were then trypsinized and plated at appropriate dilutions. After incubation at 37°C for 2 to 3 weeks, the cells were fixed and then stained with trypan blue. Colonies containing 15 cells or more were counted.

Long-Term XP Lymphoblast Lines

Biochemical studies are now being performed on each of the known genetic forms of XP. Unfortunately, it is often difficult to obtain sufficient numbers of fibroblasts for studies of this kind. Partly to alleviate this problem, we have attempted to establish long-term lymphoblast lines from the peripheral blood of XP patients. Such long-term lines grow rapidly in suspension to high density and are therefore a ready source of large numbers of cells.

We previously reported the establishment of lymphoblast lines from an XP patient in complementation group C (Andrews, Robbins, Kraemer, and Buell, 1974). These lines were shown to have increased sensitivity to the

TABLE 2. *Incorporation of ³HTdR into DNA of lymphoblast lines*

Treatment		[³H]TdR incorporation (cpm ± S.E.)		Significance of [³H]TdR incorporation
HU	UV	Normal line C3BE-L1	XP line XP1BE-L1	
−	−	171,195 ± 2,158	176,641 ± 4,053	S-phase synthesis
−	+	54,452 ± 554	41,222 ± 911	UV-resistant S-phase synthesis plus repair
+	−	2,996 ± 45	3,295 ± 253	HU-resistant S-phase synthesis
+	+	11,500 ± 153	4,167 ± 90	Repair plus HU- and UV-resistant S-phase synthesis

HU, hydroxyurea; UV, ultraviolet radiation; −, absent, +, present

Lymphoblasts were cultured in RPMI 1715 containing 20% fetal calf serum and transferred to RPMI 1640 containing 3% human plasma 24 hr post-irradiation. Log-phase cells, suspended in a 1-mm layer of the latter culture fluid at a concentration of 10^6 cells/ml, were irradiated with an incident dose of 250 erg/mm². Hydroxyurea, at a final concentration of 2×10^{-2} M, was added just prior to the time of irradiation. Approximately 5 min after irradiation, ³HTdR was added, and four replicate 0.2-ml aliquots of each cell suspension were incubated for 2 hr at 37°C in an air:CO_2 incubator. The cells were then harvested and washed on chromatography paper, and the retained radioactivity was determined in a liquid scintillation spectrometer and expressed as the cpm/2×10^5 cells (±SEM for the four replicate samples).

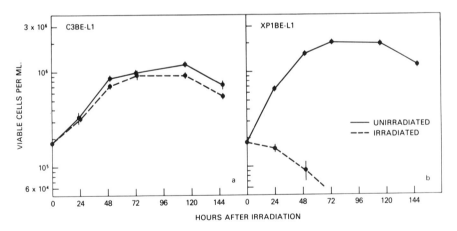

FIG. 5. Concentration of viable cells in suspensions of a non-XP (C3BE-L1) and of an XP lymphoblast line at various times after irradiation with an incident UV dose of 50 erg/mm². Each symbol represents the average (vertical line, the range) of the number of viable (trypan blue-excluding) cells in two replicate samples. This experiment utilized aliquots of the cell suspensions used in the experiment of Table 2 and was begun on the same day. Cells were suspended at a concentration of 10^6 cells per milliliter in a 1-mm layer of medium RPMI 1640 with 20% fetal calf serum. Cells were then irradiated, diluted to 1.8×10^5 cells/ml with fresh medium, and incubated at 37°C in an air:CO_2 incubator.

killing effects of UV radiation. We have more recently established lines from another patient in group C and have been able to demonstrate that XP lymphoblasts have decreased UV-induced ^{3}HTdR incorporation (Table 2) as well as increased sensitivity to UV radiation (Fig. 5). We are currently attempting to establish such lines for each of the genetic forms of XP.

DISCUSSION

In the relatively short time since Cleaver (1968) demonstrated that XP involved defective repair of UV-damaged DNA, it has been found that there are at least six genetic forms of XP, i.e., the variant form(s) and the five different excision-deficient complementation groups.

It is clear, therefore, that to derive useful information from studies of XP cells it is necessary to know the form(s) of XP being studied. Knowledge of the genetic heterogeneity of XP has already been usefully applied in a number of studies. For instance, although the cutaneous manifestations of XP are present in all forms of the disease (Robbins, Kraemer, Lutzner, Festoff, and Coon, 1974), associated neurological abnormalities appear only in patients from groups A and D (Table I, Column I). In addition, it has been found that each of the forms of XP has its own distinctive rate of UDS (Table 1, Column II). Day (1974) has shown that the ability of XP fibroblasts to perform host-cell reactivation of UV-irradiated adenovirus 2 is also related to their complementation group assignment (Table 1, column III). The work carried out to date on post-UV (Kraemer, Barrett, and Robbins, 1974; Maher, Birch, Otto, and McCormick, 1975) (Table 1, Column IV) and post-aromatic amide carcinogen (Maher, Birch, Otto, and McCormick, 1975) (Table 1, Column V) colony-forming ability has also demonstrated characteristic abilities for each of the complementation groups studied. It is interesting to note that the characterisic UDS rates of the six forms of XP correlate with the results of functional repair assays, such as post-UV colony-forming ability and host-cell reactivation of UV-irradiated adenovirus 2, with the notable exception of group D. This group has a UDS rate greater than that of group C, but its functional repair capacity is less than that of group C and is as severely defective as that of group A (see, for example, Column II in comparison with Columns III and IV of Table 1). These findings suggest that the degree of impairment in UDS, at least in the case of group D, does not accurately reflect the severity of the defect in functional repair capacity. Thus, the genetic defect in members of group D may have rendered the excision repair system unusually error-prone.

It is perhaps not unexpected to find that the only forms of XP with associated neurological abnormalities are those with the most defective repair as measured in functional assays, such as UV survival and host-cell reactivation. DNA repair is almost certainly required to maintain the metabolic integrity of the nervous system, the neurons of which must function for the lifetime of the organism while being subjected to any number of endogenous or exogenous substances that may be DNA damaging.

The fact that there are five different complementation groups among the excision-deficient XP strains suggests that five different gene products may be required for excision repair and that they are defective among these strains. Identification of the defective gene products must await definitive biochemical studies of the repair enzymes in each of the complementation groups. An interesting study in this regard is that of Sutherland, Rice, and Wagner (1975) reporting decreased or absent photoreactivating enzyme in strains from all five excision-deficient XP groups. Although photoreactivating enzyme monomerizes pyrimidine dimers in the presence of suitable light in prokaryotes and in eukaryotes up to the placental mammals (Cook, 1972; Howard-Flanders, 1973), its function in human cells is still unclear. The long-term lymphoblast lines we are developing from each of the six forms of XP will provide a convenient source of large quantities of cells for the additional biochemical studies required to delineate the precise nature of the XP repair defects.

One clue to the nature of such defects is that X-ray-induced DNA damage consisting of single-strand breaks is repaired normally in cells from the four forms of XP tested (Cleaver, 1969; Kleijer, De Weerd-Kastelein, Sluyter, Keijzer, DeWit, and Bootsma, 1973 (Table 1, Column VI). The defects in these cells must be in gene products, which, although required for the repair of DNA damage caused by UV or certain chemicals, are not required for the repair of X-ray damage. Thus, early steps in the DNA excision repair scheme, including the recognition of damaged segments and the incision of intact strands near such damage, are suspected sites for at least some of the defects among the excision-deficient XP groups.

The finding that post-replication repair is markedly defective in the XP variants and is defective to a lesser degree in most of the excision-deficient XP groups allows us to propose that defects in DNA repair may indeed be causally related to the clinical signs, including skin cancer, of all known genetic forms of XP. Such a relationship could be explained by either of at least two simple models, both of which invoke the somatic mutation theory of carcinogenesis. The first proposes that there are certain gene products common to both the excision repair and post-replication repair systems and other products unique to one system or the other. Excision-deficient strains that also exhibit partially deficient post-replication repair would have defects in gene products common to both systems, the group E strains would have a defect in a gene product unique to the excision repair system, whereas the variants would have a defect in a gene product, or products, unique to the post-replication repair system. Mutations occurring as a result of inadequate repair by either repair system would be responsible for the clinical abnormalities of XP. In the other model (Lehmann, 1974), it is proposed that post-replication repair is an error-prone repair system even in normal cells and that either a defect that enhances the error-making potential of the system itself (as would be the case for the XP variants) or a defect that significantly increases the number of lesions presented to the system (as would be the case for excision-deficient cells) would result in more errors, and therefore more mutations, than in normal cells.

REFERENCES

Andrews, A. D., Robbins, J. H., Kraemer, K. H., and Buell, D. N. (1974): Xeroderma pigmentosum long-term lymphoid lines with increased ultraviolet sensitivity. *J. Natl. Cancer Inst.,* 53:691–693.

Bootsma, D., DeWeerd-Kastelein, E. A., Kleijer, W. J., and Keijzer, W. (1975): Complementation analysis of xeroderma pigmentosum. In: *Molecular Mechanisms for the Repair of DNA,* edited by P. C. Hanawalt and R. B. Setlow, Plenum Press, New York.

Burk, P. G., Lutzner, M. A., Clarke, D. D., and Robbins, J. H. (1971): Ultraviolet-stimulated thymidine incorporation in xeroderma pigmentosum lymphocytes. *J. Lab. Clin. Med.,* 77:759–767.

Burk, P. G., Yuspa, S. H., Lutzner, M. A., and Robbins, J. H. (1971): Xeroderma pigmentosum and DNA repair. *Lancet,* 1:601.

Cleaver, J. E. (1968): Defective repair replication of DNA in xeroderma pigmentosum. *Nature,* 218:652–656.

Cleaver, J. E. (1969): Xeroderma pigmentosum: A human disease in which an initial stage of DNA repair is defective. *Proc. Natl. Acad. Sci. USA,* 63:428–435.

Cleaver, J. E. (1972): Xeroderma pigmentosum: Variants with normal DNA repair and normal sensitivity to ultraviolet light. *J. Invest. Dermatol.,* 58:124–128.

Cook, J. S. (1972): Photoenzymatic repair in animal cells. In: *Molecular and Cellular Repair Process; Fifth International Symposium on Molecular Biology,* edited by R. F. Beer, R. M. Herriott, and R. C. Tilghman, pp. 79–94. The Johns Hopkins University Press, Baltimore.

Day, III, R. S. (1974): Studies on repair of adenovirus 2 by human fibroblasts using normal, xeroderma pigmentosum, and xeroderma pigmentosum heterozygous strains. *Cancer Res.,* 34:1965–1970.

Day, III, R. S. (1975): Xeroderma pigmentosum variants have decreased repair of ultraviolet-damaged DNA. *Nature,* 253:748–749.

Day, III, R. S., Kraemer, K. H., and Robbins, J. H. (1975): Complementing xeroderma pigmentosum fibroblasts restore biological activity to UV-damaged DNA. *Mutat. Res.,* 28:251–255.

De Sanctis, C., and Cacchione, A. (1932): L'Idiozia xerodermica. *Riv. Sper. Freniatr.,* 56:269–292.

DeWeerd-Kastelein, E. A., Keijzer, W., and Bootsma, D. (1972): Genetic heterogeneity of xeroderma pigmentosum demonstrated by somatic cell hybridization. *Nature,* 238:80–83.

DeWeerd-Kastelein, E. A., Keijzer, W., and Bootsma, D. (1974): A third complementation group in xeroderma pigmentosum. *Mutat. Res.,* 22:87–91.

DeWeerd-Kastelein, E. A., Kleijer, W. J., Sluyter, M. L., and Keijzer, W. (1973): Repair replication in heterokaryons derived from different repair-deficient xeroderma pigmentosum strains. *Mutat. Res.,* 19:237–243.

Howard-Flanders, P. (1973): DNA repair and recombination. *Br. Med. Bull.,* 29:226–235.

Kleijer, W. J., DeWeerd-Kastelein, E. A., Sluyter, M. L., Keijzer, W., DeWit, J., and Bootsma, D. (1973): UV-induced DNA repair synthesis in cells of patients with different forms of xeroderma pigmentosum and of heterozygotes. *Mutat. Res.,* 20:417–428.

Kraemer, K. H., Barrett, S. F., and Robbins, J. H. (1974): Differences in colony forming ability of ultraviolet-irradiated xeroderma pigmentosum fibroblasts. *Clinical Res., 22*:690A.

Kraemer, K. H., Coon, H. G., Petinga, R. A., Rahe, A. E., and Robbins, J. H. (1975): Genetic heterogeneity in xeroderma pigmentosum: Complementation groups and their relationship to DNA repair rates. *Proc. Natl. Acad. Sci. USA, 72*:59–63.

Kraemer, K. H., Coon, H. G., and Robbins, J. H. (1973): Cell-fusion analysis of different inherited mutations causing defective DNA repair in xeroderma pigmentosum fibroblasts. *J. Cell Biol., 59*:176a.

Kraemer, K. H., DeWeerd-Kastelein, E. A., Robbins, J. H., Petinga, R. A., Barrett, S. F., and Bootsma, D. (1975): Five complementation groups in xeroderma pigmentosum. *Mutat. Res. (In press.)*

Lehmann, A. R. (1974): Postreplication repair of DNA in mammalian cells. *Life Sci., 15*:2005–2016.

Lehmann, A. R., Kirk-Bell, S., Arlett, C. F., Patterson, M. C., Lohman, P. H. M., DeWeerd-Kastelein, E. A., and Bootsma, D. (1975): Xeroderma pigmentosum cells with normal levels of excision repair have a defect in DNA synthesis after UV-irradiation. *Proc. Natl. Acad. Sci. USA, 72*:219–223.

Maher, V. M., Birch, N., Otto, J. R., and McCormick, J. J. (1975): Cytotoxicity of carcinogenic aromatic amides in normal and xeroderma pigmentosum fibroblasts with different DNA repair capabilities. *J. Natl. Cancer Inst., 54*:1287–1294.

Patterson, M. C., Lohman, P. H. M., and Sluyter, M. L. (1973): Use of a UV-endonuclease from *Micrococcus luteus* to monitor the progress of DNA repair in UV-irradiated human cells. *Mutat. Res., 19*:245–256.

Patterson, M. C., Lohman, P. H. M., Westerveld, A., and Sluyter, M. L. (1974): DNA repair monitored by an enzymatic assay in multinucleate xeroderma pigmentosum cells after fusion. *Nature, 248*:50–52.

Regan, J. D., Setlow, R. B., and Ley, R. D. (1971): Normal and defective repair of damaged DNA in human cells: A sensitive assay utilizing the photolysis of bromodeoxyuridine. *Proc. Natl. Acad. Sci. USA, 68*:709–712.

Robbins, J. H., and Burk, P. G. (1973): Relationship of DNA repair to carcinogenesis in xeroderma pigmentosum. *Cancer Res., 33*:929–935.

Robbins, J. H., and Kraemer, K. H. (1972a): Abnormal rate and duration of ultaviolet-induced thymidine incorporation into lymphocytes from patients with xeroderma pigmentosum and associated neurological complications. *Mutat. Res., 15*:92–97.

Robbins, J. H., and Kraemer, K. H. (1972b): Prolonged ultraviolet-induced thymidine incorporation into xeroderma pigmentosum lymphocytes: Studies on its duration, amount, localization and relationship to hydroxurea. *Biochim. Biophys. Acta, 277*:7–14.

Robbins, J. H., Kraemer, K. H., and Flaxman, B. A. (1975): DNA repair in tumor cells from the variant form of xeroderma pigmentosum. *J. Invest. Dermatol., 64*:150–155.

Robbins, J. H., Kraemer, K. H., Lutzner, M. L., Festoff, B. W., and Coon, H. G. (1974): Xeroderma pigmentosum: An inherited disease with sun sensitivity, multiple cutaneous neoplasms, and abnormal DNA repair. *Ann. Intern. Med., 80*:221–248.

Robbins, J. H., Levis, W. R., and Miller, A. E. (1972): Xeroderma pigmentosum epidermal cells with normal UV-induced thymidine incorporation. *J. Invest. Dermatol., 59*:402–408.

Sutherland, B. M., Rice, M., and Wagner, E. K. (1975): Xeroderma pigmentosum cells contain low levels of photoreactivating enzyme. *Proc. Natl. Acad. Sci. USA, 72*:103–107.

Biology of Radiation Carcinogenesis, edited by
J. M. Yuhas, R. W. Tennant, and J. D. Regan.
Raven Press, New York © 1976.

Effect of DNA Repair on the Cytotoxicity and Mutagenicity of UV Irradiation and of Chemical Carcinogens in Normal and Xeroderma Pigmentosum Cells

Veronica M. Maher and J. Justin McCormick

Biology Department, Michigan Cancer Foundation, Detroit, Michigan 48201

Cellular repair enzymes are known to be able to modulate damage caused by lesions induced in DNA of cells by physical and chemical agents. For example, bacterial cells deficient in the ability to carry out excision repair of pyrimidine dimers exhibit greatly increased susceptibility to the cytotoxic and mutagenic effect of UV-irradiation (Witkin, 1969). Using an *in vitro* bacterial transforming DNA system, we have presented evidence that such bacterial DNA repair capabilities operate not only on UV damage, but also on lesions in DNA caused by covalent attachment of such carcinogenic chemicals as aromatic amide derivatives (Maher et al., 1968; Maher et al., 1970; Maher and Reuter, 1973), or polycyclic hydrocarbons (Maher et al., 1971, 1974) to alter the potential loss of transforming activity and the frequency of the mutations induced.

Evidence that human cells possess similar, genetically determined repair capabilities comes from recent studies on cells of xeroderma pigmentosum (XP) patients. Cells from most XP patients are abnormally sensitive to UV-irradiation and are deficient in excision repair of UV-induced thymine dimers (Cleaver, 1969; for reviews, see Robbins, 1974; Cleaver, 1974). It is now known that after exposure to low doses of UV, normal human cells excise up to 80% of the pyrimidine dimers introduced into their DNA by UV within 24 hr, but that cells from XP patients fail to do so (Robbins, 1974; Cleaver, 1974; Lehmann et al., 1975). The excision repair process involves the introduction of a single-strand break; the removal of a large number of nucleotides, including dimer; the introduction of new nucleotides, using the intact opposite strand as a template; and finally, rejoining of the repaired strand. In bacteria, it has been shown that this excision repair process is essentially "error-free" and that mutations arise as a result of unexcised damage (Witkin, 1969). The present studies with cultured skin fibroblasts were undertaken to determine whether cells from XP patients exhibit an increased sensitivity to the cytotoxic and mutagenic effects of exposure to UV-irradiation or to chemical carcinogens that bind covalently to DNA (Maher et al., 1968, 1974), distort the symmetry of the helix (Maher,

1968), and are repaired in a manner similar to UV induced lesions (Setlow and Regan, 1972; Stich et al., 1972; Stich and San, 1973; Regan and Setlow, 1974). We also wished to determine if such an increased cytotoxicity and mutagenicity in XP strains would correspond to a decreased capacity for DNA repair. For this reason, three strains of XP cells, two deficient in excision repair (Robbins, 1974) and another deficient in post-replication repair (Lehmann et al., 1975), were compared with normal skin fibroblasts, for survival (cloning capacity) and frequency of UV-induced mutations to azaguanine resistance after exposure to such agents.

MATERIALS AND METHODS

Carcinogenic Compounds

The aromatic amide carcinogens were prepared or obtained as described (Maher and Wessel, 1975). The hydrocarbon "K-region" epoxides were prepared and provided by Dr. Peter Sims and Dr. Philip Grover of the Chester Beatty Research Institute, London, England. The 7-bromomethyl derivative was provided by Dr. Peter Brookes of the Chester Beatty Research Institute.

CELL CULTURES

Strains of normally repairing human fibroblasts derived from foreskins were initiated, cultured, and stored until use as described (Maher and Wessel, 1975; Maher et al., 1975b). Fibroblasts derived from skin biopsies of XP patients, a Lesch-Nyhan patient and a 15-year-old normal male, obtained from American Type Culture Collection, were similarly cultured. All cells used were from stocks in the 6th to the 18th passage.

MEDIUM

Media used for culturing and cloning the cells and for selecting and culturing mutant cells resistant to 8-azaguanine (2×10^{-5} M) have been described previously (Maher and Wessel, 1975). Serum currently in use is from GIBCO. Gentamycin (Schering Corp. Pt. Reading, N.J.) at 50 μg/ml replaces penicillin and streptomycin for culturing stock cultures.

CYTOTOXICITY ASSAY (SURVIVAL OF CLONING ABILITY)

The cytotoxic effect of exposure to UV or the carcinogens was determined as described previously (Maher and Wessel, 1975; Maher et al., 1975b, 1976a) (see diagram, Fig. 1A). Upon incubation for 10 hr for cell attachment, the culture medium was removed by aspiration. For irradiation, cells

A. CYTOXICITY

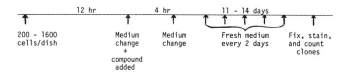

B. MUTAGENESIS

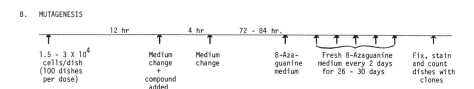

FIG. 1. Human fibroblasts. Protocols for the determination of (A) cytotoxicity and (B) induction of 8-aza-guanine-resistant mutants by N-AcO-AAF. (From Maher and Wessel, 1975.)

were rinsed in 0.9% saline and exposed to the specified doses of UV as described (Maher et al., 1975b, 1976); culture medium was then replaced. For carcinogen treatment, serum-free medium was added to the cells, and the carcinogen was introduced at the specified final concentrations from freshly prepared solutions as described (Maher and Wessel, 1975; Maher et al., 1975b). Aromatic amide compounds were dissolved in 95% ethanol, the hydrocarbons in anhydrous acetone. All operations were carried out in almost total darkness because the chemical carcinogens are light-sensitive. Cells were protected from photoreactivation from the time of exposure to the mutagenizing agent until they had undergone several cell divisions. Exposure of the cells to carcinogens was terminated by replacing the medium with fresh culture medium containing 15% fetal calf serum. This medium should inactivate any remaining electrophylic reactants (carcinogens), as proteins are strong nucleophiles. Clones were allowed to develop, and the cytotoxicity was determined as described (Maher and Wessel, 1975; Maher et al., 1975b.)

INDUCTION OF MUTATIONS

The generalized protocol for the mutagenicity assay is diagrammed in Fig. 1B. After incubation for 10 hr for cell attachment, the medium was removed, and the cells were exposed to UV-irradiation or to carcinogen as described above. The treated cells were allowed sufficient time to permit approximately three cell divisions to occur in order to overcome phenotypic lag of cellular expression of azaguanine resistance and allow for the fixing of the mutation before selection was begun. This critical period of time, which varied with the cell strain and dose administered, was determined as described previously (Maher and Wessel, 1975). A control population of 1.0 to 1.5 × 10⁶ cells in 100 dishes was included with every experiment to correct for background mutation frequency.

RECONSTRUCTION EXPERIMENTS TO DETERMINE THE EFFICIENCY OF RECOVERY OF MUTANTS

Since overcrowding of cells in the dishes results in an apparent reduction in mutation frequency caused by metabolic cooperation (Maher and Wessel, 1975; Subak-Sharpe et al., 1969), in every experiment a known number of azaguanine-resistant Lesch-Nyhan cells were seeded into a series of the control and experimental dishes to provide an estimate of the efficiency of recovery of mutants under the particular conditions employed.

DETERMINING THE FREQUENCY OF INDUCED MUTATIONS

The method used to quantitate the frequency of mutations has been described previously (Maher and Wessel, 1975; Albertini and DeMars, 1973). In summary, this consists of determining the probability of a mutational event occurring per experimental culture dish from the number of culture dishes containing no clones: $P(0) = \exp(-x)$, where x is probability of a mutant event per dish. For each experiment this value is corrected first, for the efficiency of recovery of mutants, and second, for the small contribution of the background frequency, and then calculated per 10^5 survivors.

MEASURING REPAIR REPLICATION IN PARENTAL STRANDS USING ALKALINE CsCl GRADIENT CENTRIFUGATION OF LABELED DNA

The procedures used for detecting excision repair in cells following exposure to UV or carcinogens by measuring the incorporation of tritiated thymidine into parental DNA in the absence of normal DNA synthesis has been described (Maher et al., 1975b).

MEASURING POST-REPLICATION REPAIR BY DETERMINING RATE OF INCREASE IN SIZE OF NEWLY REPLICATED DNA USING ALKALINE SUCROSE GRADIENTS

The procedures for measuring ability of cells to increase the size of newly replicated DNA synthesized from damaged templates using radioactive pulse-chase experiments have been described (Lehmann et al., 1975). Cells ($\sim 2.5 \times 10^5$) are lysed for 2 hr at 25°C in a solution containing 0.02 M EDTA, 2% sodium dodecylsulfate, and 0.95 M NaOH on top of a 5 to 20% alkaline sucrose gradient. This gives reproducible gradients without the need to break the DNA by X-irradiation. The rest of the procedure is as described (Lehmann et al., 1975).

RESULTS AND DISCUSSION

Survival of the Cloning Ability of the Cell Strains as a Function of Dose of Irradiation or Carcinogen

As can be seen in Fig. 2, the cloning ability of the XP2BE strain, from complementation group C, is more sensitive to UV-irradiation than that of normal cells. We compared the survival of the cloning ability of these two strains following exposure to four series of carcinogenic aromatic amide

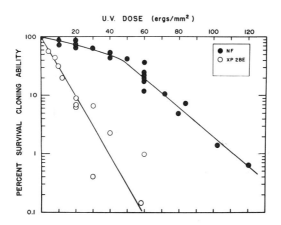

FIG. 2. Percent survival of the cloning ability, as a function of UV irradiation, of normal human fibroblasts and of the XP2BE strain from complementation group C.

derivatives: 4-acetylaminobiphenyl (AABP), 2-acetylaminofluorene (AAF), 2-acetylaminophenanthrene (AAP), and 4-acetylaminostilbene (AAS). Figure 3 compares the percent survival of the cloning capacity of these four series of related compounds as a function of dose. The N-hydroxy derivatives and the N-acetoxy and N-sulfate ester derivatives caused significant loss of the ability of the cells to form clones, whereas the parent compounds, which are known to require a two-step metabolic activation into the N-hydroxy and ester forms (Maher et al., 1970; Maher and Reuter, 1973; Miller and Miller, 1969) did not prove cytotoxic even at doses two to ten times higher. The strongest cytotoxicity was exhibited by the stilbene derivations (Fig. 3D). The XP2BE cells consistently exhibited a two- to threefold greater sensitivity to the various active derivatives of each series than did the cells taken from normal individuals.

The survival of the cloning ability of these two strains was then com-

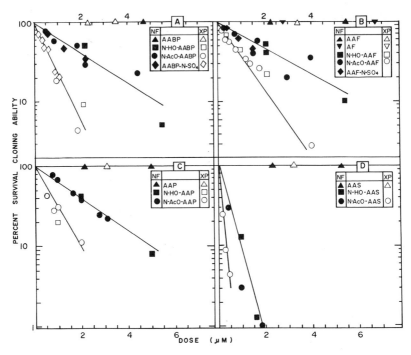

FIG. 3. Comparison of the cytoxicity (loss of cloning ability) produced in normal human fibroblasts and XP2BE cells by exposure (4 hr) to the indicated concentrations of aromatic amides: (A) AABP, (B) AAF (C) AAP, (D) AAS, and their respective N-hydroxy and N-acetoxy ester derivatives. The N-sulfate ester of N-HO-AAF and N-HO-AABP are included in their series, as is the amine, 2-aminofluorene (AF). (From Maher et al., 1975b.)

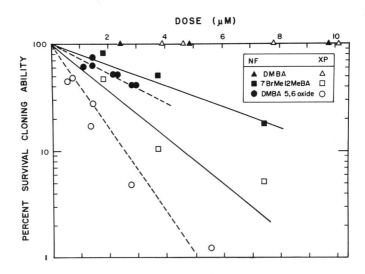

FIG. 4. Comparison of the cytoxicity (loss of cloning ability) in normal and XP2BE cells following exposure (3 hr) to the indicated concentrations of DMBA, its K-region epoxide, and its 7-bromomethyl derivative.

pared after exposure to a series of active derivatives of the hydrocarbon, 7,12-dimethylbenz(a)anthracene (DMBA). As can be seen in Fig. 4, the cloning ability of the XP2BE strain consistently exhibited a two- to three-fold greater sensitivity to the various active derivatives than did that of the normal cells.

To determine if this difference in cell survival reflected capacity for DNA repair, the cytotoxic effect of active derivatives of such chemical carcinogens on the survival of a series of XP strains was determined. The XP strains selected were chosen on the basis of the different ability of the cultured

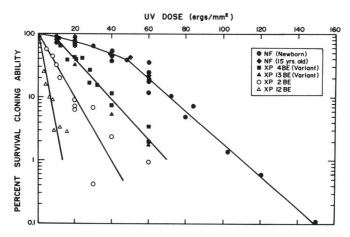

FIG. 5. Percent survival of the cloning ability, as a function of UV-irradiation, of strains of human skin fibroblasts with different DNA repair capabilities. Cloning efficiencies ranged from 15 to 35% for the normal cells, 10 to 20% for the XP2BE; XP13BE and XP4BE cells, and 5 to 15% for XP12BE. The exponential portion of these survival curves were drawn using the least-squares method. Each symbol represents the survival of the cloning efficiency averaged from a series of 8 to 12 replicate dishes and the data are drawn from a large number of experiments. (From Maher et al., 1975b.)

lymphocytes and fibroblasts obtained from various XP patients to incorporate thymidine in repair of DNA following UV-irradiation (Robbins, 1974). Thus, XP12BE from genetic complementation group A is reported to incorporate less than 2% of the amount of thymidine normal cells incorporate during the first 3 hr after exposure to UV-irradiation (Robbins, 1974); XP2BE, from Group C, to incorporate 15 to 25% of normal (Burk et al., 1971), and XP4BE 100% of normal (Cleaver, 1972). The latter XP patient, whose excision repair rate appears normal, has been designated an XP variant (Cleaver, 1972). It has recently been shown to be defective in postreplication repair (Lehmann et al., 1975; Maher et al., 1975a) and in host cell reactivation of UV-damaged virus (Day, 1974, 1975).

Figure 5 compares, as a function of UV irradiation, the survival of four XP strains with that of normal cells. (A second XP variant, XP13BE, is

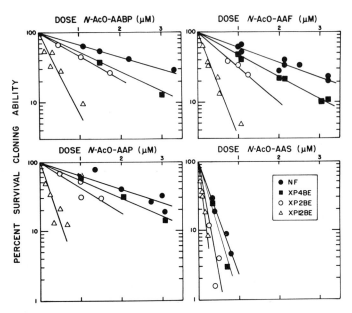

FIG. 6. Percent survival of the cloning ability of the four strains as a function of the dose of the N-acetoxy ester derivative of the carcinogenic aromatic amide administered. Each symbol represents the survival of the cloning ability averaged from a series of 8 to 10 replicate dishes. The lines are drawn using the least-squares method. (From Maher et al., 1975b.)

included for comparison. Cells from a biopsy of a 15-year-old normal male are included with the normal cells prepared from newborns to determine if a difference in survival could be caused by age of the donor.) The normal cells exhibit a shoulder on the UV survival curve, which suggests DNA repair. A smaller shoulder is seen for the XP variant cells and the exponential portion of their survival curve has a slope approximately 1.3-fold steeper than that of normal cells. The slope of the XP2BE cells is 1.9-fold steeper than that of normal, but because it lacks a shoulder it requires only 8 erg/mm² to reduce the survival level to 37% of the untreated control, compared with approximately 48 erg/mm² for normal. Strain XP12BE is still more sensitive to the killing effect of UV. The slope of its survival curve is 5.8 times steeper than that of the linear portion of the curve for normal cells. A dose of only approximately 3 erg/mm² lowers the survival to 37% of the control.

The survival of the three XP strains, compared to that of normal, was then determined as a function of the concentration of N-acetoxy ester derivatives of four aromatic amide carcinogens (Fig. 6) or of K region epoxide derivatives of three carcinogenic hydrocarbons (Fig. 7). No shoulder was detected in these survival curves. For each carcinogen derivative, the ratio between the slope of the curve for the particular XP strain and that measured for the normal fibroblasts was similar and approximately equal to the

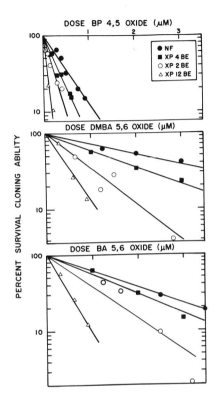

FIG. 7. Percent survival of the cloning ability of the four strains as a function of the dose of K-region epoxide derivative of the carcinogenic hydrocarbon administered.

ratio of the slopes for the exponential portion of the corresponding UV survival curves. Thus, for the aromatic amides, the curve for the XP4BE variant was 1.2- to 1.7-fold steeper than that of the normal cells; for XP2BE, 1.8- to 2.3-fold steeper, and for XP12BE, 3.1- to 8.9-fold steeper than that of normal cells (Maher et al., 1975*b*). For the hydrocarbons, the curve for the variant was 1.25- to 1.5-fold steeper; that for XP2BE, 2.1- to 3.1-fold steeper; and for XP12BE, 5.0- to 6.0-fold steeper than that of normal cells (Maher et al., 1976*b*).

PHYSICOCHEMICAL EVIDENCE OF DNA REPAIR

The ability of these strains to carry out excision repair of DNA following exposure to N-AcO-AAF was determined using incorporation of tritiated thymidine into preexisting parental strands of DNA as a measure of excision repair (Cleaver, 1973; Maher et al., 1975*b*). Figure 8 compares the incorporation of [3H]-labeled TdR into the [14C]-labeled (light density) parental strand of the DNA of untreated control cells (1st and 3rd rows, A–F) and of cells exposed to 50 μm N-AcO-AAF for 1 hr (2nd and 4th rows). As can be seen, a substantial amount of incorporation of [3H]-TdR into unreplicated

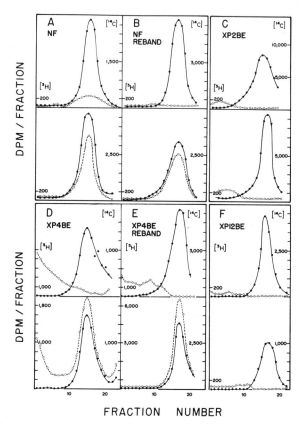

FRACTION   NUMBER

FIG. 8. Physicochemical evidence of DNA excision repair by human fibroblasts following exposure to N-AcO-AAF. The DNA of the cells was prelabeled with ^{14}CTdR (*filled circles*) for 20 hr. Fresh, serum-free medium supplemented with BrdUrd (10 μg/ml) was given for 1 hr to density-label any replicating DNA molecules. Cells were then exposed to 0.4% ethanol (control cells, 1st and 3rd rows) or 0.4% ethanol containing 50 μM N-AcO-AAF (2nd and 4th rows) for 1 hr in serum-free medium with hydroxyurea present during the last 20 min to stop normal DNA replication. The cells were given fresh medium containing 15% fetal calf serum hydroxyurea and BrdUrd and allowed 3 hr to incorporate ^{3}HTdR (*open circles*). The DNA of the cells was extracted and centrifuged to equilibrium in alkaline CsCl gradients: (A) normal cells, (B) reband of the major peak in (A), (C) XP2BE cells, (D) XP4BE, (E) reband of the major peak in (D), (F) XP12BE. The ^{14}C-label locates the unreplicated light parental DNA strands at density 1.700 g/cm^2. Centrifugation is from the right to left. (From Maher et al., 1975b.)

(light) parental strands took place when normal (A) and XP4BE cells (D) were allowed to incubate in the presence of BrdUrd, HU, and ^{3}HTdR for several hours following attack by N-acetoxy 2-acetylaminofluorene (N-ACO-AAF). This incorporation persisted even after rebanding in a second gradient (B) and (E). Such incorporation represents DNA repair, since any DNA replication that took place in spite of the HU block would be density-labeled by the BrdUrd in the medium. In contrast, the XP12BE and XP2BE cells did not exhibit detectable levels of incorporation during the incubation period although, given sufficient time, cells from XP2BE might have been expected to carry out some DNA repair (Robbins, 1974). The fact that no incorporation was detected in this strain may reflect the insensitivity of the scintillation counter in detecting low levels of ^{3}H in the presence of high levels of ^{14}C or that, given the high concentration of administered carcinogen, repair was not taking place in the time during which repair was being measured.

We undertook to determine, as reported by Lehmann (1975) for two other XP variants, if XP4BE and XP13BE exhibit abnormally slow rates of converting initially low-molecular weight DNA synthesized in UV-irradiated cells into high-molecular weight DNA similar in size to that found in untreated cells. Figure 9 shows that this is indeed the case for XP4BE. We found the same profile with XP13BE (data not shown); Buhl et al. (1972) reported that the former strain forms normal size DNA after 8 hr. Recently Lehmann et al. (1975) reported a similar profile for XP4BE and showed that this process of lengthening the size of newly synthesized DNA in XP variants is extremely sensitive to caffeine. This process of lengthening the

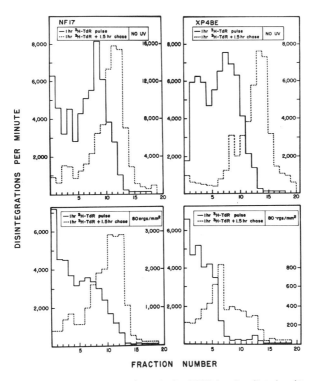

FIG. 9. Alkaline sucrose gradient profiles of newly synthesized DNA in unirradiated and irradiated normal cells and variant XP4BE cells. Unirradiated cells (*upper frames*) and UV-irradiated cells (*bottom frames*) were pulse-labeled for 60 min with [^{3}H]dT (100 μC/ml) 1 hr after exposure to 80 erg/mm^2 (*solid curve*). Cells were harvested, lysed, and centrifuged on alkaline sucrose gradients immediately following the pulse, or after a 3.5-hr chase in unlabeled medium (*dotted curve*).

DNA is attributed to filling, by means of *de novo* DNA synthesis (Lehmann et al., 1975; Buhl et al., 1972; Rupp and Howard-Flanders, 1968), gaps caused by replication past unexcised dimers (Rupp and Howard-Flanders, 1968).

COMPARING THE FREQUENCY OF MUTATIONS INDUCED BY UV OR BY CARCINOGENS IN NORMAL AND XP STRAINS

As can be seen from Fig. 10, exposure of the two excision-defective XP strains and the normal strain to low doses of UV-irradiation results in a dose-dependent increase in the frequency of induced mutations to 8-azaguanine resistance. The XP2BE strain (excision rate, 15 to 25% of normal) shows an approximately fivefold greater mutagenic response to irradiation than do the normal cells. The XP12BE strain (excision rate $\sim 2\%$) shows approximately a 16-fold greater mutagenic response to UV than do the normal cells. The dose of UV, in erg/mm^2, which results in a mutation frequency of ten azaguanine resistant colonies per 10^5 survivors is ~ 3 for XP12BE, ~ 8 for XP2BE, and ~ 48 for normal cells. From the data in Fig. 5, it will be seen that these doses cause similar survival levels in the three strains (viz., 37%). When the increase in mutation frequency per survivor induced by UV in these strains with different rates of excision repair is analyzed as a function of the lethal effect of UV, as shown in Fig. 11, it is apparent that the muta-

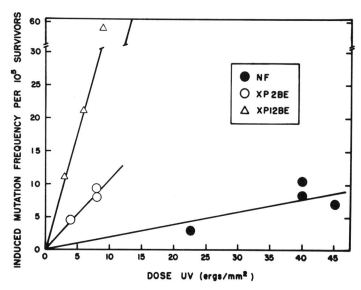

FIG. 10. Mutagenic effect of UV-irradiation in three strains of human fibroblasts as a function of the dose of UV administered. Lines are calculated by the method of least squares. (From Maher et al., 1976a.) See Maher and Wessel (1975) and Maher et al. (1976a) for details on the method of quantitating induced mutation frequency.

genicity of the UV is directly related to its cytotoxicity and both effects are directly related to the capacity for excision repair of UV-induced lesions.

The cytotoxicity and mutagenicity results of this comparative study (Figs. 5,10,11) provide strong evidence for error-free excision repair of UV damage in human cells (Maher et al., 1976a). If excision repair were introducing errors (mutations), the normal strain, which received the highest UV dose and which has repeatedly been demonstrated to carry on more extensive excision repair than the two XP strains (Cleaver et al., 1969, 1974; Robbins, 1975), would be expected to exhibit a higher frequency of in-

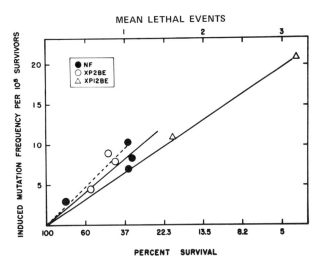

FIG. 11. Mutagenic effect of UV-irradiation in three strains of human fibroblasts as a function of the percent survival of the cells following irradiation. By the Poisson distribution function, if 37% of the population survives, the average number of lethal events per cell (hits) is one. A survival of 13.5% corresponds to two mean lethal events; 5% survival, three mean lethal hits, etc. The data are drawn from that shown in Figs. 5 and 10. (From Maher et al., 1976a.)

duced mutations per survival level. Figure 11 clearly shows that this is not the case.

A hypothesis that would explain our data, and which is consistent with what is known about UV repair and mutagenesis in mammalian cells (Cleaver, 1974; Trosko and Chu, 1975), is that the three strains, although receiving very different UV doses, nevertheless, because of their different rates of DNA excision repair, contain, on the average, the same number of unrepaired lesions at the time of some critical event. It is these *unrepaired lesions* present in the DNA at this critical time that are directly or indirectly responsible for both the mutagenic and lethal effect of the irradiation. We postulate that the critical cellular event is DNA replication, because the unexcised dimers present at the time of DNA synthesis could lead to errors in the newly replicated DNA.

It is known that bacterial cells can survive the presence of at least some unexcised dimers (Witkin, 1969). Evidence suggests that in such cells, replication past the dimer occurs, resulting in "gaps," which are by-passed by means of recombinational repair (Rupp and Howard-Flanders, 1968). In mammalian cells, evidence (Buhl et al., 1972*a,b*; Lehmann 1972, Lehmann et al., 1975) suggests that similar gaps, formed by replication past unexcised dimers, are subsequently filled in by *de novo* DNA synthesis (gap-filling) from a faulty template that still contains the dimer. This process could result in the introduction of error. If one assumes that such a post-replication repair process varies only in the amount of time required by these three strains, the fact that even the classic XP cells take somewhat longer than normal cells to complete the rejoining process (Lehmann, 1975) need not increase the cytotoxic or mutagenic effect of the presence of gaps resulting from unexcised dimers as long as this process is completed before a second round of DNA synthesis begins. We have found that the cell doubling time of these two classic XP strains is approximately one and one-half times longer than that of our normal fibroblasts, which is consistent with this hypothesis.

An extensive study of mutation frequencies induced in normal cells and in XP2BE cells by K region epoxides of hydrocarbons give us additional evidence that the process (excision repair) that results in a higher survival in normal cells than XP2BE cells after exposure to such reactive compounds is also error-free (Maher et al., 1976*b*). (see Fig. 12.)

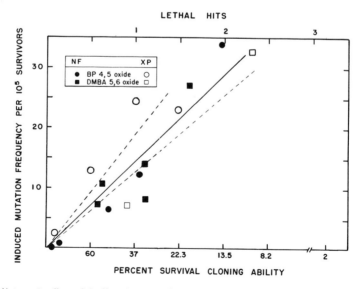

FIG. 12. Mutagenic effect of the K-region epoxides of two carcinogenic hydrocarbons in normal and XP strains of human fibroblasts as a function of the percent survival of the cells following exposure. By the Poisson distribution function, if 37% of the population survives, the average number of lethal events per cell (hits) is one. (Data from Maher er al., 1976*b*.)

Studies of the frequency of mutations induced in XP variants by UV or other such carcinogens are of obvious importance for understanding the mechanisms of mutations. We are currently carrying out such studies.

SUMMARY

The cytotoxic and mutagenic action of ultraviolet (UV) irradiation and of aromatic amides or polycyclic hydrocarbons was quantitatively compared in normally repairing strains of human cells and in several excision-repair deficient or post-replication repair–deficient xeroderma pigmentosum (XP) strains.

The survival of the cloning capacity of the various excision-defective XP strains following exposure to UV or the carcinogens reflected the excision capacity of the particular strain tested. Cells from XP variants showed lower survival than normal cells after exposure to these agents. In addition, they exhibited a markedly reduced capacity for post-replication repair (gap-filling) of UV lesions.

An excision-defective XP strain from complementation group A and group C were compared with normal cells for the frequency of mutations induced by various doses of UV. The XP strains showed an increased frequency of mutations, which correlated with their sensitivity to UV and their capacity for excision repair of UV-induced lesions. The induced mutation frequency of the two XP strains and the normal strain, examined as a function of the percent survival (cytotoxicity) of the particular strain, are equal. This is evidence of an error-free excision repair process in human cells.

The frequency of mutations induced in normal cells and in the group C XP strain by active aromatic carcinogens were compared. For each compound, the XP strain exhibited a significantly higher mutation frequency than that of the normal. These mutation frequencies, examined as a function of percent survival of the strains, are equal.

ACKNOWLEDGMENTS

We thank Nancy Birch, Marilyn Mittlestat, James Otto, Thomas Schnur, and Susan Van Hoeck for excellent technical assistance. This work was supported by USPH NIH Grants CA 13058 and CA 14680 and Research Contract NOI-CP-33226 and by an Institutional Grant to the Michigan Cancer Foundation by the United Foundation of Greater Detroit.

REFERENCES

Albertini, R. J., and DeMars, R. (1973): Somatic cell mutation detection and quantification of x-ray-induced mutation in cultured, diploid human fibroblasts. *Mutat. Res.*, 18:199–224.

Buhl, S. N., Stillmann, R. M., Setlow, R. B., and Regan, J. D. (1972a): DNA chain elongation and joining in normal and xeroderma pigmentosum cells after ultraviolet irradiation. *Biophys. J.,* 12:1183–1191.

Buhl, S. N., Stillmann, R. M., Setlow, R. B., and Regan, J. D. (1972*b*): Steps in DNA chain elongation and joining after ultraviolet irradiation of human cells. *Int. J. Radiat. Biol.,* 22:417–423.

Burk, P. G., Lutzner, M. A., Clarke, D. D., and Robbins, J. H. (1971): Ultraviolet-stimulated thymidine incorporation in xeroderma pigmentosum lymphocytes. *J. Lab. Clin. Med.,* 77:759–767.

Cleaver, J. E. (1969): Xeroderma pigmentosum: A human disease in which an initial stage of DNA repair is defective. *Proc. Natl. Acad. Sci. USA,* 63:428–435.

Cleaver, J. E. (1972): Xeroderma pigmentosum: Variants with normal DNA repair and normal sensitivity to ultraviolet light. *J. Invest. Dermatol.,* 58:124–128.

Cleaver, J. E. (1973): DNA repair with purines and pyrimidines in radiation- and carcinogen-damaged normal and xeroderma pigmentosum human cells. *Cancer Res.,* 33:362–369.

Cleaver, J. E. (1974): Repair processes for photochemical damage in mammalian cells. In: *Advances in Radiation Biology,* Vol. 4, edited by J. T. Lett, H. Adler, and M. Zelle, Academic Press, New York, 1974, pp. 1–75.

Day, R. (1974): Studies on repair of adenovirus 2 by human fibroblasts using normal, xeroderma pigmentosum, and xeroderma pigmentosum heterozygous strains. *Cancer Res.,* 34:1965–1970.

Day, R. (1975): Xeroderma pigmentosum variants have decreased repair of ultraviolet-damaged DNA. *Nature,* 253:748–749.

Lehmann, A. R. (1972): Postreplication repair of DNA in ultraviolet irradiated mammalian cells. *J. Mol. Biol.,* 66:319–337.

Lehmann, A. R. (1975): Postreplication repair of DNA in UV-irradiated mammalian cells. In: *Molecular Mechanisms for Repair of DNA.* Squaw Valley ICN-UCLA 1974 Symposium, pp. 617–623. Plenum Press, New York.

Lehmann, A. R., Kirk-Bell, S., Arlett, C. F., Paterson, M. C., Lohman, P. H. M., de Weerd-Kastelein, E. A., and Bootsma, D. (1975): Xeroderma pigmentosum cells with normal levels of excision repair have a defect in DNA synthesis after UV irradiation. *Proc. Natl. Acad. Sci. USA,* 72:219–223.

Maher, V. M., Birch, N., Mittlestat, M., Otto, J., Ouellette, L., Schnur, T., and McCormick, J. J. (1975*a*): Effect of excision and post-replication repair on the cytotoxicity and mutagenicity of UV in human skin fibroblasts. *Proc. Am. Ass. Cancer Res.,* 16:630.

Maher, V. M., Birch, N., Otto, J. R., and McCormick, J. J. (1975*b*): Cytotoxicity of carcinogenic aromatic amides in normal and xeroderma pigmentosum fibroblasts with different DNA repair capabilities. *J. Natl. Cancer Inst.,* Vol. 54.

Maher, V. M., Douville, D., Tomura, T., and Van Lancker, J. L. (1974): Mutagenicity of reactive derivatives of carcinogenic hydrocarbons: Evidence of repair. *Mutation Res.,* 23:113–128.

Maher, V. M., Lesko, S. A., Jr., Straat, P. A., and Ts'o, P. O. P. (1971): Mutagenic action, loss of transforming activity, and inhibition of deoxyribonucleic acid template activity *in vitro* caused by chemical linkage of carcinogenic polycyclic hydrocarbons to deoxyribonucleic acid. *J. Bacteriol.,* 108:202–212.

Maher, V. M., McCormick, J. J., Grover, P. L., and Sims, P. (1976*b*): (*Manuscript in preparation.*)

Maher, V. M., Miller, J. A., Miller, E. C., and Summers, W. C. (1970): Mutations and loss of transforming activity of *Bacillus subtilis* DNA after reaction with esters of carcinogenic *N*-hydroxy aromatic amides. *Cancer Res.,* 30:1473–1480.

Maher, V. M., Miller, E. C., Miller, J. A., and Szybalski, W. (1968): Mutations and decreases in density of transforming DNA produced by derivatives of the carcinogens 2-acetylaminofluorene and *N*-methyl-4-aminoazobenzene. *Mol. Pharmacol.,* 4:411–426.

Maher, V. M., Curren, R. D., and McCormick, J. J. (1976*a*): Effect of DNA repair on the frequency of mutations induced in normal human skin fibroblasts and in strains of xeroderma pigmentosum by ultraviolet irradiation. *Proc. Natl. Acad. USA* (Submitted for publication.)

Maher, V. M., and Reuter, M. (1973): Mutations and loss of transforming activity of DNA caused by the O-glucuronide conjugate of the carcinogen N-hydroxy-2-amino-fluorene. *Mutation Res.,* 21:63–71.

Maher, V. M., and Wessel, J. E. (1975): Mutations to azaguanine resistance induced in cultured diploid human fibroblasts by the carcinogen, N-acetoxy-2-acetylamino-fluorene. *Mutat. Res.,* 28:277–284.

Miller, J. A., and Miller, E. C. (1969): Metabolic activation of carcinogenic aromatic amines and amides via N-hydroxylation and N-hydroxy-esterification and its relation-ship to ultimate carcinogens as electrophilic reactants. In: *The Jerusalem Symposia on Quantum Chemistry and Biochemistry. Physicochemical Mechanisms of Carcino-gens,* edited by E. D. Bergmann and B. Pullman, Vol. I, pp. 237–261. Israel Aca. Sci. Human, Jerusalem.

Regan, J. D., and Setlow, R. B. (1974): Two forms of repair in the DNA of human cells damaged by chemical carcinogens and mutagens. *Cancer Res.,* 34:3318–3325.

Rupp, W. D., and Howard-Flanders, P. (1968): Discontinuities in an excision-defective strain of *Escherichia coli* following ultraviolet irradiation. *J. Mol. Biol.,* 31:291–304.

Setlow, R. B., and Regan, J. D. (1972): Defective repair of N-acetoxy-2-acetylamino-fluorene-induced lesions in the DNA of xeroderma pigmentosum cells. *Biochem. Biophys. Res. Commun.,* 46:1019–1024.

Stich, H. F., and San, R. H. C. (1973): DNA repair synthesis and survival of repair deficient human cells exposed to the K-region epoxide of benz(a)anthracene. *Proc. Soc. Exp. Biol. Med.,* 142:155–158.

Stich, H. F., San, R. H. C., Miller, J. A., and Miller, E. C. (1972): Various levels of DNA repair synthesis in xeroderma pigmentosum cells exposed to the carcinogens, N-hydroxy and N-acetoxy-2-acetylaminofluorene. *Nature* [New Biol.], 238:9–10.

Subak-Sharpe, H., Burk, R. R., and Pitts, J. D. (1969): Metabolic cooperation between biochemically marked mammalian cells in tissue culture. *J. Cell. Sci.,* 4:353–367.

Trosko, J. E., and Chu, E. H. Y. (1975): The role of DNA repair and somatic muta-tion in carcinogenesis. *Adv. Cancer Res.,* 21:391–425.

Witkin, E. M. (1969): Ultraviolet-light-induced mutation and DNA repair. *Ann. Rev. Microbiol.,* 23:487–510.

Robbins, J. H., et al. (1974): Xeroderma pigmentosum—an inherited disease with sun sensitivity multiple cutaneous neoplasms, and abnormal DNA repair. *Ann. Inter. Med.,* 80:221–248.

Biology of Radiation Carcinogenesis, edited by
J. M. Yuhas, R. W. Tennant, and J. D. Regan.
Raven Press, New York © 1976.

The Metabolic Activation of Chemical Carcinogens to Reactive Electrophiles

James A. Miller and Elizabeth C. Miller

*McArdle Laboratory for Cancer Research, University of Wisconsin Medical Center, Madison, Wisconsin
53706*

Ionizing radiations and ultraviolet light constitute the principal known *physical* carcinogens. Likewise, a great variety and large number of chemicals and over 50 DNA and RNA viruses comprise the known *chemical* and *viral* carcinogens. These three categories of carcinogenic agents include the great majority of extrinsic agents known to induce cancer in mammals. Man is clearly susceptible to the action of physical and chemical carcinogens and, indeed, was the first species in which the activities of some of these agents were demonstrated. It seems certain that viral carcinogenic information is involved in the etiology of at least some human tumors, but ethical and methodological problems have made it difficult to obtain unequivocal data. Given the long availability of experimental carcinogens of these three classes, there is surprisingly little known of their interrelationships in the production of cancer in experimental animals. The objective of this brief review is to present some salient aspects of experimental chemical carcinogenesis and an analysis of how some of these features relate to the mechanisms of action of radiation carcinogens.

THE GROSS NATURE OF CHEMICAL CARCINOGENS AND CARCINOGENESIS

At present the term "carcinogen" is unavoidably broad and includes all agents that cause malignant tumors to develop in mammalian and other hosts in incidences significantly greater than would occur spontaneously. Regardless of how these agents may differ in their mechanisms of action, they give rise to or select for cells with heritable and at least quasi-permanent defects in growth control. Natural selection among these altered cells and their progeny for those with proliferative advantages favors the progression and growth of these cells into gross neoplasms. These neoplastic processes can also occur in cell cultures under the influence of chemical carcinogens

* The work of the authors has been supported by funds from CA 07175 and CA 15785 of the National Cancer Institute, USPHS.

and radiation (Borek and Sachs, 1968; Borek and Hall, 1973; Heidelberger, 1973).

Chemical (and physical) carcinogens induce changes in cells that can then progress independently and give rise to gross tumors, which frequently appear long after administration of a required amount of the carcinogen has ceased. Clear dose-response relationships have been observed for many of these agents (Druckrey, 1967). The administration of larger doses of carcinogen in experimental animals leads to more tumor-bearers sooner and a higher total number of tumors, until the toxic effects of the carcinogen intervene. The latent period for gross tumor formation is generally an appreciable fraction of the life-span and in man and rodents usually consists of periods of many years and months, respectively.

Carcinogenesis is generally conceived to be a multi-step process, and at least two qualitatively different steps are recognized in the action of chemicals in several tissues. This was first noted many years ago in the initiation and promotion steps in chemical carcinogenesis in mouse skin (Berenblum and Shubik, 1947; Boutwell, 1974; Van Duuren et al., 1975). Initiation denotes an initial, largely irreversible change in certain cells, which predisposes them to be precursors of tumors. This can be achieved by single non-carcinogenic doses of carcinogenic hydrocarbons, for example. At present, the changed cells cannot be recognized microscopically or biochemically, and they become evident as gross tumors after a subsequent and reversible step of promotion is induced with specific proliferative agents, especially certain phorbol esters (Hecker and Schmidt, 1974). Recently, long-term administration of phenobarbital, which causes hypertrophy of the liver, has been found to markedly increase the incidence of hepatic tumors in rats previously fed initiating doses of 2-acetylaminofluorene (Peraino et al., 1973). Similarly, initiation and promotion steps in the chemical induction of mammary tumors in rats and liver and of lung tumors in mice have been described (Armuth and Berenblum, 1972, 1974). Chemical carcinogenesis in cell culture also appears divisible into these two steps (Mondal et al., 1975), and much progress can be expected from studies in such quantifiable systems of chemical carcinogenesis (Heidelberger, 1973).

THE VARIETY OF CHEMICAL CARCINOGENS

It is now a central fact in chemical carcinogenesis that chemical carcinogens are structurally very diverse and consist of numerous, non-viral, non-radioactive compounds capable of inducing tumors in a wide range of tissues and species. Most of these compounds have molecular weights of less than 500, and most of them are organic compounds and generally lipid-soluble. Some inorganic carcinogens are known, but most classes of inorganic compounds have yet to be tested for their carcinogenic potentials. The structural diversity of chemical carcinogens became evident first among the com-

TABLE 1. *Chemicals and crude chemical mixtures recognized as carcinogens in the human (and experimental animals)*

Agents or mixtures	Target organs
2-Naphthylamine, benzidine, 4-aminobiphenyl	Urinary bladder
4-Nitrobiphenyl	Urinary bladder
N,N-bis(2-Chloroethyl)-2-naphthylamine	Urinary bladder
bis(2-Chloroethyl)sulfide	Respiratory tract
Diethylstilbestrol	Vagina
Chloromethyl methyl ether and bis(chloromethyl)ether	Lungs
Vinyl chloride	Liver
Certain soots, tars, oils	Skin, Lungs
Cigarette smoke	Lungs, urinary bladder
Betel nuts	Buccal mucosa
Chromium compounds	Lungs
Nickel compounds	Lungs, nasal sinuses
Asbestos (a "physical" carcinogen?)	Lungs,[a] pleura
Arsenic compounds (inactive in rodents)	Skin, lungs

[a] Usually in workers who smoked cigarettes.

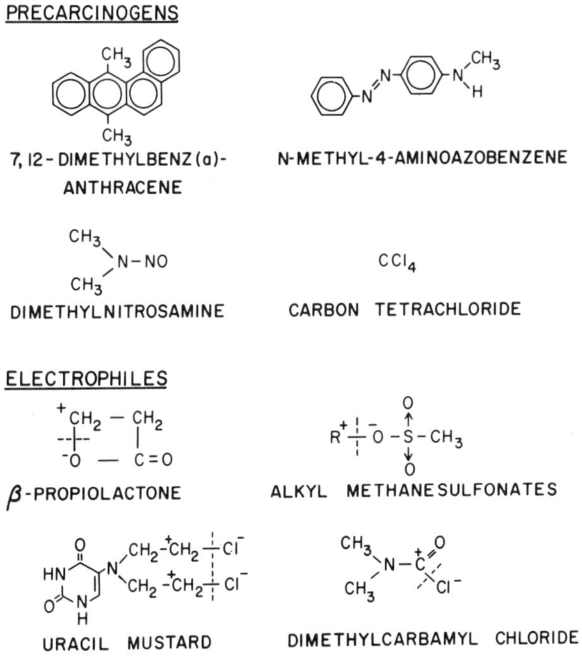

FIG. 1. Some synthetic chemical carcinogens. The precarcinogens undergo metabolic activation to reactive electrophiles. The carcinogenic electrophiles are generally alkylating agents, but some acylating carcinogens (i.e., dimethylcarbamyl chloride) and arylating and arylamidating carcinogens (i.e., 2-acetylaminofluorene-N-sulfate) (see text) are known.

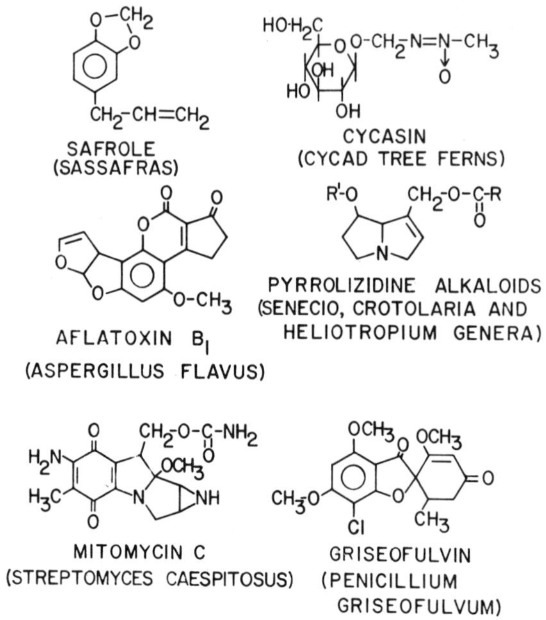

FIG. 2. The structures and properties of some carcinogenic green plant and fungal metabolites.

pounds recognized as carcinogenic in man, and today the list of these agents (Table 1) shows the wide range of structures active in our species. Most of these agents were discovered in small population groups exposed in industrial and some medical situations to large amounts of these compounds for prolonged times. Except for cigarette smoke, these agents account for only a small percentage of all human cancers. But, as a result of studies in cancer epidemiology in recent decades (Higginson, 1969; Higginson and Muir, 1973), chemicals in the general environment, both man-made and naturally occurring, are under great suspicion as playing a major role in the etiology of much cancer in man. These putative chemical carcinogens for man (in foods, drugs, air, water, etc.) will surely range widely in structure. The diversity of chemical carcinogens is further seen in the agents active in experimental animals. Figure 1 shows several kinds of synthetic chemical carcinogens. Figure 2 shows the structures of some naturally occurring carcinogens, which are primarily metabolites of certain fungi and green plants (J. A. Miller, 1970). No common structural features are evident between the various classes of chemicals that are carcinogenic in man and experimental animals.

THE INTERACTIONS OF CHEMICAL CARCINOGENS
WITH CELLULAR MACROMOLECULES *IN VIVO*

The transformation of normal cells into tumor cells appears to require at least a quasi-permanent alteration in phenotype. Thus, carcinogens must interact directly or indirectly with one or more informational macromolecules in cells involved in the control of growth. Neither the critical macromolecule(s) nor the critical modification(s) have yet been demonstrated unequivocally in the mechanism of action of any physical, chemical, or viral carcinogen. In approaches to such a demonstration in chemical carcinogenesis, considerable attention has been directed to the characterization of the reactive forms of chemical carcinogens, to the natures of their interactions with macromolecules, and to the relations of these interactions to tumor formation.

In early studies, the covalent binding *in vivo* of carcinogenic aminoazo dyes (E. C. Miller and J. A. Miller, 1947) and the polycyclic aromatic hydrocarbons (E. C. Miller, 1951) to proteins were noted in tissues susceptible to their carcinogenic action. Subsequently, many covalent bindings of residues of chemical carcinogens with both nucleic acids and proteins of tumor-susceptible tissues *in vivo and in vitro* have been observed (E. C. Miller and J. A. Miller, 1966; J. A. Miller, 1970). The amounts of these carcinogens bound *in vivo* are of the order of one carcinogen residue per 10^4 to 10^7 monomer residues in these macromolecules. In several cases, fair to good correlations appear to exist between the amounts of certain macromolecular bindings and carcinogenicity (J. A. Miller and E. C. Miller, 1953; Brookes and Lawley, 1964; Heidelberger, 1964; Colburn and Boutwell, 1968). In other cases, the correlations of carcinogenicity with the level of bound carcinogen are poor (Swann and Magee, 1968; Den Engelse et al., 1969/1970; Swann and Magee, 1971; Lijinsky et al., 1973). Although non-carcinogenic structures related to chemical carcinogens generally bind at only low levels, exceptions exist in which weak or apparently inactive compounds bind appreciably (J. A. Miller and E. C. Miller, 1953; Heidelberger, 1964), and some binding of chemical carcinogens may occur in apparently non-target tissues (Sarrif et al., 1975). But, no exceptions are known in which an adequately studied chemical carcinogen has failed to exhibit covalent binding to macromolecules in its target tissue *in vivo*. As noted below, there are multiple sites of binding in cellular macromolecules, and some of the more complex chemical carcinogens are metabolized to more than one reactive form. So it is to be expected that only a few of the macromolecular bound forms will be critical in the initiation of the carcinogenic process in any instance.

THE METABOLIC ACTIVATION AND REACTIVITIES OF CHEMICAL CARCINOGENS

In recent years, the nature of the interactions *in vivo* of chemical carcinogens with tissue macromolecules has become much clearer. It is now evident that the majority of chemical carcinogens are *precarcinogens,* which must be converted *in vivo* to *ultimate carcinogens;* these conversions are usually mediated by enzymes and may involve the formation of intermediate metabolites or *proximate carcinogens* (Fig. 3). Furthermore, an important generalization has been made in the past few years that most, if not all, chemical carcinogens have ultimate carcinogenic forms that are strong electrophilic reactants (J. A. Miller and E. C. Miller, 1969; J. A. Miller, 1970). That is, the ultimate carcinogens contain relatively electron-deficient atoms that can react covalently with electron-rich or nucleophilic atoms in cellular components, especially in such macromolecules as the nucleic acids and proteins. Thus, chemical carcinogens, which have no common structural features per se, are converted metabolically into strong electrophilic reactants or, as in the case of the carcinogenic alkylating and acylating agents, they already exist in this state.

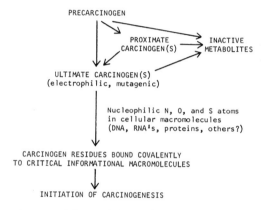

FIG. 3. General aspects of the metabolism and reactivities of chemical carcinogens.

These ultimate reactive forms are presumably also the ultimate carcinogenic forms of chemical carcinogens. This is clearly the case for the carcinogenic alkylating and acylating agents (Fig. 1). These agents are structurally very diverse, but they have in common the ability to act as carcinogens and to act as electrophiles in the alkylation or acylation of cellular nucleophiles. The identification of an ultimate reactive electrophilic metabolite as an ultimate carcinogenic form has also been possible for the aromatic amide 2-acetylaminofluorene (see below). Although the identity of certain ultimate reactive electrophiles with ultimate carcinogens is expected for chemical carcinogens in general, more evidence is needed on this point for many of these agents.

The electrophilic nature of ultimate chemical carcinogens and the related fact that no reactive nucleophilic form of a carcinogen has been noted so far appear to be the consequence of the structures of cellular components. Nucleic acids, proteins, and many other molecules in cells contain many more strongly nucleophilic centers (certain N, S, and O atoms) than electrophilic centers. Multitudinous covalent bond-breaking and bond-making events occur in cell metabolism. The physiologic electrophiles and nucleophiles formed and joined in these reactions are under tight and highly ordered control at enzyme surfaces and do not enter into reactions at random. In contrast, the strongly reactive electrophilic forms of chemical carcinogens attack cellular nucleophiles with little apparent discrimination and, as far as known, without the aid of enzymes. Although some of these attacks evidently initiate malignant transformation of cells, the critical molecular targets and the molecular processes that ensue in chemical carcinogenesis have not been identified unequivocally.

The problem of identifying the critical targets of chemical carcinogens in carcinogenesis is complex. One of the complicating factors is the multiplicity of bound derivatives formed from a single carcinogen. Thus, on treatment with alkylating agents, reactions occur *in vitro* or *in vivo* at a number of sites on the bases in the nucleic acids. Although the N-7 position of guanine is the major site of attack, alkylation also occurs at O-6 of guanine, at the N-1, N-3, and N-7 positions of adenine, and at N-3 of cytosine (Lawley, 1972). Evidence has been obtained that O-6 alkylation of guanine in nucleic acids *in vivo* may be of special importance in the induction of mutations and tumors (Loveless, 1969; Lawley, 1972; Gerchman and Ludlum, 1973; Goth and Rajewsky, 1974; Nicoll et al., 1975). With the electrophilic metabolites of aromatic arylamines and arylamides, the major reaction of the nucleic acids occurs at the 8-position of guanine (J. A. Miller, 1970; Irving, 1973; E. C. Miller and J. A. Miller 1974; Kriek, 1974; Lin et al., 1975*b;* Lin et al., 1975*a*). Reaction of alkylating agents or arylamine derivatives on the tertiary phosphate groups of nucleic acids also occurs (Price et al., 1968; Bannon and Verly, 1972; Lawley, 1973; Singer and Fraenkel-Conrat, 1975; King et al., 1975), and this substitution can lead to breaks in the sugar-phosphate backbone. Similarly, the binding of chemical carcinogens *in vivo* occurs at a number of sites in proteins. Among the products noted so far are derivatives resulting from reactions of carcinogenic electrophiles with methionyl, cysteinyl, histidyl, and tyrosyl residues in these macromolecules (J. A. Miller, 1970; E. C. Miller and J. A. Miller, 1974).

As expected, different precarcinogenic structures are often converted *in vivo* to electrophilic reactants by different enzymatic routes. Many of these reactions are oxidative in nature and occur in the endoplasmic reticulum of cells. This lipid-rich organelle is a principal site of activation and inactivation of a variety of foreign lipid-soluble molecules. It contains inducible cytochrome P-450 and flavoprotein oxidases that require NADPH and O_2 and oxidize a wide range of foreign and physiologic lipid-soluble molecules. Recent work with some of the more structurally complex chemical carcinogens has shown that several of these compounds are metabolized to more than one electrophilic reactant. These aspects of chemical carcinogenesis are illustrated in the following examples.

It is now established that the carcinogenicity of aromatic amines, amides, and nitro compounds in liver and other tissues depends on their conversion to *N*-hydroxy derivatives as proximate carcinogens (J. A. Miller, 1970; E. C. Miller and J. A. Miller, 1974). Further metabolism converts these *N*-hydroxy metabolites to electrophilic reactants. The metabolic activation and inactivation of the versatile carcinogen 2-acetylaminofluorene (AAF) in rat liver is presented in Fig. 4. Its *N*-hydroxy metabolite is esterified by one or more sulfotransferases in the soluble fraction of the liver to form the very reactive and mutagenic sulfuric acid ester. The figure shows the structures of some of the covalently bound protein-methion-S-yl and nucleic acid-guan-8-yl derivatives of the carcinogen that are formed *in vivo* in the liver. The same structures are formed *in vitro* nonenzymatically from the *N*-sulfate or similar esters and these macromolecules. Close correlations between the activity of this enzymatic esterification system and the carcinogenicity and reactivity of the *N*-hydroxy metabolite in rat liver indicate that the sulfuric acid ester is a major reactive ultimate carcinogen in this organ (DeBaun et al., 1970; Weisburger et al., 1972). Other electrophilic metabolites of *N*-hydroxy-AAF may be formed enzymatically. Peroxidases form a nitroxide-free radical from this substrate, and the free radical readily dismutates to form *N*-acetoxy-AAF and 2-nitrosofluorene, both highly carcinogenic and mutagenic substances (cf. Bartsch et al., 1972*b*). This reaction may occur in liver. Similarly, a soluble

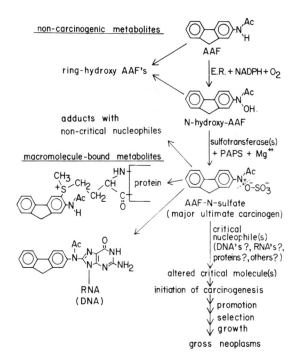

FIG. 4. The activation and inactivation of 2-acetylaminofluorene in rat liver.

acyl transferase in liver and some other tissues converts N-hydroxy-AAF into the powerful electrophile N-acetoxy-2-aminofluorene; this metabolite may also be an ultimate carcinogen at nonhepatic sites of tumor formation by AAF (Bartsch et al., 1972a; King, 1974). Even the circulatory and execretory metabolite, the O-glucuronide of N-hydroxy-AAF, has some electrophilic activity (Miller et al., 1968; Irving et al., 1969). Recent studies have demonstrated that the hepatocarcinogen N-methyl-4-aminoazobenzene is N-hydroxylated and esterified in a 3′-phosphoadenosine-5′-phosphosulfate-(PAPS)-dependent reaction in rat liver (Kadlubar et al., 1975). The resultant N-sulfate reacts with methionine and guanosine in reactions that are analogous to the reactions observed *in vitro* for the synthetic carcinogenic ester N-benzoyloxy-N-methyl-4-aminoazobenzene (Lin et al., 1975b) and for N-methyl-4-aminoazobenzene *in vivo* in rat liver (Lin et al., 1975a). Thus, the metabolic activation of this and probably other aminoazo dyes fits within the general framework observed with various aromatic amine and amide carcinogens.

Studies on the activation of the carcinogenic polycyclic aromatic hydrocarbons are under intensive investigation in many laboratories. Cells in culture and preparations of fragmented endoplasmic reticulum (microsomes) from liver and other tissues metabolize these carcinogens to a series of epoxides, dihydrodiols, phenols, and quinones. Some of the K-region epoxides are more potent than the parent hydrocarbon in inducing the malignant transformation of cells in culture (Heidelberger, 1973). The recent studies on benzo(a)pyrene, a carcinogenic constituent of coal tar and an ubiquitious environmental pollutant, typify current investigations in this field. Multiple enzymatic pathways to electrophilic reactants have been noted for this hydrocarbon (Fig. 5). The pathway recently discovered by Sims et al. (1974) may be especially relevant. These investigators noted the formation of a non-K-region epoxide, which was converted by epoxide hydrase to a dihydrodiol. The isolated double bond in the dihydrodiol ring was then epoxidized to yield a reactive dihydrodiol epoxide, which appeared to account for a major DNA-bound form of the hydrocarbon in cells in culture. Two kinds of reactive free radicals have been proposed as possible metabolites of benzo(a)pyrene. Nonenzymatic, one-electron oxidation of this hydrocarbon yields reactive free radical cations (Umans et al., 1969; Ts'o et al., 1969). Air oxidation of the 6-hydroxy metabolite of benzo(a)pyrene yields a reactive 6-oxo free radical that readily binds to DNA (Caspary et al., 1974; Nagata et al., 1974; Ts'o et al., 1974). 6-Hydroxymethylation is another novel metabolic reaction that occurs with benzo(a)pyrene; synthetic esters of the benzylic 6-hydroxymethyl metabolite are reactive and carcinogenic (Flesher and Sydnor, 1973; Sloane and Davis, 1974). It seems likely that several of these pathways may contribute to the carcinogenic action of this hydrocarbon in various tissues.

Carcinogenic natural products exhibit the same need for metabolic activa-

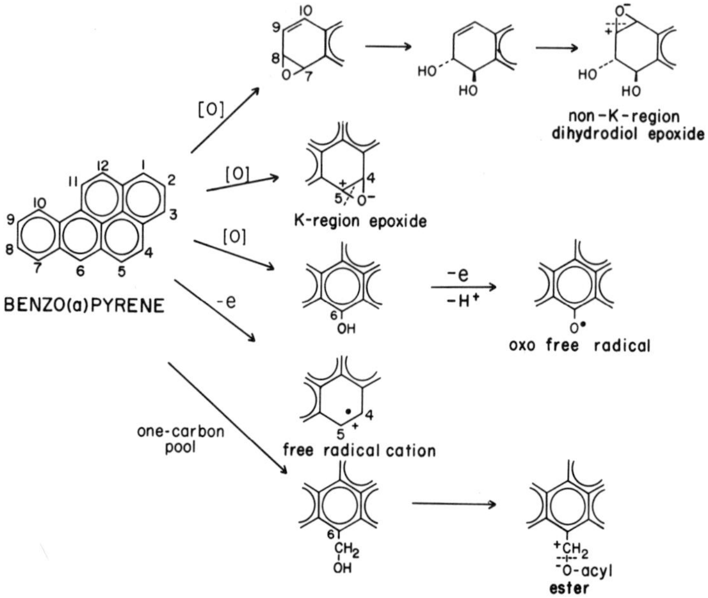

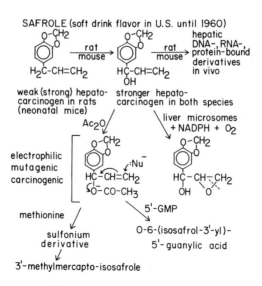

FIG. 5. The formation of multiple electrophilic reactants from benzo(a)pyrene.

tion as synthetic chemical carcinogens. The plant constituent safrole is metabolized in the rat and mouse to the proximate carcinogen 1'-hydroxysafrole (Fig. 6) (Borchert et al., 1973). The ultimate reactive and carcinogenic derivatives may include an ester of this proximate carcinogen (Borchert et al., 1973b; Borchert et al., 1973a) and other electrophilic metabolites, such as

FIG. 6. The metabolic activation of safrole.

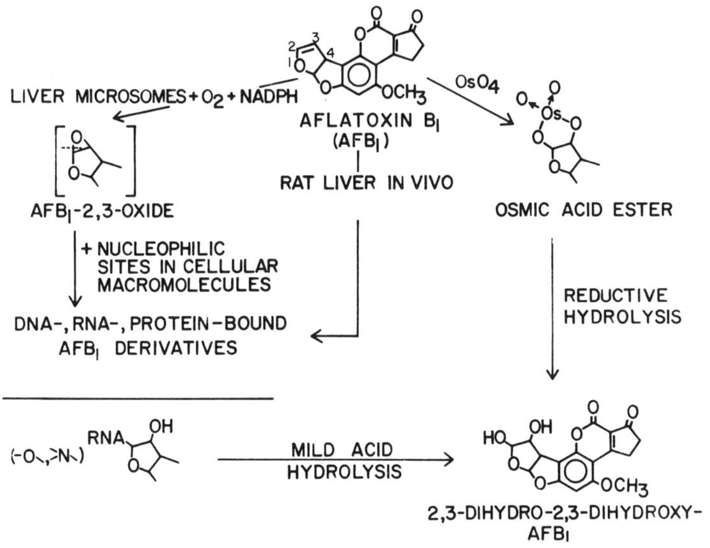

FIG. 7. The metabolic activation of aflatoxin B_1.

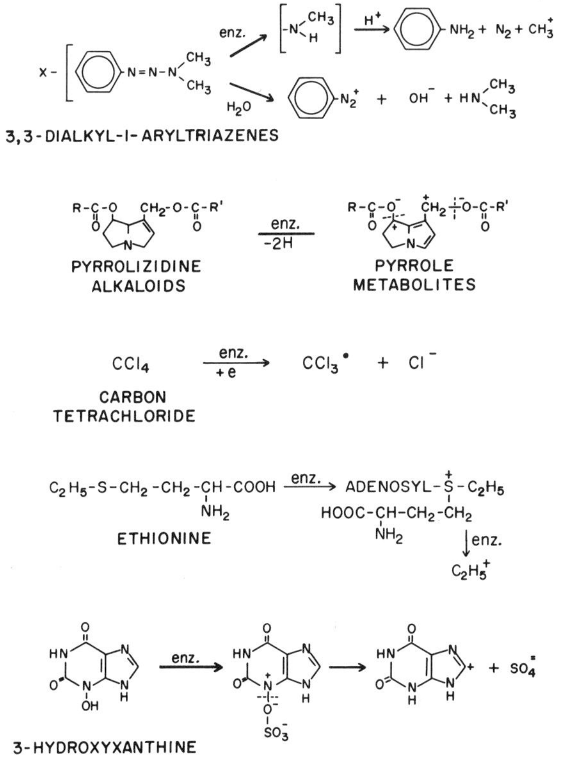

FIG. 8. Electrophilic reactive metabolites of various chemical carcinogens.

the 2′,3′-oxide (Stillwell et al., 1974; Wislocki, 1974). Similarly, the extremely potent hepatocarcinogen aflatoxin B_1 is apparently metabolized to a reactive epoxide (Fig. 7) (Swenson et al., 1973, 1974), which is probably a major ultimate carcinogenic metabolite of this mycotoxin.

This principle of metabolic activation of chemical carcinogens to reactive electrophiles applies to a very wide range of structures and further examples, including both synthetic compounds and natural products, are shown in Fig. 8 (reviewed in E. C. Miller and J. A. Miller, 1974).

CHEMICAL EVENTS IMMEDIATELY FOLLOWING THE CELLULAR ABSORPTION OF IONIZING AND ULTRAVIOLET RADIATIONS

The initial chemical events that follow the absorption of ionizing radiation by cells are complex (Myers, 1973; Pryor, 1973), and they strongly resemble those that occur in the initial steps of chemical carcinogenesis. Thus, a variety of reactive electrophilic free radicals are generated by the absorption of ionizing radiation. This may occur either directly in cellular macromolecules or indirectly in these molecules from free radicals produced in the radiolysis of water (Fig. 9). Molecular oxygen, which can assume a diradical character, can also generate and react with free radicals to form a variety of oxidation products (Demopoulos, 1973; Myers, 1973; Pryor, 1973).

Ultraviolet light, although non-ionizing, is absorbed by double bonds in nucleic acids, proteins, and other cellular components. Oxidation of cholesterol and aromatic amino acids to potentially carcinogenic compounds may result (Neckers, 1968; Black and Douglas, 1972, 1973). Pyrimidine dimer formation follows the absorption of ultraviolet light by DNA (Setlow, 1968), and

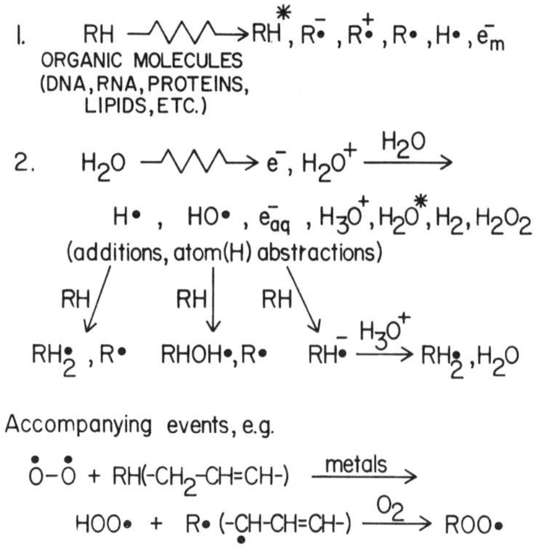

FIG. 9. Initial events in the absorption of ionizing radiations in cells.

this event appears to be related to carcinogenesis by such radiation in fish cells (Setlow and Hart, 1974).

MOLECULAR MECHANISMS OF CHEMICAL AND RADIATION CARCINOGENESIS

The paucity of definitive data on the critical cellular targets of chemical carcinogens and the difficulty of obtaining such data have led to considerable speculation on the molecular nature of chemical carcinogenesis. Similar problems are evident in studies on the molecular nature of radiation carcinogenesis. Both genetic and epigenetic models have been proposed, but these models have not yet led to decisive experiments that reveal the molecular nature of carcinogenesis by chemical or radiation carcinogens. Viruses or viral information, hormonal imbalances, immunodeficiencies, etc., have been implicated in the mechanisms of action of several chemical and radiation carcinogens, but the molecular nature of the carcinogenic processe(s) in these instances is not clear. Similarly, information on the molecular mechanisms of carcinogenesis have not yet appeared from studies on the nature of the phenotypes of tumor cells.

POSSIBLE GENETIC MECHANISMS OF CARCINOGENESIS

Genetic theories of carcinogenesis are based on the pivotal role of DNA as the heritable source of phenotypic information. Direct modification of DNA by ultimate carcinogenic electrophiles from chemicals or ionizing radiation may yield carcinogenic somatic mutations. The mutagenicity of ionizing radiation and of ultraviolet light has been evident for some time. It is now evident that the ultimate reactive electrophilic forms of chemical carcinogens also are mutagenic in a variety of test systems (Miller and Miller, 1971), including the direct modification of isolated transforming DNA (Maher et al., 1968). Repair of these lesions in DNA may play a role in these processes, if the repair is error-prone. This would be consistent with the apparent requirement that cells undergo one or two cell divisions soon after treatment with a chemical or radiation carcinogen in order to undergo malignant transformation (Borek and Sachs, 1968). Likewise, the carcinogen-induced lesions in DNA may trigger the transcription of integrated carcinogenic viral DNA or facilitate the integration and transcription of such carcinogenic information (Stich and Laishes, 1973).

Direct modification of an RNA that is replicated as DNA and then ultimately integrated into the DNA genome of cells (Temin, 1974) or modification of the polymerases that replicate these nucleic acids also provide the means for carcinogenic alterations of the genome. The existence of error-prone DNA polymerases in certain mutant phages (Speyer et al., 1966) suggested that similar, error-prone cellular DNA polymerases might result from the direct alteration of such enzymes by carcinogens (J. A. Miller and E. C. Miller, 1971; Nelson and Mason, 1972). The possible importance of this mechanism is underlined by the recent finding that some DNA polymerases from leukemic tissues are more error-prone than those of normal tissues (Loeb et al., 1974) and, especially, from the observation that treatment of a DNA polymerase *in vitro* with the carcinogen β-propiolactone reduced the fidelity with which it replicated DNA (Sirover and Loeb, 1974).

POSSIBLE EPIGENETIC MECHANISMS OF CARCINOGENESIS

The differentiation of normal tissues appears to involve repression and derepression of the expression of information in the diploid genome common to their constituent cells and does not appear to involve directed mutations in this genome (Dustin, 1972; Simnett, 1974; Gurdon, 1974). Tumor cells might also arise through similar quasi-permanent alterations in the expression of normal cell genomes (Weinstein, 1970). Support for this point of view comes from the ability of nuclei of cells from renal tumors of frogs to direct the growth and differentiation of enucleated frog eggs (Gurdon, 1974) and from the differentiation of certain tumors (Weinstein, 1970; Dustin, 1972; Simnett, 1974; Pierce, 1974).

Finally, it must be recognized that, in some situations, chemicals and radiation may induce tumor formation without directly initiating neoplastic changes in any cell. Thus, chemicals or radiation that depress immune responses or alter the hormonal balance in a particular tissue might provide the appropriate conditions for the preferential growth of pre-existing tumor cells.

PROSPECTUS

There is good reason to expect marked advances in our knowledge of carcinogenesis in the next few years. Studies in molecular biology can be expected to provide further fundamental probes on the nature of malignant transformations, especially in quantitative studies of these process in cell cultures. With these tools, more insight will be obtained on the molecular mechanisms by which chemical, physical, and viral carcinogens alter growth controls in cells.

REFERENCES

Armuth, V., and Berenblum, I. (1972): Systemic promoting action of phorbol in liver and lung carcinogenesis in AKR mice. *Cancer Res.,* 32:2259–2262.

Armuth, V., and Berenblum, I. (1974): Promotion of mammary carcinogenesis and leukemogenic action by phorbol in virgin female Wistar rats. *Cancer Res.,* 34:2704–2707.

Bannon, P., and Verly, W. G. (1972): Alkylation of phosphates and stability of phosphate triesters in DNA. *Europ. J. Biochem.,* 31:103–111.

Bartsch, H., Dworkin, M., Miller, J. A., and Miller, E. C. (1972a): Electrophilic N-acetoxyaminoarenes derived from carcinogenic N-hydroxy-N-acetylaminoarenes by enzymatic deacetylation and transacetylation in liver. *Biochim. Biophys. Acta,* 286: 272–298.

Bartsch, H., Miller, J. A., and Miller, E. C. (1972*b*): *N*-Acetoxy-*N*-acetyl aminoarenes and nitrosoarenes. One-electron non-enzymatic and enzymatic products of various carcinogenic aromatic acethydroxamic acids. *Biochim. Biophys. Acta,* 273:40–51.

Berenblum, I., and Shubik, P. (1947): A new, quantitative, approach to the study of the stages of chemical carcinogenesis in the mouse's skin. *Brit. J. Cancer,* 1:383–391.

Black, H. S., and Douglas, D. R. (1972): A model system for the evaluation of the role of cholesterol α-oxide in ultraviolet carcinogenesis. *Cancer Res.,* 32:2630–2632.

Black, H. S., and Douglas, D. R. (1973): Formation of a carcinogen of natural origin in the etiology of ultraviolet light-induced carcinogenesis. *Cancer Res.,* 33:2094–2096.

Borchert, P., Miller, J. A., Miller, E. C., and Shires, T. K. (1973*a*): 1′-Hydroxysafrole, a proximate carcinogenic metabolite of safrole in the rat and mouse. *Cancer Res.,* 33:590–600.

Borchert, P., Wislocki, P. G., Miller, J. A., and Miller, E. C. (1973*b*): The metabolism of the naturally occurring hepatocarcinogen safrole to 1′-hydroxysafrole and the electrophilic reactivity of 1′-acetoxysafrole. *Cancer Res.,* 33:575–589.

Borek, C., and Hall, E. J. (1973): Transformation of mammalian cells *in vitro* by low doses of x-rays. *Nature,* 243:450–453.

Borek, C., and Sachs, L. (1968): The number of cell generations required to fix the transformed state in x-ray-induced transformation. *Proc. Natl. Acad. Sci., USA,* 59:83–85.

Boutwell, R. K. (1974): The function and mechanism of promoters of carcinogenesis. *CRC Crit. Rev. Toxicol.,* 2:419–443.

Brookes, P., and Lawley, P. D. (1964): Reaction of some mutagenic and carcinogenic compounds with nucleic acids. *J. Cell. Comp. Physiol.,* 64 (Suppl. 1):111–120.

Caspary, W., Lesko, S., Lorentzen, R., and Ts'o, P. O. P. (1974): Properties and formation of 6-oxo-benzo(a)pyrene radical. *Fed. Proc.,* 33:1500.

Colburn, N. H., and Boutwell, R. K. (1968): The binding of β-propiolactone and some related alkylating agents to DNA, RNA, and protein of mouse skin; relation between tumor-initiating power of alkylating agents and their binding to DNA. *Cancer Res.,* 28:653–660.

DeBaun, J. R., Miller, E. C., and Miller, J. A. (1970): *N*-Hydroxy-2-acetylaminofluorene sulfotransferase: Its probable role in carcinogenesis and in protein-(methion-S-yl) binding in rat liver. *Cancer Res.,* 30:577–595.

Demopoulos, H. B. (1973): The basis of free radical pathology. *Fed. Proc.,* 32:1859–1861.

Den Engelse, L., Bentvelzen, A. J., and Emmelot, P. (1969/70): Studies on lung tumors. Methylation of deoxyribonucleic acid and tumor formation following administration of dimethylnitrosamine to mice. *Chem.-Biol. Interact.,* 1:395–406.

Druckrey, H. (1967): Quantitative aspects in chemical carcinogenesis. In: *Potential Carcinogenic Hazards from Drugs,* edited by R. Truhaut, UICC Monograph, Vol. 7, pp. 60–78. Springer-Verlag, New York.

Dustin, P., Jr. (1972): Cell differentiation and carcinogenesis: A critical review. *Cell Tissue Kinet.,* 5:519–533.

Flesher, J. W., and Sydnor, K. L. (1973): Possible role of 6-hydroxymethylbenzo(a)-pyrene as a proximate carcinogen of benzo(a)pyrene and 6-methylbenzo(a)pyrene. *Int. J. Cancer,* 11:433–437.

Gerchman, L. L., and Ludlum, D. B. (1973): The properties of O^6-methylguanine in templates for RNA polymerase. *Biochim. Biophys. Acta,* 308:310–316.

Goth, R., and Rajewsky, M. F. (1974): Persistence of O-6-ethylguanine in rat-brain DNA: Correlation with nervous system-specific carcinogenesis by ethylnitrosourea. *Proc. Natl. Acad. Sci., USA,* 71:639–643.

Gurdon, J. B. (1974): *The Control of Gene Expression in Animal Development.* 160 pp. Harvard University Press, Cambridge.

Hecker, E., and Schmidt, R. (1974): Phorbolesters—the irritants and cocarcinogens of Croton Tiglium L. In: *Progress in the Chemistry of Organic Natural Products,* edited by W. Herz, H. Grisebach, and G. W. Kirby, Vol. 31, pp. 377–467. Springer-Verlag, New York.

Heidelberger, C. (1964): Studies on the molecular mechanism of hydrocarbon carcinogenesis. *J. Cell. Comp. Physiol.,* 64 (Suppl. 1):129–148.

Heidelberger, C. (1973): Chemical oncogenesis in culture. *Adv. Cancer Res.,* 18:317–336.

Higginson, J. (1969): Present trends in cancer epidemiology. *Canad. Cancer Conf.,* 8:40–75.

Higginson, J., and Muir, C. S. (1973): Epidemiology. In: *Cancer Medicine,* edited by J. F. Holland and E. Frei, III, Chapter IV, pp. 241–306, Lea and Febiger, Philadelphia.

Irving, C. C. (1973): Interactions of chemical carcinogens with DNA. In: *Methods in Cancer Research,* edited by H. Busch, Vol. 7, pp. 190–244. Academic Press, New York.

Kadlubar, F. F., Miller, J. A., and Miller, E. C. (1975): The metabolic activation of N-methyl-4-aminoazobenzene by rat liver. *Proc. Am. Assoc. Cancer Res.,* 16:14.

King, C. M. (1974): Mechanism of reaction, tissue distribution, and inhibition of arylhydroxamic acid acyltransferase. *Cancer Res.,* 34:1503–1515.

King, C. M., Shayman, M. A., and Thissen, M. R. (1975): Reaction of arylhydroxylamines with phosphate of RNA: Cleavage of the nucleic acid chain. *Proc. Am. Assoc. Cancer Res.,* 16:119.

Kriek, E. (1974): Carcinogenesis by aromatic amines. *Biochim. Biophys. Acta,* 355:177–203.

Lawley, P. D. (1972): The action of alkylating mutagens and carcinogens on nucleic acids: N-methyl-N-nitroso compounds as methylating agents. In: *Topics in Chemical Carcinogenesis,* edited by W. Nakahara, S. Takayama, T. Sugimura, and S. Odashima, pp. 237–258, University of Tokyo Press, Tokyo.

Lawley, P. D. (1973): Reaction of N-methyl-N-nitrosourea (MNUA) with ^{32}P-labelled DNA: Evidence for formation of phosphotriesters. *Chem. Biol. Interact.,* 7:127–130.

Lijinsky, W., Keefer, L., Loo, J., and Ross, A. E. (1973): Studies of alkylation of nucleic acids in rats by cyclic nitrosamines. *Cancer Res.,* 33:1634–1641.

Lin, J.-K., Miller, J. A., and Miller, E. C. (1975a): Structures of hepatic nucleic acid-bound dyes in rats given the carcinogen N-methyl-4-aminoazobenzene. *Cancer Res.,* 35:844–850.

Lin. J.-K., Schmall, B., Sharpe, I. D., Miura, I., Miller, J. A., and Miller, E. C. (1975b): N-Substitution of carbon 8 in guanosine and deoxyguanosine by the carcinogen N-benzoyloxy-N-methyl-4-aminoazobenzene *in vitro. Cancer Res.,* 35:832–843.

Loeb, L. A., Springgate, C. F., and Battula, N. (1974): Errors in DNA replication as a basis of malignant changes. *Cancer Res.,* 34:2311–2321.

Loveless, A. (1969): Possible relevance of O-6 alkylation of deoxyguanosine to mutagenicity and carcinogenicity of nitrosamines and nitrosamides. *Nature,* 223:206–207.

Maher, V. M., Miller, E. C., Miller, J. A., and Szybalski, W. (1968): Mutations and decreases in density of transforming DNA produced by derivatives of the carcinogens 2-acetylaminofluorene and N-methyl-4-aminoazobenzene. *Mol. Pharmacol.,* 4:411–428.

Miller, E. C. (1951): Studies on the formation of protein-bound derivatives of 3,4-benzpyrene in the epidermal fraction of mouse skin. *Cancer Res.,* 11:100–108.

Miller, E. C., Lotlikar, P. D., Miller, J. A., Butler, B. A., Irving, C. C., and Hill, J. T. (1968): Reactions *in vitro* of some tissue nucleophiles with the glucuronide of the carcinogen N-hydroxy-2-acetylaminofluorene. *Mol. Pharmacol.,* 4:147–154.

Miller, E. C., and Miller, J. A. (1947): The presence and significance of bound aminoazo dyes in the livers of rats fed p-dimethylaminoazobenzene. *Cancer Res.,* 7:468–480.

Miller, E. C., and Miller, J. A. (1966): Mechanisms of chemical carcinogenesis: Nature of proximate carcinogens and interactions with macromolecules. *Pharmacol. Rev.,* 18:805–838.

Miller, E. C., and Miller, J. A. (1971): The mutagenicity of chemical carcinogens: Correlations, problems, and interpretations. In: *Chemical Mutagens: Principles and Methods for Their Detection,* edited by A. Hollaender, Vol. 1, pp. 83–119, Plenum Press, New York.

Miller, E. C., and Miller, J. A. (1974): Biochemical mechanisms of carcinogenesis. In:

The Molecular Biology of Cancer, edited by H. Busch, pp. 377–402, Academic Press, New York.

Miller, J. A. (1970): Carcinogenesis by chemicals: An overview—G. H. A. Clowes Memorial lecture. *Cancer Res.,* 30:559–576.

Miller, J. A. (1973): Naturally occurring substances that can induce tumors. In: *Toxicants Occurring Naturally in Foods,* pp. 508–549, National Academy of Sciences, Washington, D.C.

Miller, J. A., and Miller, E. C. (1953): The carcinogenic aminoazo dyes. *Adv. Cancer Res.,* 1:339–396.

Miller, J. A., and Miller, E. C. (1969): Metabolic activation of carcinogenic aromatic amines and amides via N-hydroxylation and N-hydroxy-esterification and its relationship to ultimate carcinogens as electrophilic reactants. In: *The Jerusalem Symposia on Quantum Chemistry and Biochemistry. Physicochemical Mechanisms of Carcinogenesis,* edited by E. D. Bergmann and B. Pullman, Vol. 1, pp. 237–261, Israel Academy of Sciences, Jerusalem.

Miller, J. A., and Miller, E. C. (1971): Chemical carcinogenesis: Mechanisms and approaches to its control. *J. Natl. Cancer Inst.,* 47:V–XIV.

Mondal, S., Peterson, A. R., and Brankow, D. W. (1975): Initiation and promotion in ocogenesis in cell cultures. *Proc. Am. Assoc. Cancer Res.,* 16:74.

Myers, L. S., Jr. (1973): Free radical damage of nucleic acids and their components by ionizing radiations. *Fed. Proc.,* 32:1882–1894.

Nagata, C., Tagashira, Y., and Kodama, M. (1974): Metabolic activation of benzo(a)-pyrene: Significance of the free radical. In: *The Biochemistry of Disease,* Vol. 4, *Chemical Carcinogenesis,* Part A, edited by P. O. P. Ts'o and J. A. DiPaolo, pp. 87–111. Marcel Dekker, New York.

Neckers, D. C. (1973): Photochemical reactions of natural macromolecules. Photoreactions of proteins. *J. Chem. Educ.,* 50:164–168.

Nelson, R. L., and Mason, H. A. (1972): An explicit hypothesis for chemical carcinogenesis. *J. Theor. Biol.,* 37:197–200.

Nicoll, J. W., Swann, P. F., and Pegg, A. E. (1975): Effect of dimethylnitrosamine on persistence of methylated guanines in rat liver and kidney DNA. *Nature,* 254:261–262.

Peraino, C., Fry, R. J. M., Staffeldt, E., and Kisieleski, W. E. (1973): Effects of varying the exposure of phenobarbital on its enhancement of 2-acetylaminofluorene-induced hepatic tumorigenesis in the rat. *Cancer Res.,* 33:2701–2705.

Pierce, G. B. (1974): Neoplasms, differentiations, and mutations. *Am. J. Pathol.,* 77:103–114.

Price, C., Gaucher, G. M., Koneru, P., Shibakawa, R., Sowa, J. R., and Yamaguchi, M. (1968): Relative reactivities for monofunctional nitrogen mustard alkylation of nucleic acid components. *Biochim. Biophys. Acta,* 166:327–359.

Pryor, W. A. (1973): Free radical reactions and their importance in biochemical systems. *Fed. Proc.,* 32:1862–1869.

Sarrif, A. M., Bertram, J. S., Karmarck, M., and Heidelberger, C. (1975): The isolation and characterization of polycyclic hydrocarbon-binding proteins from mouse liver and skin cytosols. *Cancer Res.,* 35:816–824.

Setlow, R. B. (1968): The photochemistry, photobiology, and repair of polynucleotides. *Prog. Nucleic Acid Res. Mol. Biol.,* 8:257–295.

Setlow, R. B., and Hart, R. R. (1974): Direct evidence that damaged DNA results in neoplastic transformation—A fish story. *Proc. 5th International Congress of Radiation Research (in press.)*

Simnett, J. D. (1974): Nuclear differentiation in the development of normal and neoplastic tissues. In: *Neoplasia and Cell Differentiation,* edited by G. V. Sherbet, Karger, Basel, pp. 1–26.

Sims, P., Grover, P. L., Swaisland, A., Pal, K., and Hewer, A. (1974): Metabolic activation of benzo(a)pyrene proceeds by a diol-epoxide. *Nature,* 252:326–328.

Singer, B., and Fraenkel-Conrat, H. (1975): Reactions of oncogenic alkylating agents with nucleic acids. *Proc. Am. Assoc. Cancer Res.,* 16:81.

Sirover, M. A., and Loeb, L. A. (1974): Erroneous base-pairing induced by a chemical carcinogen during DNA synthesis. *Nature,* 252:414–416.

Sloane, N. H., and Davis, T. K. (1974): Hydroxymethylation of the benzene ring.

Microsomal hydroxymethylation of benzo(a)pyrene to 6-hydroxymethylbenzo(a)-pyrene. *Arch. Biochem. Biophys.*, 163:46–52.

Speyer, J. F., Karam, J. D., and Lenny, A. B. (1966): On the role of DNA polymerase in base selection. *Cold Spring Harbor Symp. Quant. Biol.*, 31:693–697.

Stich, H. F., and Laishes, B. A. (1973): DNA repair and chemical carcinogens. In: *Pathobiology Annual*, edited by H. L. Ioachim, Vol. 3, pp. 341–376, Appleton-Century-Crofts, New York.

Stillwell, W. G., Carman, M. J., Bell, L., and Horning, M. G. (1974): The metabolism of safrole and 2′,3′-epoxysafrole in the rat and guinea pig. *Drug Metab. Disposition*, 2:489–498.

Swann, P. F., and Magee, P. N. (1968): Nitrosamine-induced carcinogenesis. The alkylation of nucleic acids of the rat by N-methyl-N-nitrosourea, dimethylnitrosamine, dimethylsulfate, and methyl methanesulfonate. *Biochem. J.*, 110:39–47.

Swann, P. F., and Magee, P. N. (1971): Nitrosamine-induced carcinogenesis. The alkylation of N-7 of guanine of nucleic acids of the rat by diethylnitrosoamine, N-ethyl-N-nitrosourea, and ethyl methanesulfonate. *Biochem. J.*, 125:841–847.

Swenson, D. H., Miller, E. C., and Miller, J. A. (1974): Aflatoxin B_1-2,3-oxide: Evidence for its formation in rat liver *in vivo* and by human liver microsomes *in vitro*. *Biochem. Biophys. Res. Commun.*, 60:1036–1043.

Swenson, D. H., Miller, J. A., and Miller, E. C. (1973): 2,3-Dihydro-2,3-dihydroxy-aflatoxin B_1: An acid hydrolysis product of an RNA-aflatoxin B_1 adduct formed by hamster and rat liver microsomes *in vitro*. *Biochem. Biophys. Res. Commun.*, 53: 1260–1267.

Temin, H. M. (1974): On the origin of the genes for neoplasia—G. H. A. Clowes Memorial lecture. *Cancer Res.*, 34:2835–2841.

Ts'o, P. O. P., Lesko, S. A., and Umans, R. S. (1969): The physical binding and the chemical linkage of benzpyrene to nucleotides, nucleic acids, and nucleohistones. In: *The Jerusalem Symposia on Quantum Chemistry and Biochemistry. Physicochemical Mechanisms of Carcinogenesis*, edited by E. D. Bergmann and B. Pullman, Vol. 1, pp. 106–135, Israel Academy of Sciences, Jerusalem.

Ts'o, P. O. P., Caspary, W. J., Cohen, B. I., Leavitt, J. C., Lesko, S. A., Jr., Lorentzen, R. J., and Schectman, L. M. (1974): Basic mechanisms in polycyclic hydrocarbon carcinogenesis. In: *The Biochemistry of Disease*, Vol. 4, *Chemical Carcinogenesis*, Part A, edited by P. O. P. Ts'o and J. A. DiPaolo, Marcel Dekker, New York, pp. 113–147.

Umans, R. S., Lesko, S. A., Jr., and Ts'o, P. O. P. (1969): Chemical linkage of carcinogenic 3,4-benzpyrene to DNA in aqueous solution induced by peroxide and iodine. *Nature*, 221:763–764.

Van Duuren, B. L., Sivak, A., Katz, C., Seidman, I., and Melchionne, S. (1975): The effect of aging and interval between primary and secondary treatment in two-stage carcinogenesis in mouse skin. *Cancer Res.*, 35:502–505.

Weinstein, I. B. (1970): Modifications of transfer RNA during chemical carcinogenesis. In: *Genetic Concepts and Neoplasia*, edited by University of Texas M. D. Anderson Hospital and Tumor Institute, pp. 380–408, Williams & Wilkins, Baltimore.

Weisburger, J. H., Yamamoto, R. S., Williams, G. H., Grantham, P. H., Matsushima, T., and Weisburger, E. K. (1972): On the sulfate ester of N-hydroxy-2-fluorenylacetamide as a key ultimate hepatocarcinogen in the rat. *Cancer Res.*, 32:491–500.

Wislocki, P. G. (1974): On the proximate and ultimate carcinogenic metabolites of precarcinogens: Safrole and certain N-alkylaminoazobenzene dyes. Ph.D. Thesis, University of Wisconsin.

Biology of Radiation Carcinogenesis, edited by
J. M. Yuhas, R. W. Tennant, and J. D. Regan.
Raven Press, New York © 1976.

Comparison of Alkylating Agent and Radiation Carcinogenesis: Some Aspects of the Possible Involvement of Effects on DNA

P. D. Lawley

Institute of Cancer Research, Royal Cancer Hospital, Pollards Wood Research Station, Nightingales Lane, Chalfont St. Giles, Bucks, England

The concept that DNA is a significant cellular target of carcinogens relates to the somatic mutation hypothesis of carcinogenesis and, in particular, to the view that initiation of carcinogenesis involves (largely) irreversible change in the genetic material of the target cell. Subsequent promotional effects would then include a stimulus to division of initiated cells.

It has proved possible, mainly by the use of isotopically labeled chemical carcinogens, to measure the extent of chemical damage to DNA of target organs at carcinogenic dose levels of alkylating agents and other carcinogens. In this chapter, we refer to some studies in progress on induction of thymoma in mice.

In order to interpret the possible significance of these measurable extents of chemical modification of DNA, recourse to other biological test objects was taken, objects with which effects thought to be related to carcinogenesis could be determined, again in quantitative relationship to the chemical effects on DNA.

In several instances, the effects of radiation on these test systems have been investigated, and comparisons between radiation and chemicals can thus be made.

In the present short review of some relevant comparisons, reference is made to a selected group of chemical agents, chosen to illustrate the influence of chemical structure and reactivity on biological effects. For the selected methylating agents, reactivity by Ingold's S_N1 mechanism increases, the Swain-Scott substrate factor s decreases, and the relative ability to alkylate O-atom sites in DNA increases, through the series, from methyl methanesulfonate (MMS) [closely similar to dimethyl sulfate (DMS)] to N-methyl-N-nitrosourea (MNUA) [which, like its analogue, N-methyl-N'-nitro-N-nitrosoguanidine (MNNG), methylates through the highly reactive methyldiazonium ion, $CH_3 N_2^+$]. With the ethylating agents, ethyl methanesulfonate (EMS) has more S_N1 character than does its analogue MMS, and N-ethyl-N-nitrosourea (ENUA) is correspondingly more reactive in this sense than is MNUA. The reactivities of these compounds are compared in Table 1. It should be noted that the relative alkylation of phosphodiester groups in DNA increases through this series in parallel to O-6 alkylation of guanine.

As reviewed in more detail elsewhere (Lawley, 1975), alkylating agents can serve as models for other carcinogens that require metabolic activation for carcinogenic activity. Thus, the products found in DNA of target cells *in vivo* following alkylation may be identical with those following administration of another carcinogen, which is not itself reactive *in vitro*. This would show that the reactive metabolites of the second carcinogen include alkylating molecular species identical with those from the first.

As an example, the pattern of DNA methylation products from the carcinogen dimethylnitrosamine (DMN) *in vivo* is closely similar to, if not identical

TABLE 1. *Relative extents of O-alkylation in nucleic acids in relation to reactivity of alkylating agents expressed as the Swain-Scott s factor*[a]

Agent	s	Ratio O-6:N-7 alkylation of DNA guanine
MMS	0.83	0.004
EMS	0.67	0.03
MNUA	0.42	0.1
MNNG	0.42	0.1
ENUA	0.26	0.7

[a] Detailed references to the sources of these data are given in Lawley (1974), except for s of MNNG (Osterman-Golkar, 1974) and ethylation of DNA by ENUA (Lawley and Warren, 1975).

with, that from MNUA, supporting the view that DMN methylates through the $CH_3N_2^+$ species (O'Connor et al., 1973; Craddock, 1973).

CORRELATIONS BETWEEN MODE OF ALKYLATION OF DNA AND MUTAGENIC EFFECTS OF ALKYLATING AGENTS

An important reason for studying the series of alkylating carcinogens listed in Table 1 follows from the work of Loveless (1969) and Loveless and Hampton (1969). It showed that the ability of alkylating agents to react with deoxyguanosine at the extranuclear O-6 atom (see Fig. 1) was positively correlated with the ability to induce mutation in T2 bacteriophage by extracellular alkylation.

Krieg (1963) had previously suggested that the mechanism of alkylation-induced mutagenesis in this type of system principally involved miscoding of alkylated guanine in DNA. A possible reason suggested at the time was that, in the main alkylated deoxyribonucleoside residue, 7-alkyldeoxyguanosine, the proton attached to the N-1 atom ionized more readily than in deoxyguanosine. The ionized form could then be envisaged to miscode with thymine (Lawley and Brookes, 1961). This mechanism was unsatisfactory because of the observed lack of correlation between alkylation at N-7 of guanine and mutagenesis.

But, the required anomalous tautomeric form of guanine lacking the —NH— group at N-1 is "fixed" by alkylation at O-6 (Fig. 1), and therefore O^6-alkylguanines are expected to be miscoding residues in the Watson-Crick sense. Studies with poly (O^6-methylguanylic acid) templates provided direct support for this concept (Gerchman and Ludlum, 1973).

It should be noted that mutagenesis resulting from direct miscoding of

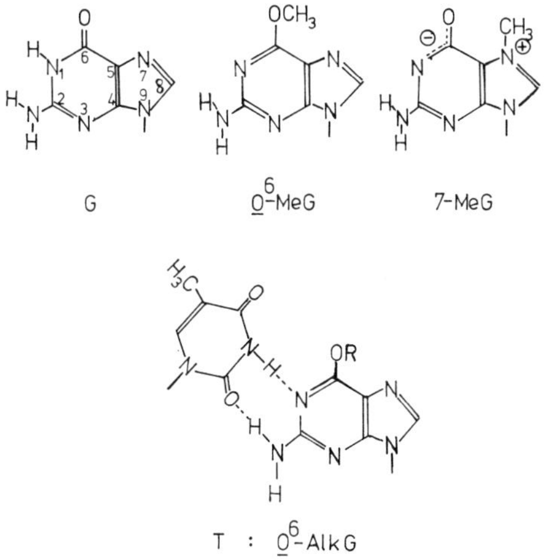

FIG. 1. Guanine, O^6-methylguanine, and 7-methylguanine residues in DNA. Miscoding of O^6-alkylguanine.

alkylated bases in DNA is not the only mechanism of alkylation mutagenesis. For example, in *Escherichia coli,* although the *O*-alkylating mutagens (in the sense defined here) are more efficient as inducers of GC→AT transition mutations, errors in base-pairing can follow from "error-prone" repair of alkylated DNA (cf. Lawley, 1974). Thus, in *E. coli* reversions, provided the *exr* repair pathway is available, MMS can be mutagenic through base-pairing errors during repair, for which the stimulus is indicated to be, for both MMS and X-rays, the induction of single-strand breaks in DNA (Bridges et al., 1973). Also, the aralkylating agent 7-bromomethylbenz(*a*)anthracene (7-BrMBA) can be mutagenic in this system; not only is the *exr* function required, but defect in *uvr* function enhances mutagenicity in this case (Venitt and Tarmy, 1972).

Whereas with *E. coli,* induction of single-strand breaks by MMS can lead to mutation, the available evidence from studies of the T4 phage alkylated extracellularly indicates that mutagenesis results from miscoding of alkylated bases, as already noted (cf. Krieg, 1963), with hydrolytic depurination of alkylated bases leading to inactivation of phage (Brookes and Lawley, 1963).

As a beginning to studies relating extent of DNA alkylation with mutagenesis, Lawley and Martin (1975) have correlated ethylation of DNA in T4 rII AP 72 with induced reversion, believed to involve GC→AT transition at a single site (Krieg, 1963). On the assumption that ethylations are random, it was calculated that ethylation of a specific guanine base in phage DNA at O-6 would correspond to a rate of induced reversion of approximately one-third.

Analogous studies relating extent of alkylation of DNA and mutagenesis have been started using the system of induction of azaguanine resistance in V79 Chinese hamster cells (Roberts et al., 1971; Roberts and Sturrock, 1973; Roberts and Ward, 1973; Roberts et al., 1974; Fox, 1975). Here no obvious correlations between O-alkylation and mutagenesis emerged. For MMS, MNUA, MNNG, and X-rays, the induced mutation frequencies at 10% survival of cells were all around 10^{-3}, and the overall extents of methylation of DNA were very similar for all three methylating agents (Roberts et al., 1974; Fox, 1975).

It was concluded by Roberts et al. (1974) that the major cause of mutation was "inadequate repair of secondary damage introduced during replication of DNA on a methylated DNA template." This type of mechanism also appeared to be involved in mutagenesis in V79 by 7-BrMBA (Duncan and Brookes, 1973).

Some correlation with O-alkylation of DNA was discerned, however, in that the human tumor cell line HeLa was markedly more sensitive to the cytotoxic action of MNUA and MNNG than to that of MMS. This was ascribed to the absence in HeLa of a caffeine-sensitive, post-replicative repair system, which was operative in V79 cells (Roberts and Ward, 1973).

ALKYLATION OF DNA AND "EXCISION REPAIR" PHENOMENA

Another relevant aspect of the consequences of O-alkylation of DNA *in vivo* concerns the specific removal of alkylated purines from DNA. It is well established that the principal alkylated bases, 7-alkylguanine and 3-alkyladenine, are lost relatively slowly from alkylated DNA by spontaneous hydrolysis of the N-glycosidic linkages to the macromolecular chain. Thus, the half-life of 7-methylguanine in DNA at neutral pH and 37°C is about 150 hr and that of 3-methyladenine about 30 hr (Lawley and Brookes, 1963). As noted, this could contribute to the toxic action of monofunctional alkylating agents, and furthermore could be a source of single-strand breaks in DNA.

But, the possibility that such depurinations could be enzymatically mediated was raised by the observations of Lawley and Orr (1970) on specific losses of methylpurines from DNA of E. coli treated with MNNG. The rate of loss of 3-methyladenine in growing cultures was much more rapid than *in vitro*, and furthermore, O^6-methylguanine, a base stable to hydrolysis from DNA, was removed within about a generation time.

Subsequently, Kirtikar and Goldthwait (1974) found that the enzyme endonuclease II (or another enzyme coisolated with this) could remove 3-methyladenine and O^6-methylguanine from MNUA-alkylated DNA.

Several reports of analogous specific removals of methylated bases from carcinogen-methylated DNA *in vivo* have appeared in the last few years [see, for example, O'Connor et al. (1973), for rat liver using DMN]. A notable point of interest is that tissue-specific differences have emerged in certain cases, particularly for "excision" of O^6-alkylguanine. These differences have been correlated with susceptibility of tissues to carcinogenesis by alkylating agents, in the sense that more susceptible tissues "excise" O^6-alkylguanine relatively less rapidly than less susceptible tissues. For example, in rat brain, the rate of excision of O^6-alkylguanine was less than for liver, following administration of MNUA (Kleihues and Margison, 1974) or ENUA (Goth and Rajewsky, 1974). For kidney of rats treated with DMN, removal of O^6-methylguanine was more rapid at a low dose (2.5 mg/kg DMN) than at a higher dose (20 mg/kg) (Magee et al., 1975). The possible significance of these findings is that O^6-alkylguanine residues must persist in cellular DNA through the replication of DNA, in order to induce transition mutations (Lawley and Orr, 1970) possibly essential for tumor initiation.

It should be noted here that the "excision" of alkylated bases by the depurination pathway would involve an enzyme different from that associated with excision repair of uv-induced thymine dimers. It is possible that the depurination pathway is the starting point of that type of repair denoted "short, ionizing-radiation type" by Regan and Setlow (1974).

The methylating and ethylating agents considered here would thus differ from aralkylating agents, such as 7-BrMBA, which attach relatively large aralkyl groups at the extranuclear amino groups of DNA bases (Dipple et al., 1971) and evoke a *uvr*-type repair response in *E. coli* (Venitt and Tarmy, 1972).

CORRELATIONS BETWEEN MODE OF ALKYLATION OF DNA AND INDUCTION OF THYMOMA IN MICE

Empirical correlations between the ability to induce O^6-alkylguanine in DNA of target organs and the carcinogenic potency of alkylating agents can be discerned in several instances. For example, the order of carcinogenic potency of alkylating carcinogens in rat kidney was found to be MNUA > EMS > MMS (Swann and Magee, 1969). Frei (1971) found that the same order of potency applied to induction of thymic lymphoma and pulmonary adenoma in Swiss mice.

More recently, in collaboration with Dr. Frei, correlations between DNA alkylation and thymoma induction have begun to be studied in more detail in C57B1 mice. Some relevant data are reported in Table 2. At the time of writing, studies of dose-response with respect to either alkylation of DNA or tumor induction are incomplete, but some correlations are already apparent. The response of C57B1 mice has so far been found to be closely similar to that of CFW/D mice (Joshi and Frei, 1971). The lack of carcinogenic activity of MMS following a single intraperitoneal injection at doses of up to 1.2 mmol/kg (i.e., about 75% of the LD_{50} dose) observed for Swiss mice of the CFW/D strain (Frei, 1971) has been confirmed for C57B1 mice. The extent of alkylation of DNA achieved in thymus was 110 μmole 7-methylguanine/mole DNA-P at about 2 hr after injection of MMS at 1.0 mmole/kg. The extent of alkylation at O-6 of guanine was expected to be small, and in order to detect this, DNA from pooled organs of single mice injected with $[^{14}C]$MMS at relatively high specific radioactivity was analyzed. It was shown that in the DNA from various organs the extents of alkylation were closely similar for MMS. The value of 0.2 μmole O^6-methylguanine/mole DNA-P quoted in Table 2 is therefore based on the assumption that DNA of thymus was methylated at this position by MMS to the same relative extent as that in other organs.

With MNUA at 0.8 mmole/kg (about 60% of the LD_{50}), the corresponding extents of alkylation were somewhat higher for 7-methylguanine but were about 90-fold higher for O^6-methylguanine. This dose yielded thymomas in over 80% of a group of 30 mice in less than 250 days, whereas no tumors

TABLE 2. Comparison of X-rays and alkylating agents based on ability to induce thymoma in mice (C57B1) by a single treatment

Agent	Dose (mmole/kg)	Mice with tumors (%)	Extent of alkylation of DNA of thymus (μmole/mol DNA-P)[a]		References[b]
			7-Alkylguanine	O^6-Alkylguanine	
MMS	1.0	0	110	($\sim$0.2)	1
MNUA	0.4	37	($\sim$77)	($\sim$9)	2
	0.8	83	154	18	
MNNG	0.4	0	5	($\sim$0.5)	3
EMS	3.2	17	n.d.	n.d.	4
ENUA	0.5	n.d.	1.9	1.1	4
	2.0	43	($\sim$8)	($\sim$4)	
X-rays	400–500 rad	40	—	—	5

[a] Alkylating agents were administered by a single intraperitoneal injection in saline into 8-week-old female mice of about 20 g body weight. The values in parentheses for extents of alkylation are derived from measurements at dose levels other than those quoted on the assumption of a linear relationship between alkylation and dose; 1 μmole/mole DNA-P corresponds to about 2×10^4 alkylations in the DNA of a mouse cell; n.d., not determined.

[b] Key to references: 1, Maitra and Frei (1975); Frei and Lawley (unpublished data); 2, Frei and Lawley (1975); 3, Frei and Joshi (1974; unpublished data); 4, Frei and Lawley (unpublished data); 5, Kaplan and Brown (1952).

appeared in controls up to this time. The extent of methylation at O-6 of DNA guanine was maintained for up to 18 hr after injection in thymus, bone marrow, liver, and various other organs and the rate of "excision" of the base in the mice was evidently slower than that found in rat liver, but the dose dependence of this rate has yet to be investigated.

In order to obtain approximately 40% yield of tumors, the dose of ENUA required is about five times that of MNUA expressed as millimoles per kilogram. The extents of alkylation quoted in Table 2 are based on extrapolation from values determined at a lower dose level on the assumption of a linear dose-alkylation relationship and require confirmation at the carcinogenic dose. But, the higher ratio of O-6:N-7 alkylation of DNA guanine found for ENUA *in vitro* is also observed *in vivo,* and for this agent the extent of alkylation at N-7 of guanine in DNA will clearly be much lower at the carcinogenic dose than for MNUA. The extent of ethylation of O-6 of guanine is of the same order as that found for MNUA or perhaps somewhat lower.

The results for alkylation of DNA in various organs of mice [Frei and Lawley (1975) for MNUA] showed that similar overall extents were achieved in thymus and bone marrow and rather higher extents in liver and small bowel, with kidney, spleen, and lung intermediate. Similar distributions emerged for MMS and ENUA. But, MNNG appeared distinctive in that the DNA of thymus was methylated to a significantly lower extent than the other organs, and MNNG was also anomalous in the sense that, despite its ability to methylate O-6 of guanine in DNA *in vitro* to the same relative extent as MNUA (see Lawley, 1974), it did not yield thymomas at 0.4 mmole/kg (about 80% of the LD_{50}) (Frei and Joshi, 1974). The methylation data are therefore consistent with the concept that the thymus is the target organ in thymoma induction.

This may be too simple a view, however, since Frei and Maitra (1974) have deduced that degeneration and regeneration of both bone marrow and thymus are essential for thymoma development. Dexter et al. (1974) have deduced that the target cell for MNUA in leukemogenesis in C57B1 × DBA/2 F1 mice is the T lymphocyte, and that in this respect, this chemical carcinogen resembles X-rays.

With regard to comparisons between the chemical agents and radiation, the lack of carcinogenic effect of MMS in this system might seem at first sight rather surprising, because, as noted, MMS appears to resemble X-rays in its mutagenic effect in both *E. coli* and cultured mammalian cells, in which both agents appear to induce mutations through errors in DNA repair. The comparative carcinogenicity of the alkylating agents in this series is evidently of the same order as their mutagenic action as inducers of transition mutations in phage. This suggests, therefore, that initiation of thymomas may involve mutation by miscoding of alkylated bases, such as O^6-alkylguanines.

But, it may be questioned whether analogous miscoding of X-ray-induced modified bases could occur.

As noted by Frei (1971), induction of pulmonary adenomas in the Swiss mice also correlated positively with the ability of agents to yield O^6-alkylguanine in DNA. Taken in conjunction with the analogous correlations for tumor induction at certain sites in the rat, as already mentioned, the order of carcinogenic potency of this group of compounds seems to apply in several test systems. But, in the production of sarcoma at the site of injection in BD rats, Druckrey et al. (1970) found that MMS and DMS were moderately active, and not much less potent than diethyl sulfate. Alkylation of DNA does not appear to have been studied in this system, but it seems possible that the correlation with O^6-alkylation of guanine with induction of sarcoma might not be as marked as in the other systems mentioned. It should also be noted that certain aralkylating agents, such as 7-BrMBA, which react with DNA *in vitro* and *in vivo* in mouse skin (Rayman and Dipple, 1973) at extranuclear N-atoms of DNA, are fairly potent carcinogens, both as initiators of papilloma in mouse skin (Dipple and Slade, 1970) and as inducers of sarcoma at the site of injection in the rat. Here, then, reaction at the extranuclear O-atom of guanine in DNA is clearly not required for carcinogenesis by aralkylating agents, and it is difficult to envisage directly induced miscoding by these agents, although, as noted, they are mutagenic, both in *E. coli* and V79 hamster cells.

SUMMARY

A series of alkylating agents was classified in terms of increasing relative ability to react at O-atom sites in DNA, MMS < EMS < MNUA < ENUA. This is the order of increasing ability to induce reversion mutations, probably GC→AT transitions, in phage T4, which could accord with the concept that O^6-alkylguanines are directly miscoding bases.

This series of agents was also used in a study of comparative carcinogenicity with respect to induction of thymic lymphoma in mice, a system in which X-irradiation yields tumors. A positive correlation between ability of agents to alkylate O-6 of guanine in DNA of thymus and carcinogenic potency was found. Although MMS was not active in this system, it was noted that it can induce tumors in other systems.

The relationship between repair of alkylation and radiation induced damage in DNA was briefly discussed. The methylating agents induce single-strand breaks in DNA, and the principal repair system appears to fall into the category of "short" repair as denoted by Regan and Setlow (1974). These single-strand breaks may result from spontaneous hydrolytic depurinations of 3- and 7-methylpurines, or from enzymatic depurinations, e.g., of 3-alkyladenine and O^6-alkylguanine. Aralkylating agents, which are also carcinogens, can evoke an alternative repair response of the *uvr* type.

ACKNOWLEDGMENTS

Work from the Chester Beatty Research Institute, Institute of Cancer Research reported here was supported by grants from the Medical Research Council and the Cancer Research Campaign.

REFERENCES

Bridges, B. A., Mottershead, R. P., Green, M. H. L., and Gray, W. J. H. (1973): Mutagenicity of dichlorvos and MMS for *E. coli* WP2 and some derivatives deficient in DNA repair. *Mutat. Res.,* 19:295.

Brookes, P., and Lawley, P. D. (1963): Effects of alkylating agents on T2 and T4 bacteriophages. *Biochem. J.,* 89:138.

Craddock, V. M. (1973): Pattern of methylated purines formed in DNA of intact and regenerating liver of rats treated with the carcinogen DMN. *Biochim. Biophys. Acta,* 312:202.

Dexter, T. M., Schofield, R., Lajtha, L. G., and Moore, M. (1974): Studies on the mechanism of chemical leukemogenesis. *Br. J. Cancer,* 30:1525.

Dipple, A., and Slade, T. A. (1970): Structure and activity in chemical carcinogenesis: Reactivity and carcinogenicity of 7-BrMBA and 7-BrM-12MBA. *Eur. J. Cancer,* 6:417.

Dipple, A., Brookes, P., Mackintosh, D. S., and Rayman, M. P. (1971): Reaction of 7-BrMBA with nucleic acids, polynucleotides and nucleosides. *Biochemistry,* 10:4323.

Druckrey, H., Kruse, H., Preussmann, R., Ivankovic, S., and Landschütz, C. (1970): Cancerogene alkylierende Substanzen. III. Alkyhalogenide, -sulfate, -sulfonate und ringgespannte Heterocyclen. *Z. Krebsforsch.,* 74:241.

Duncan, M. E., and Brookes, P. (1973): Induction of azaguanine-resistant mutants in cultured Chinese hamster cells by reactive derivatives of carcinogenic hydrocarbons. *Mutat. Res.,* 21:107.

Fox, M. (1975): Factors affecting the quantitation of dose response curves for mutation induction in V79 Chinese hamster cells after exposure to chemical and physical mutagens. *Mutat. Res. (In press.)*

Frei, J. V. (1971): Tumor induction by low molecular weight alkylating agents. *Chem. Biol. Interact.,* 3:117.

Frei, J. V., and Joshi, V. V. (1974): Lack of induction of thymomas and pulmonary adenomas in inbred Swiss mice by MNNG. *Chem. Biol. Interact.,* 8:131.

Frei, J. V., and Lawley, P. D. (1975): Methylation of DNA in various organs of C57B1 mice by a carcinogenic dose of MNUA and stability of some methylation product up to 18 hours. *Chem. Biol. Interact., (In press.)*

Frei, J. V., and Maitra, S. C. (1974): Bone marrow and thymus regeneration is a condition for thymoma development. *Chem. Biol. Interact.,* 9:65.

Gerchman, L., and Ludlum, D. B. (1973): Properties of O^6-methylguanine in template for RNA polymerase. *Biochim. Biophys. Acta,* 308:310.

Goth, R., and Rajewsky, M. F. (1974): Peristence of O^6-ethylguanine in rat brain DNA: Correlation with nervous system-specific carcinogenesis by ENUA. *Proc. Natl. Acad. Sci. USA,* 71:639.

Joshi, V. V., and Frei, J. V. (1971): Effects of dose and schedule of MNUA on incidence of malignant lymphoma in adult female mice. *J. Natl. Cancer Inst.,* 45:335.

Kaplan, H. S., and Brown, M. B. (1952): Quantitative dose-response study of lymphoid-tumor development in irradiated C57 black mice. *J. Natl. Cancer Inst.,* 13:185.

Kirtikar, D. M., and Goldthwait, D. A. (1974): Enzymatic release of O^6-methylguanine and 3-methyladenine from DNA reacted with the carcinogen MNUA. *Proc. Natl. Acad. Sci. USA,* 71:2022.

Kleihues, P., and Margison, G. P. (1974): Carcinogenicity of MNUA; possible role of excision repair of O^6-methylguanine from DNA. *J. Natl. Cancer Inst.,* 53:1839.

Krieg, D. R. (1963): Specificity of chemical mutagenesis. *Prog. Nucleic Acid Res. Mol. Biol.,* 2:125.

Lawley, P. D. (1974): Some chemical aspects of dose-response relationships in alkylation mutagenesis. *Mutat. Res.*, 23:283.

Lawley, P. D. (1975): Carcinogenesis by alkylating agents. In: *Chemical Carcinogenesis*, edited by C. E. Searle, American Chemical Society, Washington D.C. (*In press.*)

Lawley, P. D., and Brookes, P. (1961): Acidic dissociation of 7:9-dialkylguanines and its possible relation to mutagenic properties of alkylating agents. *Nature*, 192:1081.

Lawley, P. D., and Brookes, P. (1963): Further studies on the alkylation of DNA and its constituent nucleotides. *Biochem. J.*, 89:127.

Lawley, P. D., and Martin, C. N. (1975): Molecular mechanisms in alkylation mutagenesis. Induced reversion of bacteriophage T4rII AP72 in relation to extent and mode of ethylation of purines in bacteriophage DNA. *Biochem. J.*, 145:85.

Lawley, P. D., and Orr, D. J. (1970): Specific excision of methylation products from DNA *E. coli* treated with MNNG. *Chem. Biol. Interact.*, 2:154.

Lawley, P. D., and Warren, W. (1975): Specific excision of ethylated purines from DNA of *E. coli* treated with ENUA. *Chem. Biol. Interact.*, (*In press.*)

Loveless, A. (1969): Possible relevance of O-6 alkylation of deoxyguanosine to mutagenicity of nitrosamines and nitrosamides. *Nature*, 223:206.

Loveless, A., and Hampton, C. L. (1969): Inactivation and mutation of coliphage T2 by MNUA and ENUA. *Mutat. Res.*, 7:1.

Magee, P. N., Nicoll, J. W., Pegg, A. E., and Swann, P. F. (1975): Alkylating intermediates in nitrosamine metabolism. *Trans. Biochem. Soc.*, 3:62.

Maitra, S. C., and Frei, J. V. (1975): Organ-specific effects of DNA methylation in the inbred Swiss mouse. *Chem. Biol. Interact.*, 10:285.

O'Connor, P. J., Capps, M. J., and Craig, A. W. (1973): Comparative studies of the hepatocarcinogen *N,N*-dimethylnitrosamine *in vivo:* Reaction sites in rat liver DNA and significance of their relative stabilities. *Br. J. Cancer*, 27:153.

Osterman-Golkar, S. (1974): Reaction kinetics of MNNG and ENNG. *Mutat. Res.*, 24:219.

Rayman, M. P., and Dipple, A. (1973): Structure and activity in chemical carcinogenesis: comparison of reactions of 7-BrMBA and 7-Br-12MBA with mouse skin DNA *in vivo. Biochemistry*, 12:1538.

Regan, J. D., and Setlow, R. B. (1974): Two forms of repair in DNA of human cells damaged by chemical carcinogens and mutagens. *Cancer Res.*, 34:3318.

Roberts, J. J., and Sturrock, J. E. (1973): Enhancement by caffeine of MNUA-induced mutations and chromosome aberrations in Chinese hamster cells. *Mutat. Res.*, 20:243.

Roberts, J. J., and Ward, K. N. (1973): Inhibition of post-replication repair of alkylated DNA by caffeine in Chinese hamster cells but not HeLa cells. *Chem. Biol. Interact.*, 7:241.

Roberts, J. J., Pascoe, J. M., Plant, J. E., Sturrock, J. E., and Crathorn, A. R. (1971): Quantitative aspects of repair of alkylated DNA in cultured mammalian cells. Effect on HeLa and Chinese hamster cell survival of alkylation of cellular macromolecules. *Chem. Biol. Interact.*, 3:29.

Roberts, J. J., Sturrock, J. E., and Ward, K. N. (1974): Enhancement by caffeine of alkylation-induced cell death, mutations and chromosomal aberrations in Chinese hamster cells, as result of inhibition of post-replication repair. *Mutat. Res.*, 26:129.

Swann, P. F., and Magee, P. N. (1969): Induction of rat kidney tumors by EMS and nervous tissue tumors by MMS and EMS. *Nature*, 223:947.

Biology of Radiation Carcinogenesis, edited by
J. M. Yuhas, R. W. Tennant, and J. D. Regan.
Raven Press, New York © 1976.

The Base Displacement Model: An Explanation for the Conformational and Functional Changes in Nucleic Acids Modified by Chemical Carcinogens

Dezider Grunberger and I. Bernard Weinstein

Departments of Biochemistry and Medicine, Institute of Cancer Research, Columbia University College of Physicians and Surgeons, New York, New York 10032

There are many types of chemical carcinogens, which differ in their structure and chemical reactivity (Miller, 1970). It seems that they have only one feature in common, that the ultimate reactive forms of these compounds are electrophilic (Miller and Miller, 1971, 1974).

With the exception of some alkylating agents, which are electrophiles by nature, the majority of chemical carcinogens require metabolic conversion to the activated form. These reactive electrophilic forms of chemical carcinogens can then react with nucleophilic centers in nucleic acids and proteins. This has been demonstrated for *N*-2-acetylaminofluorene (AAF), polycyclic aromatic hydrocarbons, nitrosoamines, aflatoxins, and synthetic as well as naturally occurring carcinogens (Miller, 1970; Heidelberger, 1973).

The covalent binding of a carcinogen to macromolecules raises the problem of structural and functional changes of modified macromolecules. It is not known which of the macromolecules, if any, is the critical target in the process by which the carcinogen converts a normal cell into a tumor cell. We favor the possibility that the nucleic acids, either DNA or RNA, rather than protein, constitute the critical target because of the widespread disturbance in gene expression that accompanies the transformation process.

Therefore, we studied the structural and functional changes that occur in a nucleic acid when a carcinogen is bound to it. For the proper function of a nucleic acid, whether it is DNA or any of the species of RNA, native conformation and structural integrity of the molecule are required. The major factors contributing to the conformation of double-strand nucleic acid molecules are the vertical hydrophobic stacking energy of the neighboring bases, the horizontal hydrogen-bonding between complementary base-pairs, and the electrostatic repulsion of the charged phosphate groups (Ts'o et al., 1963). Interference with any of these factors can impair the structure and proper function of a nucleic acid molecule. The question we asked is whether covalent binding of chemical carcinogens to nucleic acids could produce detectable changes in the physical structure and functional properties of the modified nucleic acids. Most of our studies have been with the potent liver carcinogen AAF. Miller et al. (1966) discovered that both RNA and DNA will react nonenzymatically *in vitro* with the *N*-acetoxy derivative of AAF. The major product obtained from hydrolysates of the modified nucleic acids is 8-(*N*-2-fluorenylacetamido)-guanine (Kriek et al., 1967). The same nucleic acid derivative was obtained if AAF was administered *in vivo* (Miller, 1970).

EFFECT OF AAF MODIFICATION OF GUANOSINE RESIDUES ON BASE-PAIRING

Although the C-8 position of G in nucleic acids is not involved directly in base-pairing with the complementary C residues, it was of interest to determine if G residues modified in the C-8 position with AAF could function normally in systems in which base-pairing takes place.

A direct approach was to employ the method of complementary oligonucleotide binding to transfer RNA (tRNA) as measured by equilibrium dialysis (Uhlenbeck, 1972). Previous studies had established that the single-strand portion of dihydrouracil (D) loop of tRNA is accessible for binding with complementary trinucleotides. Furthermore, as we will see later, we have shown that the same region of the D loop of certain tRNAs is exposed for binding of AAF. We have reacted *N*-acetoxy-AAF with either phenylalanine tRNA from yeast or valine tRNA from *Escherichia coli,* as both tRNAs have a common G—G—G sequence in the D loop (Fig. 1) (RajBhandary and Chang, 1968). After binding of AAF to G residues in these tRNAs and isolation of modified molecules, we compared the ability of modified and unmodified molecules to bind the complementary oligomer [³H]C—C—C. The equilibrium dialysis experiment was started by loading a solution of modified or unmodified tRNA on one side and a solution of radioactive oligonucleotide on the other side of a dialysis chamber, and the system was placed

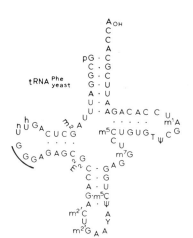

FIG. 1. Primary structure of phenylalanine-tRNA of yeast with underlined G—G—G sequence. The primary structure is taken from RajBhandary and Chang (1968).

at 0°C. Equilibrium had been achieved after 70 hr when the oligomer concentration on each side of the membrane did not change. The molar association constant (K) of C—C—C binding to G—G—G sequence is related to the ratio of [³H]C—C—C counts in the chamber containing the tRNA to the counts in the other chamber by the relation: $R = 1 + K(\text{tRNA})$. The results in Table 1 show that [³H]C—C—C was bound significantly to G—G—G sequences in control Phe-tRNA as well as in control Val-tRNA. On the contrary, there was no binding of [³H]C—C—C to modified tRNA molecules. The lack of binding of [³H]C—C—C to modified G—G—G sequences is most easily interpreted in terms of direct impairment of base-pairing be-

TABLE 1. Binding of [³H]C—C—C to G—G—G sequence in D loop of tRNA

tRNA	Source of tRNA	R	K (M⁻¹)
Val	E. coli	1.13	7263
Val^{AAF}	E. coli	0.99	—
Phe	Yeast	1.11	6330
Phe^{AAF}	Yeast	1.00	—

The equilibrium dialysis was started at 0°C by loading on one side of the chamber a 30 μM solution of tRNA in 100 μl of 0.02 M phosphate buffer, pH 6.9, 0.5 M NaCl, and 0.01 M MgCl₂, and on the other side of the chamber 100 μl of 0.3 μCi of [³H]-C—C—C (final concentration 0.5 μM) in the same buffer. To measure the oligomer concentration at different time intervals, 5-μl samples were withdrawn in triplicate from each side of the chamber, diluted to 100 μl with water, and the radioactivity was measured in a liquid scintillation spectrometer. Equilibrium was reached after 70 hr. The molar association constant (K) of C—C—C binding to G—G—G on the tRNA molecule is related to the ratio (R) of oligomer counts in the chamber containing the tRNA to the counts in the other chamber by the relation: $R = 1 + K[\text{tRNA}]$.

tween modified G and C residues. These results predict that AAF binding to nucleic acids can block the participation of the affected molecules in all processes in which hydrogen-bonding takes place.

EFFECT OF AAF ON TRANSLATION OF SYNTHETIC mRNA

Since in the course of protein synthesis the specificity of translation of messenger RNA (mRNA) depends on base-pairing between complementary bases in the anticodon region of tRNA and the corresponding bases in trinucleotide codons of mRNA (Nirenberg and Leder, 1964), we examined the functional properties of G-containing codons modified with AAF in stimulating the binding of aminoacyl-tRNAs to ribosomes (Grunberger and Weinstein, 1971). The results of these experiments are summarized in Fig. 2.

The effects of modification were twofold: the first effect was that if the G residue to which AAF was covalently bound was part of a codon, then that codon was inactive. This was the case with the Lys codon: AAG, the Val codon: GUU, or the Glu codon: GAA. With these triplets, complete in-activation of their function and no miscoding were observed. The second effect was that if there was an A residue adjacent, either at the 5′ or 3′ side of the modified G, the codon containing the residue was partially impaired in terms of its ability to stimulate ribosomal binding of the corresponding aminoacyl-tRNA (Grunberger et al., 1974). This was observed with the tetramers GAAA and AAAG, when the modification of G residues with the carcinogen led to an approximately 50% reduction of the recognition of the AAA codon by lysyl-tRNA. This inhibition diminished when pentamers

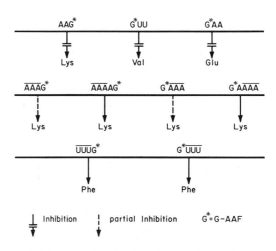

FIG. 2. Effect of AAF modification on codon function.

containing an additional A residue, GAAAA or AAAAG, were modified with AAF, suggesting that the inhibitory effect was limited mainly to the base immediately adjacent to the modified G residue.

In contrast to these effects, the ability of UUU to function as a codon for phenylalanine was not influenced if an AAF-modified G residue was present on either the 5′ or the 3′ side of the UUU triplet (Grunberger et al., 1974).

MECHANISM OF N-HYDROXY-AAF INHIBITION OF RAT LIVER RIBONUCLEIC ACID SYNTHESIS

If the base-pairing ability of modified G residues in oligonucleotides was blocked during translation, then similar effects should be observed during transcription of an AAF-modified DNA template. This possibility was examined by testing the acute effect of N-OH-AAF administration on hepatic nuclear RNA synthesis in rats (Grunberger et al., 1973).

Hepatic nucleolar RNA synthesis was significantly inhibited within 30 min after the injection of N-OH-AAF, and it reached a peak of maximum in-hibition of 90% after 1 hr (Fig. 3). The DNA-dependent RNA polymerase activity then slowly approached normal but, even 48 hr after injection, it was still markedly inhibited. Presumably, the slow restoration of template function was due to excision and repair processes, which replaced modified guanine moieties with their unaltered counterparts.

Using the nucleolar fraction from livers of rats treated with N-OH-AAF, poly [d(A-T)] as an exogenous template, and actinomycin D to inhibit endogenous template functions, we obtained evidence that the inhibitory effect of the carcinogen upon RNA polymerase activity was due to its effect upon

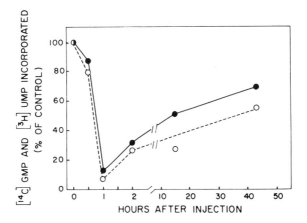

FIG. 3. Time course of the inhibition of liver nucleolar RNA polymerase activity after a single injection of N-hydroxy-2-acetylaminofluorene. (For details see Grunberger et al., 1973). [^{14}C]GMP incorporation (O------O); [^{3}H]UMP incorporation (●———●).

the DNA template and not to the polymerase that transcribed it. Other in-vestigators have interpreted the inhibition of RNA synthesis as due to an effect of AAF on the RNA polymerase enzyme (Zieve, 1972). A result consistent with our conclusion was obtained by Millette and Fink (1975) who found that when AAF-modified phage T7 DNA was used as a template for transcription by E. coli RNA polymerase, initiation of transcription was not inhibited, but chain elongation was arrested at sites of AAF modification, thus resulting in the release of the polymerase enzyme and the appearance of short pieces of the RNA product. Recent cell culture studies indicate that the carcinogen causes preferential inhibition of the transcription of the 45 S ribosomal RNA precursor (Kaplan and Weinstein, unpub.).

CONFORMATIONAL CHANGES IN NUCLEIC ACIDS MODIFIED WITH AAF

We have demonstrated in our experiments with translation and transcrip-tion that covalent binding of AAF to the C-8 position of G residues interfered with the base-pairing between guanosine and cytosine residues. As the C-8 position of G is not directly involved in base-pairing, we assumed that attachment of the bulky AAF molecules to G residues is associated with conformational alterations of the modified nucleic acids.

Molecular model building of oligonucleotides, circular dichroism (CD) and proton magnetic resonance spectra (pmr), and computer-generated molecular models provided evidence that introduction of the carcinogen at the C-8 position of guanosine residues resulted in dramatic conformational changes in the modified oligonucleotides (Grunberger et al., 1970; Nelson et al., 1971). On the basis of analyses of the conformational properties of AAF-containing dinucleoside monophosphates, we proposed a specific, three-dimensional conformation, which we have called the "base displacement model" (Levine et al., 1974; Weinstein and Grunberger, 1974).

THE BASE DISPLACEMENT MODEL

In nucleic acids with Watson-Crick geometry, the sugar residues occupy a position with respect to the base residue referred to as "anti." In this conformation, there is considerable crowding at the C-8 position of purine residues. Therefore, the attachment of the bulky AAF residue requires rotation of the guanine moiety about the glycosidic bond (N_9-C_1) to a position referred to as "syn." Similar conclusions were reached by Kapuler and Michelson (1971) and Tavale and Sobell (1970), based on studies with guanosine residues modified by either Br or AAF at the C-8 position. Computer display studies, CD and pmr data obtained with AAF-modified oligonucleotides suggested additional conformational changes (Nelson et al., 1971). This structure is depicted in Fig. 4. In addition to the "anti" to "syn" change, the modified guanine residue is displaced from its normal coplanar relation with adjacent bases. The fluorene residue occupies the former position of the displaced guanine, and the fluorene is therefore stacked coplanar to an adjacent base. Results obtained by Fuchs and Daune (1972, 1974) and by our group (Levine et al., 1974; Weinstein and Grunberger, 1974) on the physical properties of AAF-modified native DNA suggest that similar conformational changes occur when the carcinogen attacks DNA. In contrast, when DNA was modified with an AAF derivative containing an iodine residue on the fluorene ring, these conformational changes were not observed, since the bulky iodine substituent would be expected to hinder insertion of the fluorene residue into the helix (Fuchs and Daune, 1973).

The conformational changes induced in nucleic acids by AAF modification and described in the base displacement model explain the mechanism by which AAF binding to G residues prevents the base-pairing of the modified bases, since they are displaced from their usual alignment with adjacent bases. Furthermore, this model could explain why we observed decreased base-pairing capacity of adenosine and not of uridine residues,

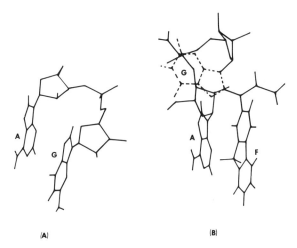

(A)   (B)

FIG. 4. Computer display of three-dimensional structures of ApG and ApG$_{AAF}$. A: The conformation of ApG with Watson-Crick type geometry. B: The base displacement model of ApG$_{AAF}$. The fluorene and adenine rings are stacked, and the displaced guanosine in syn conformation is represented by dashed lines.

adjacent to the modified guanosine residues, since our CD data indicated that the stacking interaction of a fluorene residue is much stronger with an adjacent A than with an adjacent U residue (Grunberger et al., 1974).

MODIFICATION OF SINGLE-STRAND REGIONS OF tRNA

According to the base displacement model, attachment of AAF to G residues requires rotation of the base about the glycosidic bond. Because there is less hindrance to the rotation of bases in single-strand than in double-strand regions, we could predict that G residues in single-strand regions will be more accessible to modification. The tRNAs are convenient molecules with which to test this possibility, since they have known sequences consisting of both single-strand or "loop" regions and double-strand or "stem" regions (Cramer, 1971). We found that when formyl-methionine tRNA from *E. coli,* which contains 25 G residues, was reacted with [^{14}C]acetoxy AAF, the carcinogen was bound only to the G residue at position 20 in the single-strand D loop (Fujimura et al., 1972). Similar results were obtained with AAF modification of yeast tyrosine tRNA (Pulkrabek et al., 1974). In the latter case, AAF was bound to two G residues in the D loop and also to a G residue present in the anticodon loop of this tRNA. If the modification of tyrosine tRNA was performed in the absence of Mg^{2+} and in the presence of EDTA, AAF also attacked the G-15 residue in the D loop, presumably because under these ionic conditions this region of the molecule is denatured (Fig. 5). Recent X-ray crystallography studies with yeast phenylalanine tRNA have provided information concerning the tertiary structure of tRNA molecules, which is entirely consistent with our results. According to these studies, G-20 in the D loop and bases in the anticodon loop of phenylalanine are in single-strand regions exposed on the exterior of the molecule (Kim et al., 1973; Robertus et al., 1974).

The above results with tRNA, as well as separate studies with DNA (Levine et al., 1974), confirmed the predictions of the base displacement model that single-strand regions of nucleic acid should be more susceptible to the attack by the carcinogen than double-strand regions. This suggests that *in vivo* regions of the DNA that are undergoing replication or transcription will be more susceptible to the attack by this chemical carcinogen,

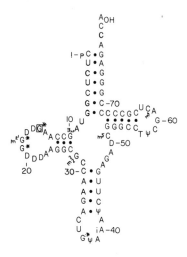

FIG. 5. Primary structure of yeast tyrosine-tRNA with sites of AAF modification. The primary structure of tRNA is taken from Madison et al. (1967). *Sites of AAF modification in the native form. □*Additional sites of modification in the denatured form.

although double-strand regions of DNA might also be susceptible, since a certain amount of cooperative "breathing" of the double-strand helix, which extends over more than one base-pair, does occur (von Hippel and Wong, 1971).

BIOLOGIC IMPLICATIONS

Our results indicate that conformational changes induced in nucleic acids by AAF modification interfere with the normal stacking interactions between neighboring bases and with the base-pairing capacity of the modified G residues. A biologic consequence of these changes is that AAF derivatives should produce frameshift mutations. Ames et al. (1972) have indeed found that, in a *Salmonella typhimurium* system, AAF derivatives are potent frameshift mutagens, as are several other planar polycyclic aromatic compounds. Frameshift mutations result from additions or deletions of one or more nucleotides from the daughter strand of DNA during its replication.

A hypothetical scheme for the mechanism of the frameshift and other types of mutations induced by AAF derivatives is depicted in Fig. 6. If, during the course of DNA replication, the replicating mechanism encounters an AAF-modified G residue on the template or (+) strand, it might simply skip that residue and then continue copying the (+) strand. This would lead to a frameshift mutation. If, instead, the replication mechanism randomly inserts a base at the site of AAF modification, this could cause a base-pair substitution. If AAF modification produces a small loop or bulge defect in the template strand, then the replication mechanism may skip the entire defect, thereby resulting in a small deletion in the daughter strand. Which one of the above processes prevails may depend on the local base sequence at the site of the AAF modification and the response of different polymerases

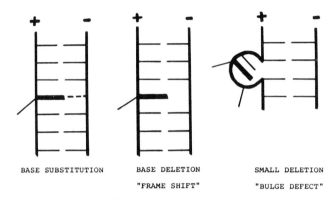

BASE SUBSTITUTION   BASE DELETION   SMALL DELETION

"FRAME SHIFT"   "BULGE DEFECT"

FIG. 6. Schematic representation of types of mutation that might occur as a consequence of the base displacement model. (+) designates a template strand to which the AAF (heavy line) is attached. (−) designates the daughter strand.

and nucleases to the distortion in conformation at the site of AAF modification.

INFERENCES FROM THE STUDY OF CONFORMATIONAL CHANGES TO RADIATION EFFECTS

Two different forms of repair to DNA damaged by radiation have been suggested (Setlow and Carrier, 1964; Painter and Young, 1972). (a) A "short repair" process triggered by ionizing radiation, which causes many single-strand breaks in DNA that are generally quickly repaired, i.e., within 30 to 60 min (Kleijer et al., 1970; Ormerod and Stevens, 1971). (b) A "long repair" process triggered by UV-radiation, which causes the formation of dimers between adjacent pyrimidine residues that are excised by a specific endonuclease. This process is associated with the excision and replacement of 50 to 100 adjacent nucleotides (Regan et al., 1968), and this type of repair takes a longer time, i.e., about 20 hr after irradiation (Regan et al., 1971).

Similar mechanisms were suggested by Regan and Setlow (1974) for the repair of DNA of human cells damaged by chemical carcinogens and mutagens. They have shown in elegant experiments that DNA damage caused by simple alkylating agents (methyl methansulfonate, ethyl methansulfonate, propane sultone) is repaired in a short time, as is the repair of single-strand breaks caused by ionizing radiation. On the other hand, lesions caused by N-acetoxy-AAF take a longer time for repair, and the process resembles the process of UV lesion repair.

Consistent with this interpretation are results obtained with cell cultures established from one form of xeroderma pigmentosum (XP). These cells show greatly reduced long repair induced by either UV-irradiation (Cleaver, 1968) or treatment of the cells with N-acetoxy-AAF (Setlow and Regan, 1972; Stich et al., 1972; Maher et al., 1975). On the other hand, these XP cells have a normal capacity for short repair after exposure to ionizing radiation or simple alkylating agents (Cleaver, 1973). Presumably, AAF (and perhaps other polycyclic carcinogens) and UV-radiation share the process in which marked conformational changes in the DNA are produced; in one case, base displacement occurs, and, in the other case, there are distortions in the symmetry of the DNA helix at regions of pyrimidine dimers. These conformational changes can lead to frameshift mutations if the replication proceeds before they are repaired, or they can be repaired by a common mechanism, which recognizes conformational distortions and excises them.

Although we have described a possible mutagenic mechanism for AAF, we must emphasize that, at present, it is not clear whether chemical carcinogens or radiation cause the conversion of normal to tumor cells by inducing mutations, by activating latent endogenous viruses or enhancing the oncogenicity of exogenous viruses, or by inducing aberrations in differentiation at the epigenetic level (Weinstein et al., 1975). New approaches employing carcinogens and radiation in cell culture systems may reveal how the structural and functional changes in nucleic acids, which we have elucidated, relate to the actual mechanism of chemical and radiation carcinogenesis.

ACKNOWLEDGMENTS

The authors wish to acknowledge the valuable contributions described in this paper made by Drs. Charles Cantor, Louis Katz, James Nelson, and Peter Pulkrabek. This research was supported by USPHS Grant CA-02332. D. G. is a Leukemia Society of America Scholar.

REFERENCES

Ames, B. N., Gurney, E. G., Miller, J. A., and Bartsch, H. (1972): Carcinogens as frameshift mutagens: Metabolites and derivatives of 2-acetylaminofluorene and other aromatic amine carcinogens. *Proc. Natl. Acad. Sci. USA,* 69:3128–3132.

Cleaver, J. E. (1968): Defective repair replication of DNA in xeroderma pigmentosum. *Nature*, 218:652–656.

Cleaver, J. E. (1973): DNA repair with purines and pyrimidines in radiation- and carcinogen-damaged normal and xeroderma pigmentosum human cells. *Cancer Res.*, 33:362–369.

Cramer, F. (1971): Three dimensional structure of tRNA. *Progr. Nucl. Acid Res. Mol. Biol.*, 11:391–421.

Fuchs, R., and Daune, M. (1972): Physical studies on deoxyribonucleic acid after covalent binding of a carcinogen. *Biochim. Biophys. Acta*, 14:2659–2666.

Fuchs, R., and Daune, M. (1973): Physical basis of chemical carcinogenesis by N-2-fluorenylacetamide derivatives and analogs. *FEBS Letters*, 34:295.

Fuchs, R., and Daune, M. (1974): Dynamic structure of DNA modified with the carcinogen *N*-acetoxy-*N*-2-acetylaminofluorene. *Biochemistry*, 13:4435.

Fujimura, S., Grunberger, D., Carvajal, G., and Weinstein, I. B. (1972): Modifications of ribonucleic acid by chemical carcinogens. Modification of *Escherichia coli* formylmethionine transfer ribonucleic acid with N-acetoxy-2-acetylaminofluorene. *Biochemistry*, 11:3629–3635.

Grunberger, D., Blobstein, S. H., and Weinstein, I. B. (1974): Modification of ribonucleic acid by chemical carcinogens. VI. Effect of *N*-2-acetylaminofluorene modification of guanosine on the codon function of adjacent nucleosides in oligonucleotides. *J. Mol. Biol.*, 82:459–468.

Grunberger, D., Nelson, J. H., Cantor, C. R., and Weinstein, I. B. (1970): Coding and conformational properties of oligonucleotides modified with the carcinogen *N*-2-acetylaminofluorene. *Proc. Natl. Acad. Sci. USA*, 66:488–494.

Grunberger, D., and Weinstein, I. B. (1971): Modifications of ribonucleic acid by chemical carcinogens. III. Template activity of polynucleotides modified by *N*-acetoxy-2-acetylaminofluorene. *J. Biol. Chem.*, 246:1123–1128.

Grunberger, G., Yu, F. L., Grunberger, D., and Feigelson, P. (1973): Mechanism of *N*-hydroxy-2-acetylaminofluorene inhibition of rat hepatic ribonucleic acid synthesis. *J. Biol. Chem.*, 248:6278–6281.

Heidelberger, C. (1973): Chemical oncogenesis in culture. *Adv. Cancer Res.*, 18:317.

Hippel, P. H., von, and Wong, K. Y. (1971): Dynamic aspects of native DNA structure: Kinetics of the formaldehyde reaction with calf thymus DNA. *J. Mol. Biol.*, 61:587–613.

Kapuler, A. M., and Michelson, A. M. (1971): The reaction of the carcinogen *N*-acetoxy-2-acetylaminofluorene with DNA and other polynucleotides and its stereochemical implications. *Biochim. Biophys. Acta*, 232:436–450.

Kim, S. H., Quigley, G. J., Suddath, F. L., McPherson, A., Sneden, D., Kim, J. J., Weinzierl, J., and Rich, A. (1973): Three dimensional structure of yeast phenylalanine transfer RNA: Folding of the polynucleotide chain. *Science*, 179:285–288.

Kleijer, W. J., Lohman, P. H. M., Mulder, M. P., and Bootsma, D. (1970): Repair of X-ray damage in DNA of cultivated cells from patients having xeroderma pigmentosum. *Mutat. Res.*, 9:517–523.

Kriek, E., Miller, J. A., Juhl, U., and Miller, E. C. (1967): 8-(N-2-fluorenylacetamide)-guanosine, an arylamidation reaction product of guanosine and the carcinogen *N*-acetoxy-*N*-2-fluorenylacetamide in neutral solution. *Biochemistry*, 6:177–182.

Levine, A. F., Fink, L. M., Weinstein, I. B., and Grunberger, D. (1974): Effect of *N*-2-acetylaminofluorene modification on the conformation of nucleic acids. *Cancer Res.*, 34:319–327.

Madison, J. T., Everett, G. A., and Kung, H. K. (1967): Oligonucleotides from yeast tyrosine transfer ribonucleic acid. *J. Biol. Chem.*, 242:1318–1323.

Maher, V. M., Birch, N., Otto, J. R., and McCormick, J. J. (1975): Cytotoxicity of carcinogenic aromatic amides in normal and xeroderma pigmentosum fibroblasts with different DNA repair capabilities. *J. Natl. Cancer Inst.*, 54:1287.

Miller, E. C., Juhl, U., and Miller, J. A. (1966): Nucleic acid guanine reaction with the carcinogen *N*-acetoxy-2-acetylaminofluorene. *Science*, 153:1125–1127.

Miller, J. A. (1970): Carcinogenesis by chemicals: An overview—G. H. A. Clowes Memorial Lecture. *Cancer Res.*, 30:559–576.

Miller, J. A., and Miller, E. C. (1971): Chemical carcinogenesis: mechanisms and approaches to its control. *J. Natl. Cancer Inst.*, 47:V.

Miller, J. A., and Miller, E. C. (1974): Some current thresholds of research in chemical carcinogenesis. In: *Chemical Carcinogenesis*, edited by P. O. P. Ts'o and J. DiPaolo, pp. 61–85. Marcel Dekker, New York.

Millette, R. C., and Fink, L. M. (1975): The effect of modification of T_7 DNA by the carcinogen *N*-2-acetylaminofluorene: Termination of transcription *in vitro*. *Biochemistry*, 14:1426–1432.

Nelson, J. H., Grunberger, D., Cantor, C. R., and Weinstein, I. B. (1971): Modification of ribonucleic acid by chemical carcinogens. IV. Circular dichroism and proton magnetic resonance studies of oligonucleotides modified with *N*-2-acetylaminofluorene. *J. Mol. Biol.*, 62:331–346.

Nirenberg, M., and Leder, P. (1964): RNA codewords and protein synthesis. *Science*, 145:1399–1407.

Ormerod, M. G., and Stevens, U. (1971): The rejoining of X-ray-induced strand breaks in the DNA of murine lymphoma cell (L5178Y). *Biochim. Biophys. Acta*, 232:72–82.

Painter, R. B., and Young, B. R. (1972): Repair replication in mammalian cells after X-irradiation. *Mutat. Res.*, 14:225–235.

Pulkrabek, P., Grunberger, D., and Weinstein, I. B. (1974): Effects of ionic environment on modification of yeast tyrosine transfer ribonucleic acid with *N*-acetoxy-2-acetylaminofluorene. *Biochemistry*, 13:2414–2419.

RajBhandary, U. L., and Chang, S. H. (1968): Studies on polynucleotides. LXXXII. Yeast phenylalanine transfer ribonucleic acid: Partial digestion with ribonuclease T_1 and derivation of the total primary structure. *J. Biol. Chem.*, 243:598–608.

Regan, J. D., and Setlow, R. B. (1974): Two forms of repair in the DNA of human cells damaged by chemical carcinogens and mutagens. *Cancer Res.*, 34:3318–3325.

Regan, J. D., Setlow, R. B., and Ley, R. D. (1971): Normal and defective repair of damaged DNA in human cells: A sensitivity assay utilizing the photolysis of bromo-deoxyuridine. *Proc. Natl. Acad. Sci. USA*, 68:708–712.

Regan, J. D., Trosko, J. E., and Carrier, W. L. (1968): Evidence for excision of ultraviolet-induced pyrimidine dimers from the DNA of human cells *in vitro*. *Biophys. J.*, 8:319–325.

Robertus, J. D., Ladner, J. E., Finch, J. T., Rhodes, D., Brown, R. S., Clark, B. F. C., and Klug, A. (1974): Structure of yeast phenylalanine tRNA at 3 Å resolution. *Nature*, 250:546–551.

Setlow, R. B., and Carrier, W. L. (1964): The disappearance of thymine dimers from deoxyribonucleic acid (DNA): An error-correcting mechanism. *Proc. Natl. Acad. Sci. USA*, 51:226–231.

Setlow, R. B., and Regan, J. D. (1972): Defective repair of *N*-acetoxy-2-acetylaminofluorene induced lesions in the DNA of xeroderma pigmentosum cells. *Biochem. Biophys. Res. Commun.*, 46:1019–1024.

Stich, H. F., San., R. H. C., Miller, J. A., and Miller, E. C. (1972): Various levels of DNA repair synthesis in xeroderma pigmentosum cells exposed to the carcinogens *N*-hydroxy- and *N*-acetoxy-2-acetylaminofluorene. *Nature [New Biol.]*, 238:9–10.

Tavale, S. S., and Sobell, H. M. (1970): Crystal and molecular structure of 8-bromoguanosine and 8-bromoadenosine, two purine nucleosides in the Syn configuration. *J. Mol. Biol.*, 48:109.

Troll, W., Belman, L., Berkowitz, E., Chmielewicz, Z. F., Ambrus, J. L., and Bardos, T. J. (1968): Differential responses of DNA and RNA caused by action of the carcinogen acetylaminofluorene *in vivo* and *in vitro*. *Biochim. Biophys. Acta*, 157:16–24.

Ts'o, P. O. P., Lesko, S. A., and Umans, R. S. (1963): The physical binding and the chemical linkage of benzpyrene to nucleotides, nucleic acids and nucleohistones. In: *The Jerusalem Symposium on Quantum Chemistry and Biochemistry. I. Physicochemical Mechanisms of Carcinogenesis*, edited by D. Bergmann and B. Pullman, pp. 106–135. Jerusalem, Israel.

Uhlenbeck, D. C. (1972): Complementary oligonucleotide binding to transfer RNA. *J. Mol. Biol.*, 65:25–41.

Weinstein, I. B., and Grunberger, D. (1974): Structural and functional changes in nucleic acids modified by chemical carcinogens. In: *Chemical Carcinogenesis,* edited by P. O. P. Ts'o and J. DiPaolo, pp. 217–235, Part A, Marcel Dekker, New York.

Weinstein, I. B., Yamaguchi, N., and Gebert, R. (1975): Use of epithelial cell cultures for studies on the mechanism of transformation by chemical carcinogens. *In Vitro,* 2:130–141.

Zieve, F. J. (1972): Inhibition of rat liver RNA polymerase by the carcinogen N-hydroxy-2-fluorenylacetamide. *J. Biol. Chem.,* 247:5987–5995.

Biology of Radiation Carcinogenesis, edited by
J. M. Yuhas, R. W. Tennant, and J. D. Regan.
Raven Press, New York © 1976.

Regulatory Genes Influencing the Response to Endogenous Leukemia Viruses

Frank Lilly

Department of Genetics, Albert Einstein College of Medicine, Bronx, New York 10461

When F_1 hybrids are produced by crossing mice of the high leukemia AKR strain with mice of various low leukemia inbred strains, the incidence of the spontaneous disease among the progeny is, in a few cases, moderate to high, but in the majority of cases it is quite low or absent. In other words, the expression of the leukemic phenotype of the AKR mouse may be either dominant or recessive, depending on the strain of mice to which it is crossed. This type of observation implies that the disease is influenced by complex genetic mechanisms. Here, I shall analyze the genetic factors governing the leukemic phenotype by reviewing some relevant studies from various laboratories in recent years and by resorting to a simplistic analogy based upon the classical concept of structural versus regulatory genes.

The etiological agent of the spontaneous leukemia of AKR mice has been identified by Gross (1951) as a virus. This virus is a C-type, RNA-containing agent, which is fairly representative of the family of murine leukemia viruses (MuLV). The MuLV strain from AKR mice is present in high titer in the tissues of all AKR mice from soon after birth (Rowe and Pincus, 1972); it is detectable and has been extensively studied by the XC plaque assay *in vitro* (Rowe et al., 1970). The virus is transmitted from parent to offspring in AKR mice by a genetic mechanism (Chattopadhyay et al., 1975). This aspect of the disease is discussed in detail by Dr. Lowy (*this volume*). It is sufficient here to consider that the MuLV genome is chromosomally located. Thus, its inheritance shows Mendelian properties, and it behaves as a dominant initiator of the disease. By a not too farfetched analogy, one might consider it to be the structural gene for the disease.

But, if the etiological agent is transmitted in a dominant Mendelian manner, how then can the disease be recessive in many crosses? The answer must lie in the existence of regulatory genes that are capable of repressing the action of the initiating agent.

The best studied crosses of AKR mice in which leukemia is a dominant trait are those with the C3Hf/Bi and C57BR strains (Aoki et al., 1968; Gross, 1970). Not only is the occurrence of the disease dominant in these hybrids, but also the pattern of early expression of MuLV in their tissues resembles that of the AKR parent (Rowe, 1972). Mice of the C3Hf/Bi and C57BR parental strains show only a low and very late incidence of spontaneous leukemia, but Gross (1970) found them to be by far the most susceptible of the strains tested to leukemogenesis by MuLV from AKR mice. It appears that the genomes of these mice do not include a functionally significant initiator gene for leukemia, but the virus, once introduced into the mice either by genetic means or by inoculation at an early age, is free to replicate and exert its pathological action unhampered by important regulatory genes.

Of the many crosses of AKR with low leukemia mouse strains, in which the disease is recessive, that with BALB/c mice has recently been examined in some detail (Lilly et al., 1975). The F_1 progeny of this cross show very little leukemia (Lilly and Duran-Reynals, 1972), and the occurrence of MuLV is also at a very low level, particularly in the first weeks of life (Rowe and Hartley, 1972). Since it is clear that the MuLV genome has been transmitted from the AKR parent to these hybrids, there must also be present a dominant regulatory gene or genes inherited from the BALB/c parent which is capable of suppressing either the viral genome or expression of the leukemia, or both.

Two such regulatory genes have been demonstrated in this AKR × BALB/c cross. One of these is $Fv-1$ (chromosome 4) and the other is closely associated with the complex $H-2$ region (chromosome 17). In the F_1 × AKR back-cross (low virus, low leukemia hybrid × high virus, high leukemia parental strain), approximately one-half the animals ($N = 335$) showed appreciable levels of MuLV at six weeks of age; those animals that showed no virus had apparently inherited the BALB/c-derived $Fv-1^b$ allele from the hybrid parent. The $Fv-1^b$ allele is capable of suppressing the expression of MuLV of the type (N-tropic) that are found in AKR mice by a mechanism yet to be determined (Lilly and Pincus, 1973). This mechanism, so far, does not appear to affect the expression of the endogenous, chromosomally located viral genome, but it is restrictive for the expression of AKR virus infecting the cell exogenously. Rowe (1973) has discussed this situation in some detail. The endogenous MuLV genome, present in all cells, has the same very low probability of undergoing spontaneous derepression in the cells of both AKR mice and BALB/c × AKR hybrids. Once this release occurs in a single cell, the virus produced can spread freely in AKR mice and infect neighboring cells until every cell of the mouse capable of producing virus is doing so. In the hybrids, however, when an endogenous MuLV genome is spontaneously derepressed in a cell, the virus the cell produces cannot spread to neighboring cells because of the restrictive $Fv-1$ type of these cells; therefore, the animal will show low levels of the virus if it shows any levels.

About one-third of the F_1 × AKR back-cross mice examined developed leukemia, and most of the leukemia (86%) occurred in mice that had been MuLV positive at six weeks of age. Furthermore, mice with high levels of virus showed a high incidence of leukemia, and mice with lower levels of virus showed a lower incidence. It thus seems clear that early virus expression is a major factor in leukemia of AKR mice. When the virus is suppressed by *Fv-1*[b], this condition is not met, and the disease occurs rarely.

The *H-2*-associated gene that influenced the occurrence of leukemia in these studies was seen to be a highly significant determinant of the incidence of the disease in homozygous *H-2*[k]/*H-2*[k] vs. heterozygous *H-2*[d]/*H-2*[k] mice of the back-cross generation. This observation is consistent with earlier observations that *H-2* type exerts a significant effect on susceptibility of mice to leukemogenesis by exogenously administered Gross virus (Lilly, 1970).

Although *H-2* type was correlated with leukemia incidence in these back-cross mice, there was *no* significant correlation between *H-2* type and the occurrence of MuLV. It is evident from this that, whatever the mechanism of *H-2*[d] interference with leukemogenesis, it does not interfere with virus expression. Rather, it appears that the *H-2* region influences the capacity of leukemic cells in mice to grow progressively to cause the death of the host, perhaps by an immunologic mechanism. This conclusion is consistent with the observation that *H-2* type plays no detectable role in the susceptibility of mouse cells *in vitro* to infection by AKR virus (Pincus et al., 1971).

Thus, both *Fv-1* and *H-2* act as dominant repressor genes with respect to leukemogenesis in mice, but they interfere with the pathological effect of the "structural" MuLV genes in completely different ways. It is not unlikely that still other categories of leukemia-repressing genes might remain to be found in other crosses.

In collaboration with Dr. M. L. Duran-Reynals, we are currently investigating another cross with AKR, which shows some promise of yielding another such repressor gene. This cross is AKR × RF/J. Here again, as in the case of AKR × BALB/c, the F_1 progeny show virtually no spontaneous leukemia, implying that a leukemia-repressing gene has been inherited from the RF/J parent. But, incomplete studies to date suggest that the occurrence of AKR virus is not suppressed in these hybrids. This then suggests that the repressor inherited from the RF/J parent does not operate by means of an effect on virus expression. This would clearly distinguish the RF/J repressor gene from *Fv-1*, but it is reminiscent of the effect of the *H-2*-associated gene. But, RF/J mice do not differ from AKR with respect to *H-2* type, so that presumably *H-2* cannot account for the repression of the disease in these hybrids.

Another factor to be considered in this set of observations is that RF/J mice are among those mouse strains that are exquisitely sensitive to the induction of leukemia by the percutaneous application of 3-methylcholanthrene (MCA) (Duran-Reynals and Cook, 1974). This susceptibility to MCA-induced leukemia is dominant in the low leukemia (AKR × RF/J) F_1 hybrids. By contrast, neither BALB/c mice nor (BALB/c × AKR) F_1 hybrids develop leukemia in response to MCA painting; these mice develop skin tumors instead.

These observations have led us to the hypothesis that the RF/J genome must include a leukemia-inducing gene, but this gene is kept largely in check by the simultaneous presence of a repressor gene. This repressor gene is dominant in crosses and is also capable of repressing the leukemia-inducing genes of the AKR genome. The repressor gene is itself susceptible to being suppressed by the action of MCA. This property clearly distinguishes the RF/J repressor from both *Fv-1* and *H-2*, the leukemia-repressing action of which is not abolished by MCA treatment.

If this hypothesis proves correct—that a leukemia-inducing gene of RF/J mice is repressed by another gene the action of which is abolished by a chemical carcinogen—then there is no reason why the hypothesis cannot be extended to encompass radiation leukemogenesis. The latent leukemia inciter of C57BL mice, for example (Lieberman and Kaplan, 1959), might be regulated by a repressor gene the action of which is weakened or abolished by X-irradiation.

This analysis of the genetic factors involved in leukemogenesis has by no means exhausted the varieties of genetic mechanisms that might play a role in the process. On the contrary, a whole new era is beginning, in which the intimate molecular details of the genetic aspects of malignant transformation will gradually be elucidated. Our intention here has been to emphasize the critical role of regulatory genes in the disease process. The day may come when genetic techniques for the control of human leukemia and other analogous diseases can be contemplated. If so, a knowledge of existing leukemia-repressing genes will be the starting point for these efforts.

ACKNOWLEDGMENT

The author's work is supported by a contract within the Virus Cancer Program of the National Cancer Institute.

REFERENCES

Aoki, T., Boyse, E. A., and Old, L. J. (1968): Wild-type Gross leukemia virus. III. Serological tests as indicators of leukemia risk. *J. Natl. Cancer Inst.*, 41:103–110.

Chattopadhyay, S. K., Rowe, W. P., Teich, N. M., and Lowy, D. R. (1975): Definitive evidence that the murine C-type virus-inducing locus *Akv-1* is viral genetic material. *Proc. Natl. Acad. Sci. USA*, 72:906–910.

Duran-Reynals, M. L., and Cook, C. (1974): Resistance to skin tumorigenesis by 3-methylcholanthrene in mice susceptible to leukemia. *J. Natl. Cancer Inst.*, 52:1001–1003.

Gross, L. (1951): "Spontaneous" leukemia developing in C3H mice following inoculation, in infancy, with AK-leukemic extracts, or AK-embryos. *Proc. Soc. Exp. Biol. Med.*, 76:27–32.

Gross, L. (1970): *Oncogenic Viruses*. Pergamon Press, Oxford.

Lieberman, M., and Kaplan, H. S. (1959): Leukemogenic activity of filtrates from radiation-induced lymphoid tumors of mice. *Science*, 130:387–388.

Lilly, F. (1970): The role of genetics in Gross virus leukemogenesis. In: *Comparative*

Leukemia Research 1969, Bibl. haemat., No. 36, edited by R. M. Dutcher, pp. 213–220. Karger, Basel.

Lilly, F., and Duran-Reynals, M. L. (1972): Combined neoplastic effects of vaccinia virus and 3-methylcholanthrene. II. Genetic factors. *J. Natl. Cancer Inst.,* 48:105–112.

Lilly, F., Duran-Reynals, M. L., and Rowe, W. P. (1975): Correlation of early murine leukemia virus titer and *H-2* type with spontaneous leukemia in mice of the BALB/c × AKR cross: A genetic analysis. *J. Exp. Med.,* 141:882–889.

Lilly, F., and Pincus, T. (1973): Genetic control of murine viral leukemogenesis. *Adv. Cancer Res.,* 17:231–277.

Pincus, T., Hartley, J. W., and Rowe, W. P. (1971): A major genetic locus affecting resistance to infection with murine leukemia viruses. I. Tissue culture studies of naturally occurring viruses. *J. Exp. Med.,* 133:1219–1233.

Rowe, W. P. (1972): Studies of genetic transmission of murine leukemia virus by AKR mice. I. Crosses with $Fv-1^n$ strains of mice. *J. Exp. Med.,* 136:1272–1285.

Rowe, W. P. (1973): Genetic factors in the natural history of murine leukemia virus infection— G. H. A. Clowes Memorial Lecture. *Cancer Res.,* 33:3061–3068.

Rowe, W. P., and Hartley, J. W. (1972): Studies of genetic transmission of murine leukemia virus by AKR mice. II. Crosses with $Fv-1^b$ strains of mice. *J. Exp. Med.,* 136:1286–1301.

Rowe, W. P., and Pincus, T. (1972): Quantitative studies of naturally occurring leukemia virus infection of AKR mice. *J. Exp. Med.,* 135:429–436.

Rowe, W. P., Pugh, W. E., and Hartley, J. W. (1970): Plaque assay techniques for murine leukemia viruses. *Virology,* 42:1136–1139.

Biology of Radiation Carcinogenesis, edited by
J. M. Yuhas, R. W. Tennant, and J. D. Regan.
Raven Press, New York © 1976.

The Chromosomal Localization of an Endogenous Murine Leukemia Viral Genome in the AKR Mouse

Douglas R. Lowy,* Sisir K. Chattopadhyay,† and Natalie Teich‡

*Department of Dermatology, Yale University School of Medicine, New Haven, Connecticut 06510; † Laboratory of Viral Diseases, National Institute of Allergy and Infectious Diseases, National Institutes of Health, Bethesda, Maryland 20014; ‡ Imperial Cancer Research Fund, London, England

Since its derivation by Furth et al. (1933), the inbred Ak mouse and its substrain AKR have played a central role in the study of murine leukemia. These mice have a very high incidence of spontaneous thymic lymphoma, which progresses to a fatal lymphoblastic leukemia (see review by Siegler, 1968). Gross (1951a) opened the field of mammalian RNA tumor virology when he demonstrated that cell-free extracts from lymphomatous AKR tissue could induce leukemia in newborn mice of a low leukemic strain. It was quickly recognized that soon after birth all AKR mice are chronically infected with this murine leukemia virus (MLV), which is a C-type RNA virus. This strain has therefore been widely used as a model for the study of spontaneous, virus-associated murine leukemia (reviewed by Gross, 1970).

The origin of the AKR MLV and the means by which the virus induces lymphomas have remained two central questions in understanding the pathogenesis of disease in the AKR mouse. The mechanism of tumor induction remains to be determined (unlike sarcoma viruses, infection by leukemia viruses does not ordinarily induce morphologic transformation of tissue culture cells). But, recent evidence, some of which will be reviewed here, indicates that the AKR MLV genome is part of the normal chromosomal genetic material of AKR cells. Endogenous viral genomes from other mouse strains are probably also chromosomal in location.

On the basis of stable host range differences, several classes of endogenous C-type viruses have recently been identified within the same mouse strain (Aaronson and Stephenson, 1973). Some viruses will not infect mouse fibroblasts exogenously, but will infect certain cells from other species—these viruses have been called "xenotropic" (Levy, 1973). A virus that infects both mouse cells and cells of other species (amphitropic virus) was recently found (J. W. Hartley, *personal communication*). The best studied class of murine C-type viruses are those that infect only mouse cells (mouse-tropic virus); it is these viruses that have been shown to induce lymphomas in susceptible

---

* *Present address:* Dermatology Branch, National Cancer Institute, National Institutes of Health, Bethesda, Maryland 20014.

mice. Within the mouse-tropic group, two host range patterns have been identified; each virus is either N-tropic or B-tropic in that it replicates most efficiently in mouse cells that are $Fv-1^n$ or $Fv-1^b$, respectively. (For a discussion of $Fv-1$, see the contributions by Lilly and by Tennant et al., *this volume*). Here we focus primarily on the classic N-tropic MLV, which is found in high titer in the AKR mouse (AKR MLV). For a broader discussion of C-type viruses, the reader is referred to several recent discussions (Temin, 1971; Rowe, 1973; Tooze, 1973; Cold Spring Harbor Symposium, 1974; Hirsch and Black, 1974; Lowy et al., 1974*b*).

VIRAL ACTIVATION

Gross's early work (1951*b*) had shown that MLV infection did not spread from animal to animal horizontally; instead, it spread vertically, from parent to offspring. Initially, Gross postulated that in the AKR mouse this transmission occurred via productive exogenous infection of the germ cells; low leukemic mice presumably did not contain the virus. In the late 1950s, however, Gross and Kaplan both showed that X-ray exposure of supposedly virus-negative, low leukemic mouse strains resulted in the appearance of virus similar to the AKR MLV followed by a high rate of leukemia (Kaplan, 1967; Gross, 1970). These experiments suggested that some low leukemic mice also contained the MLV genome but in a more repressed form than in AKR. The location and state of the virus could not be clearly defined, however. During the 1960s, additional indirect studies suggested that C-type viral genetic material was present in many, if not all, mouse strains (reviewed by Huebner and Todaro, 1969). In 1970, the important discovery that the virions of C-type viruses contain an RNA-directed DNA polymerase (reverse transcriptase) provided a possible mechanism by which an RNA virus might be present in the cell as DNA genetic material (Temin and Baltimore, 1972).

Our initial studies of the endogenous virus of the AKR mouse were made possible by the development of a quantitative tissue culture assay of infectious mouse-tropic MLV. (Klement et al., 1969; Rowe et al., 1970). If infectious virus could be activated from a virus-negative tissue culture system, it would have been demonstrated that the latent viral genome could be present intracellularly and that latency did not represent merely a low-grade carrier state of infectious virus. Procedures (such as X-irradiation) which activated MLV from low leukemic mice *in vivo*, had not been successful with cells from these same strains in tissue culture. We reasoned that it might be easier to activate MLV from tissue culture cells of a high virus, high leukemic mouse, since its high virus pattern might represent a greater probability of release of MLV.

The major experimental problem was to establish AKR cell cultures that were virus negative. But, it was known that AKR mice rarely become virus positive until late in gestation, and by seeding small numbers of cells from relatively early embryos some cell lines resulted that remained negative for MLV over many passages (Rowe et al., 1971). These mass cultures and several cloned sublines derived from them were then all shown to contain the MLV genome, since infectious virus could readily be activated from them by treatment with 5-iododeoxyuridine (IUdR) or 5-bromodeoxyuridine (Lowy et al., 1971). Other procedures, such as X-irradiation, could also activate virus, but they were much less efficient (Teich et al., 1973). These studies demonstrated that a mouse-tropic, C-type viral genome was present in AKR cells and could remain in an unexpressed stable heritable form for long periods.

Some low leukemic mouse strains have also been definitively shown to contain endogenous mouse-tropic genomes (Aaronson et al., 1971; Lieberman et al., 1973). Recently, it has been found that all mice contain endogenous xenotropic viruses (Aaronson and Stephenson, 1973; Levy, 1973; Benveniste et al., 1974).

The differences in frequency of mouse-tropic virus release between AKR and low leukemic mice permitted a genetic analysis of mouse-tropic MLV expression in AKR. Breeding experiments between AKR and permissive $(Fv-1^n)$ low leukemic mice indicated that the AKR mouse contains two unlinked autosomal chromosomal loci, either of which is sufficient to result in the appearance of MLV in weanling mice (Rowe, 1972). The linkage group of one locus has been identified. This gene *Akv-1* maps at the same location on mouse chromosome 7 (linkage group I) whether determined by spontaneous appearance of MLV in weanling mice or by IUdR activation of MLV in embryo cells. The gene order is centromere - *Akv-1* - glucose-6-phosphate isomerase *(Gpi-1)* - color *(c)* (Rowe et al., 1972).

NUCLEIC ACID HYBRIDIZATION STUDIES

These experiments suggested that *Akv-1* and the other virus-inducing locus might represent viral genetic material, but the results were also compatible with the alternative hypothesis that these loci represent genes that regulate viral activation but are not the viral genome. To determine which of these two possibilities was correct, nucleic acid hybridization techniques were applied to the AKR system and then to low leukemic mice.

In order to detect viral specific nucleic acid sequences in both cellular DNA and RNA, viral-specific DNA was used as the molecular probe. The virus-associated reverse transcriptase enables viral specific DNA to be synthesized from purified virions, using the viral RNA as template (Temin and Baltimore, 1972). The addition of actinomycin D to the reaction mixture results in a single-strand DNA probe, which is a more faithful copy of the complete viral RNA (Garapin et al., 1973). Purified AKR MLV virions were therefore used in an endogenous reverse transcriptase reaction in the presence of actinomycin D to synthesize a radioisotopically labeled single-strand DNA probe complementary to the viral RNA. Experimental details of these studies can be found in Chattopadhyay et al., (1974), and Lowy et al. (1974a).

Saturation hybridization of the DNA with viral RNA or with RNA from cells productively infected with AKR MLV resulted in hybridization of about 88% of the probe. When the viral probe was reacted in the presence of vast excess sheared AKR cellular DNA (from embryos or virus-negative cell lines), and association kinetics determined (Britten and Kohne, 1968), 88% of the probe hybridized maximally (Fig. 1a), indicating that the viral genome,

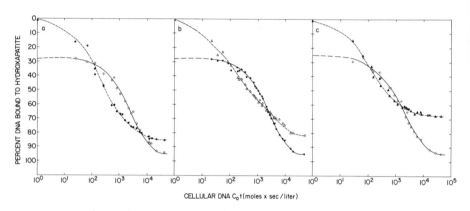

FIG. 1. Representative hybridization kinetics of AKR viral [³H]DNA probe with mouse cellular DNA from (a) a high leukemic mouse, (b) a low leukemic mouse, which contains mouse-tropic viral genome, and (c) a low leukemic mouse, which lacks mouse-tropic viral genome. The extent of hybridization was assayed by hydroxyapatite column chromatography, with the percent bound to hydroxyapatite equivalent to the percent hybridized. The C_0t is equal to the product of nucleic acid absorbancy at 260 nm and hours of incubation, divided by two. Cell-cell DNA reassociation was measured by absorbance at 260 nm (A_{260}). Probe-cell DNA association was measured by liquid scintillation counting. Association kinetics of viral [³H] DNA probe with mouse cell DNA ($\blacklozenge$, $\triangle$, $\blacktriangle$); self-association kinetics of mouse cell DNA ($\diamondsuit$, $\bullet$, $\bigcirc$) (From Lowy et al, 1974a.)

as measured by the probe, is present in the cell as DNA. Similar hybridization data were obtained with cell DNA from two other high virus, high leukemic mouse strains. DNA from mice that are congenic for *Akv-1* on an NIH genetic background hybridize 79% of the AKR viral probe.

Several interesting results were observed when the viral DNA probe was reacted with cellular DNA from low leukemic mice. Biologically, these strains can be divided into those in which mouse-tropic MLV are sometimes detected (such as BALB/c) and never detected (such as NIH Swiss). Cell DNA from strains that contain a mouse-tropic viral genome hybridize 78 to 84% of the viral probe, which is slightly less than with high leukemic DNA (Fig. 1b). Of greater interest, DNA from mice in which mouse-tropic MLV has not been isolated hybridize only 64 to 72% of the viral probe, which is significantly less than with DNA from strains that contain a mouse-tropic MLV genome

(Fig. 1c). In addition, the thermal elution profiles of the hybrids indicate significantly less homology between sequences in the AKR probe that hybridize to DNA from non-mouse-tropic mouse strains than to DNA from the mouse-tropic MLV-containing strains (Fig. 2).

To determine the number of copies of viral specific sequences in the cellular genomes, it has been useful to employ a reciprocal plot of the hybridization data (Wetmur and Davidson, 1968). In the reciprocal plot, if the data describe a single straight line, then all viral specific sequences are present in the cellular DNA in equal numbers. On the other hand, if the data form two straight lines, it implies there are two sets of viral specific sequences. The relative slope of each line is proportional to the number of copies of that set of

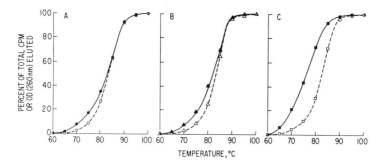

FIG. 2. Representative thermal elution profiles of the maximal hybrids formed between the AKR viral [³H]DNA probe and (A) a high leukemic mouse, (B) a low leukemic mouse, which contains mouse-tropic viral genome, and (C) a low leukemic mouse, which lacks mouse-tropic viral genome. The melting profile of the hybrids was determined by following the total A_{260} units for cell-cell hybrids and counts per minute for probe-cell hybrids. Viral [³H]DNA probe-mouse cell DNA hybrids (●, ▲, ■); self-hybridized mouse cell DNA (○, △, □). (From Lowy et al., 1974a.)

DNA sequences, and comparison of the slope of each line with that of the slope of unique cellular DNA gives an estimate of the absolute number of copies of each set of viral specific sequences per haploid cellular genome.

As seen in Fig. 3, the reciprocal plot of the data from Fig. 1 illustrates two-slope kinetics for high leukemic and mouse-tropic MLV-containing low leukemic strains. There are about 10 copies of the more rapidly associating set of sequences for both types of mice, three to four copies of the second set of sequences in the high leukemic mice, and one to two copies of the second set in the low leukemic mice. By contrast, the reciprocal plot for the low leukemic strains, which lack a mouse-tropic MLV genome, follows a single straight line, indicating only one set of sequences. The cell DNA contains about ten copies of this set. Additional hybridizations indicate that the viral probe sequences that hybridize to NIH DNA are the same as those sequences that hybridize to the more abundant set of sequences in AKR DNA. Although it is not known if these multiple copy sequences are similar in all strains, it seems the most likely hypothesis.

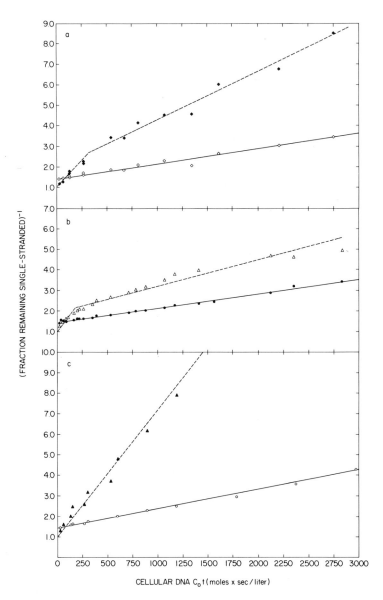

FIG. 3. Reciprocal plot of association kinetics shown in Fig. 1. a: High leukemic mouse. b: Low leukemic mouse which contains mouse-tropic viral genome. c: Low leukemic mouse which lacks mouse-tropic viral genome. The maximum observed [³H]DNA probe-cell DNA and cell DNA-cell DNA hybridizations were normalized to 100%. Symbols are the same as in Fig. 1. (From Lowy et al., 1974a.)

TABLE 1. *Summary of the hybridization results of the viral probe to the mouse DNA*

DNA from mouse strains	Maximum % of viral probe: cell DNA hybridization	Number of sets of viral specific sequences	Copies (approx.) of each set of viral specific sequences	ΔTe50 (°C)
High leukemic[a]	83–88	2	10; 3–4	0.7–2.5
Low leukemic[b] with mouse-tropic MLV	78–84	2	10; 1–2	1.0–3.0
Low Leukemic[c] without mouse-tropic MLV	64–72	1	10	5.5–7.0
AKR	83–88	2	10; 3–4	1.3
NIH	65–68	1	10	7.0
NIH congenic for *Akv-1*	79			4.5
NIH × *Akv-1* hybrid *Akv-1*[+]	80			5.0
	79			5.5
	82			5.5
	79			5.4
	79			5.0
Akv-1[−]	68			9.0
	65			8.5
	66			8.0
	73			8.3

Data from Lowy et al. (1974a) and Chattopadhyay et al. (1975)

[a] Includes AKR/J, C3H/FgLw, and C58.

[b] Includes BALB/cN, DBA/2N, C3H/HeN, and C57BL/6J.

[c] Includes NIH Swiss, C57L/J, 129/J, NZB/N, and wild mouse (mouse-tropic MLV status of wild mouse is not known).

It is concluded that the DNA from low leukemic strains that do not possess a mouse-tropic MLV genome still contain a portion of the AKR MLV genome, but they lack the less abundant set of sequences. These missing sequences apparently help confer mouse tropism to a viral genome, and their absence probably accounts for the failure to detect endogenous mouse-tropic MLV in these strains. It appears likely that at least some of the partial copies of the AKR MLV genome represent portions of xenotropic viral genomes (Callahan et al., 1974). Conversely, the presence of the less abundant set of viral sequences correlates with the presence of an endogenous mouse-tropic MLV, and high leukemic inbred mice contain more copies of this set than do the low leukemic strains. These findings are summarized in Table 1.

AKV-1 CONTAINS VIRAL SPECIFIC SEQUENCES

The observed biochemical differences between AKR and NIH DNA made possible an experiment that would indicate whether or not Akv-1 represents at least the less abundant set of viral specific sequences (Chattopadhyay et al., 1975). *Akv-1* was first isolated from the rest of the AKR genome by serial back-crossing of AKR (*Akv-1⁺, Gpi-1ᵇ,c*) to C57/Br (*Akv-1⁻,Gpi-1ᵃ, c⁺*) and NIH (*Akv-1⁻, Gpi-1ᵇ,c*). Then, a hybrid male (*Akv-1⁺, Gpi-1ᵃ, c⁺/ Akv-1⁻, Gpi-1ᵇ,c*) was mated to an NIH female to provide a three-point genetic cross. Each embryo from one litter was examined individually for the three chromosomal markers (*Akv-1, Gpi-1,* and *c*), the final extent to which its DNA hybridized the AKR viral probe, and the ΔTe50[1] of the thermal elution profile of the hybridized DNA. Five of the nine embryos were positive for *Akv-1* (as measured by IUdR induction of MLV in tissue culture), and the DNA from all five hybridized 79 to 82% of the probe (Table 1). The four embryos negative for *Akv-1* hybridized only 65 to 73% of the probe sequences. In addition, the five mice with *Akv-1* showed much smaller Te50 values than the four mice without Akv-1. These correlations were even more convincing in that five of the nine embryos were recombinants for the chromosome 7 markers, and in all cases the hybridization characteristics segregated with *Akv-1*. The *Akv-1* therefore represents at least a critical portion of the mouse-tropic AKR MLV genome and probably is the entire viral genome. Extrapolating from this finding in *Akv-1,* it appears likely that all endogenous C-type viral genomes are chromosomal genes. This hypothesis is supported by the report that viral specific DNA is associated with chromosomal DNA (Gelb et al., 1973).

CONTROL OF VIRUS ACTIVATION

Some of the factors that determine the expression of endogenous MLV genomes are now understood. Two types of cellular regulation of viral replication have been demonstrated: transcriptional control of endogenous viral DNA and cellular susceptibility to exogenous infection by endogenously activated virus.

The AKR viral DNA probe has been useful in demonstrating the transcriptional control of virus activation. Saturation hybridization with RNA from uninduced AKR cells indicates that a transcriptional block prevents virus replication, since RNA from uninduced cells hybridizes less than one-half the viral probe sequences. This block is overcome by IUdR treatment, as 24 hr after the addition of IUdR, cellular RNA hybridizes 85% of the viral probe (Chattopadhyay et al., 1974).

Restriction of spread of activated virus to other cells is also an important determinant of virus expression. Xenotropic viruses are apparently released frequently from mice and from cells in tissue culture, but exogenous infection is restricted because of the host range of xenotropic virus. In high leukemic mouse strains, the mouse-tropic MLV that is activated is permissive for the

---

[1] Te50 is the midpoint of the thermal elution profile. ΔTe50 is the difference between the Te50 of self-hybridized cell DNA molecules and that of probe-cell DNA hybrids.

host cells. If virus is released, it will quickly spread to other cells. By contrast, in the low leukemic strains, which contain a mouse-tropic viral genome, the MLV that is permissive for host cells is activated much less readily.

The molecular explanation of the differences in the probability of MLV activation remain to be determined. One possibility is that the avidity of a postulated repressor of viral RNA transcription might differ in its ability to prevent viral mRNA transcription, either because of differences between repressors in high and low leukemic mice or because of differences in the affinity of binding sites for a repressor. It is interesting that in sarcoma-transformed BALB cells, IUdR activates both mouse-tropic and xenotropic C-type virus, but protein inhibitors activate only xenotropic virus (Aaronson and Dunn, 1974).

A second possibility is that the greater number of copies of the viral genome present in high virus mice accounts for their greater likelihood of virus activation. But, mice that are congenic for *Akv-1* on an NIH background are similar to AKR in the frequency with which the mouse-tropic viral genome is activated, although they contain only one to two copies of the complete viral genome. (Table 1).

Alternatively, the particular chromosomal location of a viral genome may make activation more or less likely. Neither the high leukemic strains C3H/Fg nor C58, however, have a viral induction locus at *Akv-1* (Rowe, 1973).

Finally, AKR may possess tandem insertion of more than one MLV genome. Tandem insertion of Simian virus 40 makes activation of that virus more likely (Kelly et al., 1974).

CONCLUSION

Although many unanswered questions remain, the above studies have demonstrated that mice contain numerous C-type viral genomes, which appear to be integrated into chromosomal DNA. These results do not exclude the possibility of infection by C-type viruses from outside the organism; they do, however, provide some understanding of the epidemiological observation that, in mice, C-type virus is usually transmitted vertically. They also delineate some steps in viral replication which theoretically might be amenable to prophylactic or therapeutic intervention.

SUMMARY

Within one week of postnatal life, the high leukemic AKR mouse becomes positive for a mouse-tropic, C-type RNA virus. Several copies of this viral genome are present in AKR cellular DNA, as indicated by nucleic acid hybridization studies utilizing a single-strand DNA probe complementary to the RNA of this virus. Breeding experiments have shown that the expression of this virus is determined by classic Mendelian segregation: the chromosomal location of a virus-inducing locus (*Akv-1*) has been mapped. Combined biologic and biochemical studies demonstrate that *Akv-1* contains viral sequences. Additional studies suggest that C-type viral genetic information is present in the chromosomal DNA of many mouse strains. The cellular regulation of these viral genomes is discussed.

ACKNOWLEDGMENTS

The studies reported here were carried out in the laboratories of Dr. Wallace P. Rowe, Chief, Laboratory of Viral Diseases, National Institute of Allergy and Infectious Diseases, and Dr. Arthur S. Levine, Chief, Infectious Disease Section, National Cancer Institute. We thank Dr. Janet W. Hartley and Dr. Rowe and Dr. Levine for their indispensible advice, insight, and encouragement.

REFERENCES

Aaronson, S. A., and Dunn, C. Y. (1974): High frequency C-type virus induction by inhibitors of protein synthesis. *Science,* 183:422–424.

Aaronson, S. A., and Stephenson, J. R. (1973): Independent segregation of loci for activation of biologically distinguishable RNA C-type virus in mouse cells. *Proc. Natl. Acad. Sci. USA,* 70:2055–2058.

Aaronson, S. A., Todaro, G. J., and Scholnick, E. M. (1971): Induction of murine C-type viruses from clonal lines of virus-free Balb/3T3 cells. *Science,* 174:157–159.

Benveniste, R. E., Lieber, M. W., and Todaro, G. T. (1974): A distinct class of inducible murine type-C viruses that replicates in the rabbit SIRC cell line. *Proc. Natl. Acad. Sci. USA,* 71:602–606.

Britten, R. J., and Kohne, D. E. (1968): Repeated sequences in DNA. *Science,* 161:529–540.

Callahan, R., Benveniste, R. E., Lieber, M. M., and Todaro, G. J. (1974): Nucleic acid homology of murine type-C viral genes. *J. Virol.,* 14:1394–1403.

Chattopadhyay, S. K., Lowy, D. R., Teich, N. M., Levine, A. S., and Rowe, W. P. (1974): Qualitative and Quantitative studies of AKR-type murine-leukemia-virus (MLV) sequences in DNA of high-, low-, and non-virus-yielding mouses strains. *Cold Spring Harbor Symp. Quant. Biol.,* 39:1085–1101.

Chattopadhyay, S. K., Rowe, W. P., Teich, N. M., and Lowy, D. R. (1975): Definitive evidence that the murine C-type virus inducing locus AKV-1 is viral genetic material. *Proc. Natl. Acad. Sci. USA, (In press).*

Cold Spring Harbor Symp. Quant. Biol. (1974), 39.

Furth, J., Seibold, H. R., and Rathbone, R. R. (1933): Experimental studies on lymphomatosis of mice. *Am. J. Cancer,* 19:521–604.

Garapin, A. C., Varmus, H. E., Faras, A. J., Levinson, W. E., and Bishop, J. M. (1973): RNA-directed DNA synthesis by virions of Rous sarcoma virus: Further characterization of the templates and the extent of their transcription. *Virology,* 52:264–274.

Gelb, L. D., Milstein, J. B., Martin, M. A., and Aaronson, S. A. (1973): Characterization of murine leukemia virus-specific DNA present in normal mouse cells. *Nature [New Biol.],* 244:76–79.

Gross, L. (1951a): "Spontaneous" leukemia developing in C3H mice following inoculation, in infancy, with AK-leukemic extracts, or AK-embryos. *Proc. Soc. Exp. Biol. Med.,* 76:27–32.

Gross, L. (1951b): Pathogenic properties, and "vertical" transmission of the mouse leukemia agent. *Proc. Soc. Exp. Biol. Med.,* 78:342–348.

Gross, L. (1970): *Oncogenic viruses.* 2nd ed., pp. 286–552. Pergamon Press, New York.

Hirsch, M. S., and Black, P. H. (1974): Activation of mammalian leukemia viruses. *Adv. Virus Res.,* 19:265–313.

Huebner, R. J., and Todaro, G. J. (1969): Oncogenes of RNA tumor viruses as determinants of cancer. *Proc. Natl. Acad. Sci. USA,* 64:1087–1094.

Kaplan, H. S. (1967): On the natural history of the murine leukemias. *Cancer Res.,* 27:1325–1340.

Kelly, T. J., Jr., Lewis, A. M., Jr., Levine, A. S., and Siegel, S. (1974): Structural studies of two adenovirus 2-SV40 hybrids which contain the entire SV40 genome. *Cold Spring Harbor Symp. Quant. Biol.,* 39:409–417.

Klement, V., Rowe, W. P., Hartley, J. W., and Pugh, W. E. (1969): Mixed culture cytopathogenicity: A new test for growth of murine leukemia viruses in tissue culture. *Proc. Natl. Acad. Sci. USA,* 63:753–758.

Levy, J. A. (1973): Xenotropic viruses: Murine leukemia viruses associated with NIH Swiss, NZB, and other mouse strains. *Science,* 182:1151–1153.

Lieberman, M. O., Niwa, O., Decleve, A., and Kaplan, H. S. (1973): Continuous propagation of radiation leukemia virus on a C57BL mouse-embryo fibroblast line, with attenuation of leukemogenic activity. *Proc. Natl. Acad. Sci. USA,* 70:1250–1253.

Lowy, D. R., Chattopadhyay, S. K., Teich, N. M., Rowe, W. P., and Levine, A. S. (1974a): AKR murine leukemia virus genome: Frequency of sequences in DNA of high-, low-, and non-virus-yielding mouse strains. *Proc. Natl. Acad. Sci. USA,* 71:3555–3559.

Lowy, D. R., Rowe, W. P., Teich, N., and Hartley, J. W. (1971): Murine leukemia virus: High frequency activation *in vitro* by 5-iododeoxyuridine and 5-bromodeoxyuridine. *Science,* 175:155–156.

Lowy, D. R., Teich, N. M., and Chattopadhyay (1974b): Expression and detection of endogenous mouse C-type RNA viruses, *In Vitro.* (*In press.*)

Rowe, W. P. (1972): Studies of genetic transmission of murine leukemia virus by AKR mice. I. Crosses with Fv-1ⁿ strains of mice. *J. Exp. Med.,* 36:1272–1285.

Rowe, W. P. (1973): Genetic factors in the natural history of murine leukemia virus infection. *Cancer Res.,* 33:3061–3068.

Rowe, W. P., Hartley, J. W., and Bremner, T. (1972): Genetic mapping of a murine leukemia virus-inducing locus of AKR mice. *Science,* 178:860–862.

Rowe, W. P., Hartley, J. W., Lander, M. R., Pugh, W. E., and Teich, N. (1971): Noninfectious AKR mouse embryo cell lines in which each cell has the capacity to be activated to produce infectious murine leukemia virus. *Virology,* 46:866–876.

Rowe, W. P., Hartley, J. W., and Pugh, W. E. (1970): Plaque assay techniques for murine leukemia viruses. *Virology,* 42:1136–1139.

Siegler. R. (1968): Pathology of murine leukemia. In: *Experimental Leukemia,* edited by M. A. Rich, pp. 51–95. Appleton-Century-Crofts, New York.

Teich, N., Lowy, D. R., Hartley, J. W., and Rowe, W. P. (1973): Studies of the mechanism of induction of infectious murine leukemia virus from AKR mouse embryo cells by 5-iododeoxyuridine and 5-bromodeoxyuridine. *Virology,* 51:163–173.

Temin, H. M. (1971): Mechanism of cell transformation by RNA tumor viruses. *Ann Rev. Microbiol.,* 25:609–648.

Temin, H. M., and Baltimore, D. (1972): RNA directed DNA synthesis and RNA tumor viruses. *Adv. Virus Res.,* 17:129–186.

Tooze, J. (ed.) (1973): *The Molecular Biology of Tumor Viruses,* pp. 502–699. Cold Spring Harbor Laboratory, Cold Spring Harbor, N.Y.

Wetmur, J. G., and Davidson, N. (1968): Kinetics of renaturation of DNA. *J. Mol. Biol.,* 31:349–370.

Biology of Radiation Carcinogenesis, edited by
J. M. Yuhas, R. W. Tennant, and J. D. Regan.
Raven Press, New York © 1976.

Genetics of Cell Transformation by SV40

Carlo M. Croce

The Wistar Institute of Anatomy and Biology, 36th Street at Spruce,
Philadelphia, Pennsylvania 19104

We have recently shown that the genes for SV40 T-antigen and tumor-specific transplantation antigen (TSTA) and the SV40 genome are on the human chromosome 7 in the SV40-transformed human cell line LN-SV (Croce et al., 1973, 1974; Croce, Aden, and Koprowski, 1975; Croce, Huebner, Girardi, and Koprowski, 1975). We have also shown that somatic cell hybrids between LN-SV cells and normal human diploid fibroblasts (WI38) behave as transformed cells *in vitro* (Croce and Koprowski, 1974*b*), indicating that the transformed phenotype is dominant.

We wished to determine whether the human chromosome 7 carrying the SV40 genome coding for transforming gene products is responsible for the expression of the transformed phenotype *in vitro,* and of the tumorigenic phenotype *in vivo.* Therefore, we decided to hybridize normal mouse cells (mouse peritoneal macrophages) with SV40-transformed human cells deficient in hypoxanthine guanine phosphoribosyltransferase (HGPRT) and to select for the hybrid cells in hypoxanthine-aminopterin-thymidine (HAT) medium (Littlefield, 1964). Since the mouse peritoneal macrophages are nondividing cells (Epifanova and Terskikh, 1969) in the culture conditions used in this study (Croce and Koprowski, 1974*c,* 1975), the hybrid cells should be the only cells that can grow in HAT selective medium (Croce and Koprowski, 1974*c,* 1975). In the human chromosome 7 carrying the SV40 genome codes for transforming gene products, all the somatic cell hybrids that contain this chromosome should be transformed and tumorigenic in immunosuppressed mice.

CHARACTERIZATION OF HYBRIDS BETWEEN MOUSE PERITONEAL MACROPHAGES AND LN-SV CELLS

One hundred and sixty-eight independent hybrid cell clones derived from the fusion of mouse peritoneal macrophages (MPM) of either C57BL/6 or BALB/c origin with LN-SV cells were found to be SV40 T-antigen positive in 100% of the cells examined (Table 1). As the gene for SV40 T-antigen has been assigned to human chromosome 7 in LN-SV cells (Croce et al., 1973; Croce and Koprowski, 1974*a*), these results indicate that the human chromosome 7 carrying the SV40 genome was retained by the totality of the

TABLE 1. *Presence of SV40 T-antigen in hybrid clones between mouse peritoneal macrophages and SV40-transformed human fibroblasts*

Hybrid cells (mouse × human)	No. of hybrid clones studied	No. of clones showing the presence of SV40 T-antigen[a]
C57BL/6 × LN-SV	111	111
Balb/c × LN-SV	57	57

[a] One hundred percent of the cells of each clone were positive for SV40 T-antigen.

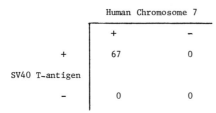

Human Chromosome 7

		+	−
SV40 T-antigen	+	67	0
	−	0	0

FIG. 1. Positive correlation between the expression of SV40 T-antigen and the presence of the the human chromosome 7 in 67 independent hybird clones between C57BL/6 and BALB/c MPM and LN-SV cells. At least one human chromosome 7 was present in all the metaphases examined.

hybrids between mouse peritoneal macrophages and LN-SV cells. In fact, karyological analysis of 67 of these hybrid clones (45 clones derived from the fusion of C57BL/6 MPM and LN-SV cells and 22 clones between Balb/c MPM and LN-SV cells) showed that the human chromosome 7 was present

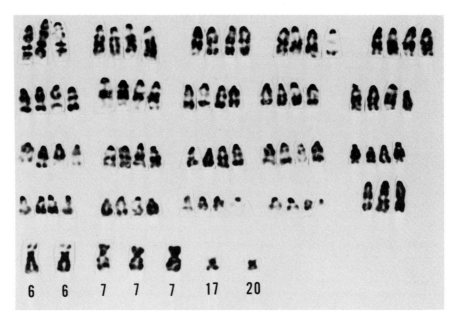

6   6   7   7   7   17   20

FIG. 2. Karyotype of a C57BL MPM × LN-SV hybrid. The human chromosomes 6, 7, 17, and 20 are present in this clone; all of the remaining chromosomes are of mouse origin. The number of mouse chromosomes present in this clone is quasi-tetraploid.

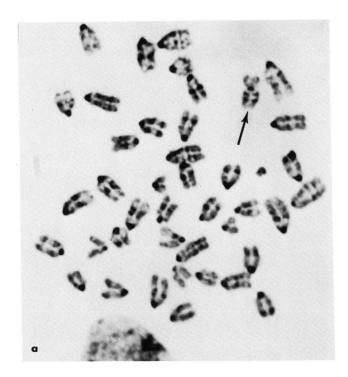

FIG. 3. a: Metaphase of a cell of a hybrid clone between BALB/c MPM and LN-SV cells. The human chromosome 7 (arrow) is the only human chromosome present in this hybrid clone, which contains a perfectly diploid number of mouse chromosomes. b: Karyotype of the chromosomes present in the hybrid cell.

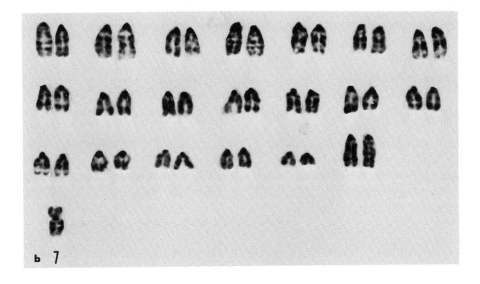

b 7

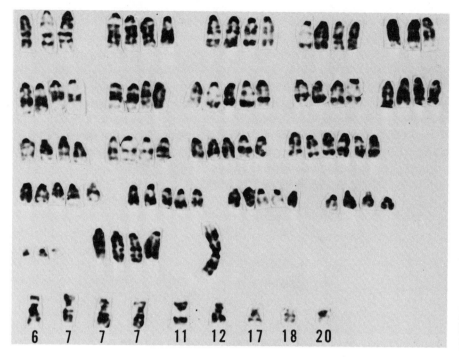

FIG. 4. Karyotype of a C57BL MPM × LN-SV hybrid cell. The human chromosomes 6, 7, 11, 12, 17, 18, and 20 are present in this hybrid. All the other chromosomes are of mouse origin. The biarmed chromosome present in the fourth row has originated by the centric fusion of two mouse chromosomes.

in all the clones examined (Figs. 1 and 2). The human chromosome 7 was present in all the metaphases examined. In 13 of the 67 hybrid cell clones, the human chromosome 7 was the only human chromosome present in the hybrid cells (Fig. 3). The other human chromosomes segregated in the various hybrid clones (Fig. 4). Approximately 75% of the hybrid clones contained a quasi-tetraploid number of mouse chromosomes (Fig. 2), and only 25% of the hybrid clones contained a diploid number of mouse chromosomes (Fig. 3). In general, the hybrid clones that contained a diploid number of mouse chromosomes contained a very reduced number of human chromosomes. The recognition of the human chromosomes is particularly easy in these hybrids as they stand out nicely against the background of the 20 pairs of mouse chromosomes. Fusion of mouse peritoneal macrophages with normal Lesch-Nyhan fibroblasts did not result in the formation of hybrid cell colonies in HAT selective medium. It is possible, however, that formation of hybrid cells occurred but that these hybrids had a limited life-span.

EXPRESSION OF THE TRANSFORMED PHENOTYPE IN THE HYBRID CELLS

None of the hybrid cell clones examined displayed the density-dependent inhibition of cell division (contact inhibition) characteristic of normal cells, and they piled up in culture. The hybrid cell clones had a saturation density five times higher than that of normal diploid human cells and four times higher than that of mouse fibroblasts (Table 2). In addition, the hybrid cells gave rise to colonies when seeded in soft agar (0.33% noble agar) (Table 3). Figure 5 summarizes the data obtained by seeding 67 hybrid cell clones in soft agar. Colony formation in soft agar is considered one of the characteristics of transformed cells (Macpherson, 1969).

TABLE 2. *Saturation density of parental and hybrid cells[a]*

Cells	Saturation density[b] ($\times 10^5$ cells/cm^2)
Lesch-Nyhan diploid fibrob'asts	0.4
LN-SV	2.0
Mouse diploid fibroblasts	0.6
Hybrid clone 1	2.0
Hybrid clone 2	2.1
Hybrid clone 6	2.3
Hybrid clone 17	1.9

[a] Parental diploid human and mouse fibroblasts and hybrid cells were counted ten days after seeding the same number (2×10^6) of cells in 75 cm^2 plastic Falcon flasks.
[b] The saturation density of mouse peritoneal macrophages was not determined, since the macrophages are nondividing cells.

TABLE 3. *Transformed phenotype in hybrids between mouse peritoneal macrophages and SV40-transformed human cells*

Cells	Colony formation in soft agar[a]
Lesch-Nyhan diploid fibroblasts	—
LN-SV	+
Mouse peritoneal macrophages	—
Mouse diploid fibroblasts	—
Hybrid clone 1	+
Hybrid clone 2	+
Hybrid clone 6	+
Hybrid clone 13	+

[a] The efficiency of colony formation in agar was between 1 and 5 colonies/100 LN-SV or hybrid cells seeded. No colonies developed from plating either Lesch-Nyhan fibroblasts or mouse macrophages or mouse diploid fibroblasts.

These experiments indicate that hybrids between normal mouse cells and SV40-transformed human cells, which retain the entire chromosome complement of the normal mouse parent, behave as transformed cells *in vitro*, confirming that the transformed phenotype is dominant in hybrids between normal and SV40-transformed cells.

Because the presence of the human chromosome 7 carrying the SV40

Human Chromosome 7

	+	−
Transformed phenotype +	67	0
−	0	0

FIG. 5. Positive correlation between the expression of the transformed phenotype as determined by growth in soft agar and the presence of the human chromosome 7 carrying the SV40 genome.

genome is the common denominator of the transformed mouse peritoneal macrophage × LN-SV cell hybrids, it can be inferred (1) that the human chromosome 7 carrying the SV40 genome contains gene(s) coding for transforming gene products and (2) that the human chromosome 7 carrying the SV40 genome is responsible for the growth of the hybrid cells (since segregant cells, which did not contain the human chromosome 7, were not found).

TUMORIGENICITY OF THE HYBRID CELLS IN NUDE MICE

To determine if the human chromosome 7 carrying the SV40 genome is responsible for the expression of the tumorigenic phenotype *in vivo,* we injected a heterogeneous population of hybrid cells and several homogeneous hybrid clones into nude mice in which heterotransplantation of human tumors can be successfully achieved (Flanagan, 1966; Rygaard and Povlsen, 1969; Visfeldt et al., 1972). The injected nude mice developed tumors [which have been extensively studied and will be reported elsewhere; H. Koprowski, D. Aden, and C. M. Croce (*unpublished*)].

Karyological analysis of cells derived from tumors induced in five nude mice by the injection of a heterogeneous population of hybrids derived from the fusion of C57BL/6 MPM and LN-SV cells (Table 4) is shown in Table 5. The human chromosome 7 carrying the SV40 genome was present in all the tumor cells examined (Table 5). All the cells derived from the five tumors were SV40 T-antigen positive.

Cells derived from the tumors induced in nude-8 and in nude-1 were reinjected into nude mice. Cells derived from a tumor obtained by the injection of nude-1 tumor cells in a nude mouse ("nude-9") were also reinjected into nude mice. Karyological analysis of the tumor cells derived from seven of such tumors is described in Table 6. The human chromosome 7 carrying the SV40 genome was retained by all the tumor cells obtained from these tumors (Table 6).

These experiments indicate that somatic cell hybrids between normal mouse cells and SV40-transformed human cells are tumorigenic in nude mice and that these hybrids retain the human chromosome 7 carrying the SV40 genome.

TABLE 4. *Presence of different human chromosomes in hybrid cells between C57BL/6 mouse peritoneal macrophages and LN-SV human cells*

Human chromosome	Frequency in hybrids (%)[a]	Human chromosome	Frequency in hybrids (%)[a]
4	5.9	13	5.9
5	60.8	14	7.8
6	70.6	15	17.6
7	100[b]	16	2.0
9	5.9	17	60.8
11	54.9	18	3.9
12	23.5	20	5.9

[a] A total of 51 metaphases was analyzed.

[b] On the average, the hybrid cells contained 2.3 chromosomes 7/cell.

TABLE 5. *Karyological analysis of cells recovered from tumors induced in nude mice by inoculation of hybrid cells*

Source of tumors	Removal (days after inoculation)	Cells showing SV40 T-antigen (%)	Human chromosomes[a]				
			5	6	7	11	17
Nude-1	22	100	8/45	35/45	45/45	0/45	0/45
Nude-2	28	100	0/30	21/30	30/30	0/30	0/30
Nude-4	42	100	0/39	25/39	39/39	1/39	15/39
Nude-7	70	100	0/26	10/26	26/26	0/26	1/26
Nude-8	76	100	0/33	3/33	33/33	0/33	0/33

[a] Number of metaphases showing presence of this chromosome over total analyzed.

TABLE 6. *Karyological analysis of cells of tumors derived from the inoculation of nude-8 and nude-9 tumor cells into nude mice*

Tumor	Removal (days after inoculation)	Cells showing SV40 T-antigen (%)	Human chromosomes[a]		
			5	6	7
Nude 8–1	40	100	0/32	0/32	32/32
Nude 8–2	40	100	0/37	0/37	37/37
Nude 8–3	56	100	0/37	0/37	37/37
Nude 9[b]	67	100	0/41	29/41	41/41
Nude 9–1	24	100	0/31	23/31	31/31
Nude 9–2	38	100	0/26	20/26	26/26
Nude 9–3	39	100	0/30	21/30	30/30

[a] Number of metaphases showing presence of this human chromosome over total analyzed. No other human chromosomes were present in the hybrid cells.

[b] Hybrid cells derived from nude-1 were inoculated into nude-9.

CONCLUSIONS

The results summarized here indicate that the integration of the SV40 genome into the human chromosome 7 results in the synthesis of transforming gene products responsible for the maintenance of the transformed phenotype. The hybridization of mouse peritoneal macrophages with SV40-transformed human cells (LN-SV) resulted in the production of somatic cell hybrids that contained, without exception, the human chromosome 7 carrying the SV40 genome. All these hybrids were transformed as indicated by their high saturation density and by their growth in soft agar.

These data confirm that the transformed phenotype is dominant in hybrids between normal and SV40-transformed cells and are in contrast with the hypothesis formulated by Harris et al. (1969, 1971) and Harris and Klein (1969), which states that, as a rule, somatic cell hybrids between transformed and normal cells behave as normal cells if the chromosomes derived from the normal parents are retained by the hybrids. We found, however, that cell hybrids between normal mouse cells and SV40-transformed human cells retain all the chromosomes of the mouse normal parent; they behave as transformed cells *in vitro;* and they can be subcultured indefinitely (Croce and Koprowski, 1974c).

In addition, these hybrids were tumorigenic when injected in nude mice (Croce, Aden, and Koprowski, 1975). Karyological analysis of the tumor cells derived from the tumors so induced indicated that they were mouse-human hybrids containing the entire complement of mouse chromosomes and a very few human chromosomes, but including the human chromosome 7 carrying the SV40 genome.

It is possible that the hybridization of mouse nondividing cells with human cancer cells could also result in the retention of a specific human chromosome responsible for the expression of the cancer phenotype. In this case, it might be feasible to identify the human cancer chromosome(s) responsible for the cancer phenotype in man.

ACKNOWLEDGMENTS

We are very grateful to Irene Kieba, Cecelia Green, Emma DeJesus, and Jean Letofsky for excellent technical assistance. This work was supported in part by USPHS Research Grants CA 10815 from the National Cancer Institute, RR 05540 from the Division of Research Resources, GM 20700 from the National Institute of General Medical Sciences, by a Basil O'Connor Starter Grant from the National Foundation, and by funds from the Commonwealth of Pennsylvania. C.M.C. is recipient of a Research Career Development Award CA 00143 from the National Cancer Institute.

REFERENCES

Croce, C. M., Aden, D., and Koprowski, H. (1975): Somatic cell hybrids between mouse peritoneal macrophages and simian virus 40 transformed human cells. II. Presence of human chromosome 7 carrying simian virus 40 genome in cells of tumors induced by hybrid cells. *Proc. Natl. Acad. Sci. USA,* 72:1397.

Croce, C. M., Girardi, A. J., and Koprowski, H. (1973): Assignment of the T-antigen gene of simian virus 40 to human chromosome C-7. *Proc. Natl. Acad. Sci. USA,* 70:3617.

Croce, C. M., Huebner, K., Girardi, A. J., and Koprowski, H. (1974): Rescue of defective SV40 from mouse-human hybrid cells containing human chromosome 7. *Virology,* 60:276.

Croce, C. M., Huebner, K., Girardi, A. J., and Koprowski, H. (1975): Genetics of cell transformation by simian virus 40. *Cold Spring Harb. Symp. Monograph,* 39:335.

Croce, C. M., and Koprowski, H. (1974a): Concordant segregation of the expression of SV40 T antigen and human chromosome 7 in mouse-human hybrid subclones. *J. Exp. Med.,* 139:1350.

Croce, C. M., and Koprowski, H. (1974b): Positive control of the transformed phenotype in hybrids between normal and SV40 transformed cells. *Science,* 184:1288.

Croce, C. M., and Koprowski, H. (1974c): Somatic cell hybrids between mouse peritoneal macrophages and SV40-transformed human cells. I. Positive control of the transformed phenotype by the human chromosome 7 carrying the SV40 genome. *J. Exp. Med.,* 140:1221.

Croce, C. M., and Koprowski, H. (1975): Assignment of gene(s) for cell transformation to human chromosome 7 carrying the simian virus 40 genome. *Proc. Natl. Acad. Sci. USA,* 72:1658.

Epifanova, O. I., and Terskikh, V. V. (1969): On the resting periods in the cell life cycle. *Cell Tissue Kinet.,* 2:75.

Flanagan, S. P. (1966): "Nude," a new hairless gene with pleiotropic effects in the mouse. *Genet. Res.,* 8:295.

Harris, H., and Klein, G. (1969): Malignancy of somatic cell hybrids. *Nature,* 224:1314.

Harris, H., Miller, O. J., Klein, G., Worst, P., and Tachibana, T. (1969): Suppression of malignancy by cell fusion. *Nature,* 223:363.

Klein, G., Bregula, U., Wiener, F., and Harris, H. (1971): The analysis of malignancy by cell fusion. *J. Cell Sci.,* 8:659.

Littlefield, J. W. (1964): Selection of hybrids from matings of fibroblasts *in vitro* and their presumed recombinants. *Science,* 145:709.

Macpherson, I. (1969): Agar suspension culture for quantitation of transformed cells. In: *Fundamental Techniques in Virology,* edited by K. Habel and N. Salzman, p. 214. Academic Press, New York.

Rygaard, J., and Povlsen, C. O. (1969): Heterotransplantation of a human malignant tumor in nude mice. *Acta Pathol. Microbiol. Scand.,* 77:758.

Visfeldt, J., Povlsen, C. O., and Rygaard, J. (1972): Chromosome analysis of human tumors following heterotransplantation of the mouse mutant "nude." *Acta Pathol. Microbiol. Scand.,* 80:169.

Wiener, F., Fenyo, E. M., Klein, G., and Harris, H. (1972): Fusion of tumor cells with host cells. *Nature [New Biol.],* 238:155.

Biology of Radiation Carcinogenesis, edited by
J. M. Yuhas, R. W. Tennant, and J. D. Regan.
Raven Press, New York © 1976.

Radiation Activation of Endogenous Leukemia Viruses in Cell Culture: Acute X-Ray Irradiation

A. Declève, O Niwa, E. Gelmann, and H. S. Kaplan

Department of Radiology, Stanford University School of Medicine, Stanford, California 94305

The activation of endogenous murine leukemia viruses (MuLV) *in vivo* has been experimentally achieved by three different types of treatment. These viruses can be extracted from radiation-induced lymphomas in mice of strains C57BL and C3H and also from radiation-induced myeloid leukemias of RF mice. MuLV may also be isolated from the same spectrum of leukemias and lymphomas after treatment of mice with carcinogenic hydrocarbons, cytotoxic alkylating agents, purine analogs, urethane, and estrogens. More recently it has been demonstrated that graft-versus-host reactions induced *in vivo* may also activate the replication of MuLV (cf. Kaplan, 1974, for review).

In vitro, the replication of endogenous viruses may be induced by X- or UV-irradiation or by treatment with the halogenated pyrimidine analogs 5-bromodeoxyuridine (BrUdR) and 5-iododeoxyuridine (IUdR) in non-virus-producing cell lines from various mouse strains (Aaronson et al., 1971; Klement et al., 1971; Lieber et al., 1973; Lowy et al., 1971; Rowe et al., 1971; Teich et al., 1973). Recently, activation of an endogenous C-type virus in mouse embryo fibroblasts and established cell lines from strain C57BL mice has been accomplished after treatment with BrUdR or IUdR (Lieberman et al., 1973b; Gelmann et al., *in preparation*). Preliminary experiments have demonstrated that an endogenous C-type virus can also be induced in C57BL cells by X-irradiation (Declève et al., 1974a). In the present report, we submit additional evidence that confirms the induction of MuLV from C57BL cells by X-irradiation and explores the influence of varying experimental conditions on this phenomenon.

MATERIALS AND METHODS

Cells. Secondary mouse embryo fibroblast (BL-MEF) cultures were prepared from C57BL/Ka mice, as previously described (Declève et al., 1970); BL-5, an established line of C57BL/Ka mouse embryo fibroblasts, has been described elsewhere (Lieberman et al., 1973). The NIH/3T3 and normal rat kidney (NRK) cells were obtained from Dr. Stuart Aaronson (National Cancer Institute, NIH, Bethesda, Md.) and have been described (Aaronson and Stephenson, 1973; Duc-Nguyen et al., 1966).

Culture medium. Cultures were grown in Eagle's minimal essential medium supplemented with 10% heat-inactivated fetal calf serum, penicillin (100 units/ml), streptomycin (100 μg/ml), and polymixin (50 units/ml). This medium will be referred to as MEM 10%.

Virus assays. Reverse XC assays and immunofluorescence (IF) assays were performed as previously described (Niwa et al., 1973; Declève et al., 1974b).

X-irradiation. Cells in plastic dishes were irradiated by a single dose of X-rays with either a 50 kVp twin beryllium window tube X-ray unit at a dose rate of 0.14 krad/sec for high doses or with a 250 kVp X-ray unit (Phillips RT250) at a dose rate of 80 rad/min for low doses. In all experiments, three to nine Petri dishes (60 mm) were used for each X-ray dose.

RESULTS

Direct Examination of the Target Cells by IF After Different X-Ray Doses

Growth curves of BL-5 cells irradiated with various doses of X-rays 1 day after seeding 2×10^5 cells/60-mm dish indicate that no growth in cell population is observed for doses over 1,000 rad (Fig. 1). From the survival curve

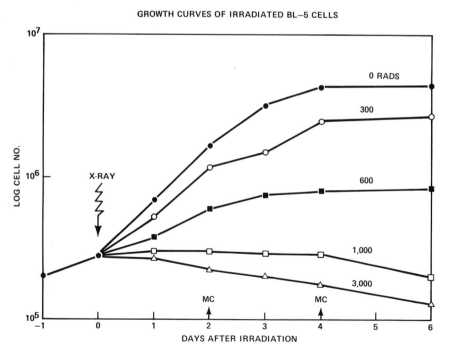

GROWTH CURVES OF IRRADIATED BL–5 CELLS

FIG. 1. Growth curves of BL-5 cell cultures treated by various single exposures to X-rays 1 day after plating. MC = medium change.

of the same cells, based on their colony-forming ability after irradiation in suspension (Fig. 2), one can observe that fewer than 1% of the cells survive doses larger than 750 rads. With this in mind, BL-5 cells were irradiated in suspension with doses ranging from 250 to 1,000 rad; 2×10^5 cells were then seeded/60-mm dish (three dishes per dose for low doses and up to 12 dishes per dose for high doses). After treatment, the cells were subcultured at 4-day intervals for at least six passages. Cell aliquots from each passage were processed for IF assay. For the high dose groups, 12 dishes yielded barely enough surviving cells to be subcultured for the first few times. In one of three replicate experiments, faint, atypical fluorescence was detected after five passages (i.e., after more than 12 cell-cycle generations) in the cytoplasm of irradiated cells (450 rad or more). Similar observations could not be made after secondary culture with C57BL BL-MEF, since such cells, even if not irradiated, would be expected to die within a few passages.

From this first set of experiments, it was concluded that overlaying the

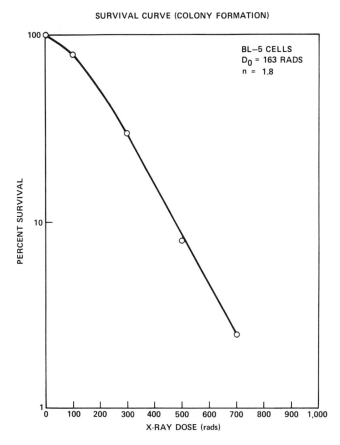

FIG. 2. Survival curve as estimated by colony-forming ability of BL-5 cells after X-ray treatment.

irradiated target cells with a detector cell inoculum would present several advantages.

1. In order to replicate virus productively, cells have to undergo several divisions (Declève et al., 1975a). An actively dividing overlay of an established cell line would fulfill this requirement.

2. The virus may be released by the target cells during the dying process and promptly infect a healthy detector cell growing nearby. Higher doses of X-ray may be studied this way, since the target cells do not have to divide.

3. The transmission of MuLV, or the spreading of viral infection, seems to be far more efficient through cell-to-cell contact than through the supernatant (Declève et al., *unpublished*). Close contact between target cells and detector cells of the overlay may, therefore, provide a better system for detection of newly induced virus particles.

4. Finally, an overlay by cells from different mouse strains or even from different species may allow typing of the induced viruses in terms of their tropisms (Pincus et al., 1971a,b; Levy, 1973).

X-Ray Induction of MuLV from C57BL Cells as Detected by Overlay Cultures

The results of ten experiments covering a dose range of 150 to 10,000 rads are given in Table 1. The BL-MEF or BL-5 cells were irradiated in suspension, plated at 2×10^5 cells/60-mm dish, and overlaid one day later with either BL-5, NIH/3T3, or NRK cells. At 4-day intervals, the cultures were subcultured and passed six to eight times. At each passage, cell suspensions

TABLE 1. *Virus induction from C57BL cells by different doses of X-ray (rad)*

	150	250–300	450–500	550–600	750–800	1,000	2,000–2,500	4,000	5,000	7,500	10,000
EXPERIMENT NUMBER	2 8	2 8 9 10	4 8 9 10	2 8 10	1 2 3 5 8 10	4 6 7 8 9	2 4 6 9	4 9	6	6 9	6
OVERLAY CELL TYPE											
BL–5	0 0	0 0 0 0	+ 0 0 +	0 0 +	+ 0 0 + 0 +	+ + + 0 +	0 + + 0	+ 0	+	+ 0	+
NIH/3T3	0 0	0 0 0 NT	NT 0 0 NT	0 0 NT	+ 0 0 + 0 NT	NT + + 0 NT	0 NT + 0	NT 0	+	+ 0	+
NRK (RAT)	NT 0	NT 0 0 NT	NT 0 0 NT	NT 0 NT	NT NT NT NT 0 NT	NT 0 + 0 NT	NT NT 0 0	NT 0	0	0 0	0
ASSAY											
REVERSE XC	√	√	√	√	√ √ √	√	√ √	√			
IF	√ √	√ √ √ √	√ √ √ √	√ √ √	√ √ √ √ √ √	√ √ √ √ √	√ √ √ √	√ √	√	√ √	√

* SCORED AFTER 20 CELL DOUBLINGS OF THE OVERLAY CELLS
NT = NOT TESTED
√ = TESTED

were made for IF and reverse XC assays. The results after 20 cell-doublings of the overlay cells indicate that a dose higher than 450 rad was necessary to induce virus at a detectable level under our experimental conditions. In the dose range from 450 to 10,000 rad, the occurrence of induction was observed in seven of the ten experiments. When MuLV was detected, it was by both of the murine detector cell cultures: BL-5 (Fv-1^{bb}) and NIH/3T3 (Fv-1^{nn}). In only one instance did the NRK cells become positive. Since the IF assay detects viral replication, by virtue of the appearance of viral antigens in the

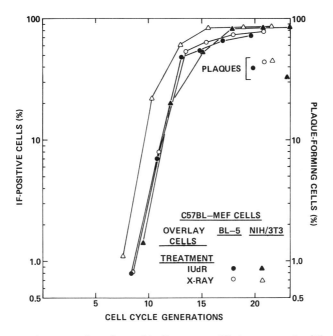

FIG. 3. Percentage of positive cells as detected by IF or reverse XC plaque assay for different cell cycle generations of the overlay cells. The original C57BL-MEF target cells were treated either by IUdR or X-ray and overlaid 1 day later with either BL-5 or NIH/3T3 cells.

cytoplasm of the overlay cells, earlier than the XC test (which requires the emergence of infectious virus), the IF test was more often used than the reverse XC test. Both tests, however, have documented the occurrence of viral replication in secondarily infected detector cell cultures after cocultivation with irradiated target cells. In Fig. 3, the progression of virus infection in the overlay cells after induction of target cells by X-ray treatment is compared to induction by IUdR. In this instance, the infected overlay cells were detected as being positive after seven to eight cell cycle generations (three passages) for both overlay cell types and after both treatments. In replicate experiments, it became evident that the number of cell generations required to detect very small numbers of positive cells varied from 6 to 15. After 20 generations, a very high (close to 100%) percentage of the overlay cells were IF positive and also could form plaques by the reverse XC assay. Additional experiments were then designed in an attempt to improve the reproducibility of virus induction as a prerequisite to the study of its mechanism.

Influence of Variations in Experimental Conditions on Virus Induction by X-Ray as Detected by IF Assay

For the following experiments, the cells were irradiated with 750 or 1,000 rad and were overlaid with 2×10^3 BL-5 cells, unless otherwise stated.

a. *Mouse embryo fibroblasts compared with an established line as target cells.* Earlier attempts to induce virus replication in non-established BL-MEF cells by halogenated pyrimidine analogues have yielded either negative (Rowe and Hartley, 1972) or transient (Stephenson and Aaronson, 1972) responses. As already mentioned, activation of an endogenous virus has been obtained by BrUdR treatment of an established cell line (Lieberman et al., 1973), BL-5, derived from BL-MEF. Accordingly, it seemed of interest to compare the two types of cultures (BL-MEF versus the established line BL-5) with respect to susceptibility to virus induction by X-irradiation. In two experiments in which BL-MEF and BL-5 cells were exposed to X-rays and overlaid with BL-5 cells, virus was induced in both types of cultures. No significant difference in percentage of positive cells was observed in the IF test.

b. *Time after plating at which X-ray dose is delivered.* Both the BL-5 and BL-MEF cell cultures were irradiated either 3 days (exponential or log phase cultures) or five days (confluent or stationary phase cultures) after plating. For one group, the cells were then subcultured into new dishes and overlaid 1 day later, whereas the target cells of another group were overlaid immediately. After three passages all groups were negative, but after six all were positive with no significant difference in the percentage of IF-positive cells. Therefore, neither the phase of the cell culture nor the subculture schedule seemed to influence the virus induction rate.

c. *Time of the cell cycle at which the X-ray dose is given.* It was postulated that the efficiency of virus induction might be increased by irradiating the cells in the G_1 or S phase of the cell cycle, since DNA synthesis is needed for transcription. The BL-5 cells (doubling time = 24 hr) were synchronized by treating the culture with thymidine (5×10^{-3} M) for 16 hr. The thymidine was replaced by fresh medium (MEM 10%) for 8 hr, and the cultures were then treated with either hydroxyurea (10^{-3} M) or again with thymidine (5×10^{-3} M) for 16 hr, after which they were washed several times and reincubated with fresh medium. Various doses of X-rays were then given at either 2 hr (S phase) or 12 hr (cells most likely to be in G_1 phase) after release of the block.

The results after five passages indicated no further increase in virus induction rates at either time interval, as compared with other experiments using non-synchronized cells.

d. *Irradiation of monolayers versus cell suspensions.* Here BL-MEF or BL-5 cells were plated at 2×10^5 cells/60-mm dish, irradiated 24 hr later, and then overlaid with BL-5 cells. Other aliquots of these cells were irradiated in suspension at 1 to 2×10^6 cells/ml and then plated at 2×10^5 cells/60-mm dish to be overlaid 24 hr later. After six passages (more than 15 doublings of the overlay), both groups were positive for X-ray doses greater than 450 rads, and no difference in the percentage of IF-positive cells was observed. Nonetheless, irradiation of cells in suspension is more convenient than irradiation of monolayers.

e. *Target cell number at the time of irradiation.* Determination of the minimal number of target cells required to detect X-ray induction of viral replication would provide the basis for an estimate of the probability of induction in a given cell population. The number of cells subjected to X-ray treatment was therefore adjusted from 100 cells/dish to 10^6 cells/dish in 10-fold steps. The IF-positive cells in the overlay were detected only when the number of target cells equaled or exceeded 10^5 cells/dish. If the overlay cell cultures were 100% efficient in detecting induced virus, Poisson statistics would suggest that a minimal estimate of the induction rate is approximately 10^{-5}.

f. *Type of overlay cell.* From earlier studies on the kinetics of replication of *in-vitro*-passaged radiation leukemia virus (RadLV) replication in non-restrictive cell cultures (Declève et al., 1975a), it was concluded that the detection of actively replicating RadLV depends on the rate of cell division. Accordingly, the replication of induced virus should be detected much earlier with BL-5 cells (doubling time = 24 hr) than with BALB/c-3T3 cells (doubling time = 35 hr). In two experiments to date, this expectation was confirmed; induction was detected with BL-5 cells but not with the BALB/c cell line.

g. *Initial density and time of overlay.* The optimal number of cells to use as an overlay was studied. Under our experimental conditions, plating efficiency varied from 10 to 50% depending on the cell line. Several concentrations of detector cells ranging from 10^2 to 2×10^5 cells/dish were overlaid on irradiated cells. For small numbers of overlay cells (100 to 1,000) the culture did not have to be subcultured before 10 days, whereas for larger numbers of overlay cells the cultures became confluent and had to be subcultured much earlier. The results indicated that at least 10^2 cells (plating efficiency taken into account) are needed to serve as efficient detector cells.

It also appeared that an overlay of 10^2 or 10^3 cells, which does not require subculture for as long as 10 days, remains in contact longer with the irradiated cells, thus increasing the chance of detection of virus released from a dying cell.

In an attempt to determine the time after irradiation at which virus could be detected, 2×10^5 target cells were overlaid at different intervals (1 to 15 days) after irradiation with 2×10^5 BL-5 cells. The results were inconclusive, since in most experiments the overlay one day after treatment became positive for viral antigens by IF, and in one experiment, virus spread was detected with an overlay as late as 12 days after treatment.

DISCUSSION

X-ray induction *in vitro* can be demonstrated in BL-MEF and BL-5 cells after single acute exposures to X-rays. The use of an overlay technique was required to detect progeny virus. Doses of X-rays greater than 450 rads were needed to achieve induction. No precise estimate of the induction rate could be made, but a minimal estimate of approximately 10^{-5} was suggested by the fact that induction could not be demonstrated when fewer than 10^5 cells were exposed. The conditions required for detection of induced virus are stringent and have not been fully optimized. It is clear, however, that detection of progeny virus requires cell-to-cell contact and extensive passage of the indicator cells, indicating that very few infectious particles are originally released. In some experiments, virus was induced at very high X-ray exposures, which would be expected to kill almost all of the target cells, suggesting that induction may occur during the process of cell death. The low induction rate (or the low efficiency of our detection methods) does not yet permit quantitative or biochemical study of the phenomenon in the light of what is now known about radiation injury to cell DNA and its repair.

Finally, the fact that the X-ray-induced virus from C57BL cells grows on both C57BL and on NIH/3T3 mouse cells, and sometimes even on NRK rat cells, leaves the question of the tropism of the induced virus unresolved. Indeed, recent experiments using IUdR as the inducing agent suggest that IUdR-induced virus from C57BL cells is N-tropic even though it is equally well propagated by both NIH/3T3 and C57BL cell overlays (Gelmann et al., *in preparation*). Accordingly, careful studies of the kinetics of replication (one-hit versus two-hit) on both $Fv-1^{bb}$ and $Fv-1^{nn}$ cells will be required before the tropism of radiation induced virus *in vitro* can be determined (Declève et al., 1975*b*).

ACKNOWLEDGMENTS

This work was supported by grants CA 03352 and CA 10372 from the National Cancer Institute, National Institutes of Health, Bethesda, Maryland.

REFERENCES

Aaronson, S. A., and Stephenson, J. R. (1973): Independent segregation of loci for activation of biologically distinguishable RNA C-type viruses in mouse cells. *Proc. Natl. Acad. Sci. USA*, 70:2055–2061.

Aaronson, S. A., Todaro, G. J., and Scolnick, E. M. (1971): Induction of murine C-type viruses in clonal lines of virus-free BALB/3T3 cells. *Science,* 174:157–158.

Declève, A., Gelmann, E., Niwa, O., and Kaplan, H. S. (1974a): X-ray induction of leukemia virus *in vitro. Radiat. Res.,* 59:90.

Declève, A., Lieberman, M., Hahn, G. M., and Kaplan, H. S. (1970): Focus formation by a murine sarcoma-leukemia virus complex. II. Quantitative aspects of the interaction between radiation leukemia virus and its murine sarcoma virus pseudo-type in strain C57BL mouse-embryo cells. *J. Virol.,* 5:437–445.

Declève, A., Niwa, O., Gelmann, E., and Kaplan, H. S. (1975a): Kinetics of propagation of B-tropic murine leukemia virus on Fv-1^b cell lines: Requirement for multiple cycles of cell replication for transformation and viral antigen expression by RadLV. *Virology,* 63:367–383.

Declève, A., Niwa, O., Gelmann, E., and Kaplan, H. S. (1975b): Replication kinetics of N and B tropic murine leukemia viruses on permissive and nonpermissive cells *in vitro. Virology,* 65:320–332.

Declève, A., Niwa, O., Hilgers, J., and Kaplan, H. S. (1974b): An improved murine leukemia virus immunofluorescence assay. *Virology,* 57:491–502.

Duc-Nguyen, H., Rosenblum, E. N., and Zeigel, R. F. (1966): Persistent infection of a rat kidney cell line with Rauscher murine leukemia virus. *J. Bacteriol.,* 92:1133–1141.

Kaplan, H. S. (1974): Leukemia and lymphoma in experimental and domestic animals. *Ser. Hematol.,* VII:94–111.

Klement, V., Nicolson, M. O., and Huebner, R. J. (1971): Rescue of the genome of focus-forming virus from rat nonproductive lines by 5'-bromodeoxyuridine. *Nature [New Biol.],* 234:12–13.

Levy, J. A. (1973): Xenotropic viruses: murine leukemia viruses associated with NIH Swiss, NZB and other mouse strains. *Science,* 182:1151–1153.

Lieber, M. M., Livingston, D. M., and Todaro, G. J. (1973a): Superinduction of endogenous type-C virus by 5-bromodeoxyuridine from transformed mouse clones. *Science,* 181:443–444.

Lieberman, M., Niwa, O., Declève, A., and Kaplan, H. S. (1973b): Continuous propagation of radiation leukemia virus on a C57BL mouse-embryo fibroblast line, with attenuation of leukemogenic activity. *Proc. Natl. Acad. Sci. USA,* 70:1250–1254.

Lowy, D. R., Rowe, W. P., Teich, N., and Hartley, J. W. (1971): Murine leukemia virus: High frequency activation *in vitro* by 5-iododeoxyuridine and 5-bromodeoxyuridine. *Science,* 174:155–156.

Niwa, O., Declève, A., Lieberman, M., and Kaplan, H. S. (1973): Adaptation of plaque assay methods to the *in vitro* quantitation of the radiation leukemia virus (RadLV). *J. Virol.,* 12:68–73.

Pincus, T., Hartley, J. W., and Rowe, W. P. (1971a): A major genetic locus affecting resistance to infection with murine leukemia viruses. I. Tissue culture studies of naturally occurring viruses. *J. Exp. Med.,* 133:1219–1233.

Pincus, T., Rowe, W. P., and Lilly, F. (1971b): A major genetic locus affecting resistance to infection with murine leukemia viruses. II. Apparent identity to a major locus described for resistance to Friend murine leukemia virus. *J. Exp. Med.,* 133:1234–1241.

Rowe, W. P., and Hartley, J. W. (1972): Studies of genetic transmission of murine leukemia virus by AKR mice. II. Crosses with Fv-1^b strains of mice. *J. Exp. Med.,* 136:1286–1301.

Rowe, W. P., Hartley, J. W., Lander, M. R., Pugh, W. E., and Teich, N. (1971): Noninfectious AKR mouse embryo cell lines in which each cell has the capacity to be activated to produce infectious murine leukemia virus. *Virology,* 46:866–876.

Stephenson, J. T., and Aaronson, S. A. (1972): Genetic factors influencing C-type RNA virus induction. *J. Exp. Med.,* 136:175–184.

Teich, N., Lowy, D. R., Hartley, J. W., and Rowe, W. P. (1973): Studies of the mechanism of induction of infectious murine leukemia virus from AKR mouse embryo cell lines by 5-iododeoxyuridine and 5-bromodeoxyuridine. *Virology,* 51:163–173.

Biology of Radiation Carcinogenesis, edited by
J. M. Yuhas, R. W. Tennant, and J. D. Regan.
Raven Press, New York © 1976.

Cellular Factors That Regulate Radiation Activation and Restriction of Mouse Leukemia Viruses

Raymond W. Tennant, James A. Otten, John M. Quarles,
Wen-Kuang Yang, and Arthur Brown*

*Carcinogenesis Program, Biology Division, Oak Ridge National Laboratory, Oak Ridge, Tennessee 37830 and *Department of Microbiology, University of Tennessee, Knoxville, Tennessee 37916*

Radiation has been demonstrated to induce thymic lymphomas in mice, and oncornaviruses recovered from these lymphomas have been shown to induce the same disease in the absence of radiation (Kaplan, 1957; Gross, 1958; Upton, 1962). It has been proposed that radiation serves to activate endogenous leukemia viruses, which induce tumor development, but activation of such viruses in cultured mouse cells by acute doses of X-rays was shown to be relatively inefficient compared to activation by halogenated pyrimidines (Rowe et al., 1971). Activation of oncornavirus by halogenated pyrimidines, however, has been shown to depend upon two discrete events associated with cell division (Teich et al., 1973; Ihle et al., 1974). During exposure to the drug, cell division is apparently required for incorporation of halogenated pyrimidines into cellular DNA. Incorporation of the drug results in the formation of a stable "activation intermediate" or provirus. The expression of the activated provirus, however, also depends on an event associated with a second cell-division cycle (Ihle et al., 1974).

EXPERIMENTAL RESULTS

Radiation Activation of Leukemia Virus

We used three sources of radiant energy to activate virus, and on the assumption that radiation activation in cell culture may also depend on cell division, experiments were performed with actively proliferating cells. The cultures were held in a 37°C incubator with the cell surface of the flask perpendicular to the source; they were exposed to relatively low dose rates of γ-radiation or neutrons. X-rays were delivered at a relatively high dose rate at ambient temperature, but care was taken not to affect cell division.

The cell cultures used in all experiments were AKR mouse embryo cells obtained from Dr. Wallace P. Rowe, National Institutes of Health. These cells have been demonstrated to carry at least two complete endogenous leukemia viruses, one of which has been genetically mapped and can be activated by exposure of the cells to 5-iododeoxyuridine (IdUrd) or 5-bromodeoxyuridine (BrUrd) (Rowe, 1973). After irradiation, the culture medium was changed, and 3 days later the cells were subcultured. After 4 or 8 days, the cells were tested for virus activation by direct plaque (XC) assay (Rowe et al., 1970).

The effects of relatively low dose rate γ-radiation (17.5 rad/hr) and neutron radiation (5.7 rad/hr) were compared with acute X-irradiation (100 to 191 rad/min) and, as shown in Table 1, virus activation was detected. All exposures were done with actively dividing cells, but γ- and neutron radiation were delivered to cells while they were in an incubator. Gamma radiation appeared to be the most efficient activator, and was less destructive to cells, but no direct comparison between the various radiation types and dose rates was possible; it is also possible that the most efficient dose rates were not used for each type.

TABLE 1. Comparison of activation rates of AKR cells by different forms of radiation

Radiation type	Dose rate	Exposure time	Total dose (R)	PFU[a]
Gamma	17.5 rad/hr	20 hr	350	13
	17.5 rad/hr	40 hr	700	40
X-ray	100 rad/min	4 min	400	0
	100 rad/min	8 min	800	3
	191 rad/min	1 min, 18 sec	250	1.5
	191 rad/min	2 min, 36 sec	500	2.0
Neutron	5.7 rad/hr[b]	20 hr	148	0.5
		40 hr	296	3.5

[a] Plaque-forming units.

[b] Additional component, 1.7 rad/hr γ-irradiation.

Besides our experiments, acute X-irradiation was also reported by Rowe et al. (1971) and Declève et al. (1976) to be inefficient in virus activation. The lower efficiency could either be due to some differences in the physical nature of the form of radiation or result from a low dose-rate exposure of the actively dividing cells. In order to test the role of cell division, the cultures were deprived of serum for 16 hr before irradiation, which significantly reduces the rate of division (Ihle et al., 1974). The cells were exposed for 20 hr in the absence of serum, but fresh medium that contained serum was added immediately after exposure. Because of the deleterious effect of longer periods of serum deprivation, it was possible to use only the 20-hr irradiation period. Table 2 shows that serum starvation significantly reduced the rate of activation, which suggests that cell proliferation may be an essential component in the activation process. Examination of the effects of irradiation and serum starvation on cell division showed that irradiation alone had little effect— shown mainly as a transient delay in cell division or the loss of some cells. Serum starvation inhibited cell division during the period of deprivation, but

TABLE 2. *Activation of virus from AKR Cells by γ-irradiation*

Dose (rad)	Serum	PFU[a]
0	—	0
0	+	0
350	—	1.0
350	+	13.0
700	+	39

[a] Plaque-forming units.

cells resumed division when serum was added. The absence of serum during irradiation resulted in the progressive loss of cells (up to 2×10^5), but upon the addition of serum cell division resumed. These results show that active cell division occurred during irradiation and that exposure to 350 or 700 rad resulted only in a transient delay in multiplication. The loss of serum-deprived cells during irradiation could reflect the selective destruction of virus-activated cells and could therefore account for the absence of virus activation. We believe that this is unlikely, but experiments to test the radiosensitivity of activated cells are in progress.

The frequency of virus activation as a function of viable cells is presented in Table 3. Although cell viability, determined by trypan blue exclusion, showed relatively little proportional decrease in viability between the 350- and 700-rad groups, we found that the plating efficiency of the cells exposed to 700 rad was significantly decreased. Since the assay of virus-activated cells involves plating the cells within 3 days of exposure, the activation frequency was corrected for plating efficiency. These limited data suggest that the activation frequency is proportional to total radiation dose. The efficiency of activation, expressed as activated cells per total cells per dose, was comparable for both the 350- and 700-rad groups exposed during active cell division, but was significantly reduced in the 350-rad group exposed during serum deprivation.

These results demonstrate that irradiation can activate the synthesis of infectious endogenous leukemia virus in cultured cells. The efficiency of acti-

TABLE 3. *Virus activation by γ-irradiation as a function of viable cells*

Total dose (rads)	PFU[a]	Plating efficiency (% control)	Virus activated/ total cells ($\times 10^{-5}$)	Activations per cell per rad
350	12	96	4.6	0.013
700	36	67	8.6	0.012
0 (20 hr)	—	100	—	—

[a] Plaque-forming units.

vation depends on cell division during irradiation, and the results of serum-deprivation experiments suggest that cell division during irradiation is required for virus expression. If cell division functioned only to transiently double the size of a molecular target (presumably the DNA provirus) population, exposure of actively dividing cells to acute irradiation would be expected to approximate the efficiency of low dose-rate exposure, which was not seen.

The results suggest, therefore, either that the ability of irradiated cells to express viral functions depends on the ability of the cells to divide within a short period of time after irradiation or that some event associated with cell division during exposure is required. It is not possible to distinguish between these alternatives on the basis of the data presented. But, the demonstrated requirement of two discrete events related to cell division for virus activation by halogenated pyrimidines (Teich et al., 1973; Ihle et al., 1974) suggests that these cellular functions may involve a mechanism common to both chemical and radiation activation. Further analysis of this system should contribute to our understanding of how cells normally control the expression of integrated endogenous leukemia viruses.

Fv-1 Locus Restriction of Mouse Leukemia-Virus Infection

The mouse Fv-1 locus is the major determinant of susceptibility to most naturally occurring strains of leukemia virus (Lilly and Pincus, 1973). Unlike the avian tumor viruses (Crittenden, 1968) and most other nononcogenic animal viruses, the resistance specified by the Fv-1 locus is expressed as a dominant trait, both *in vivo* and in cultured cells (Lilly and Pincus, 1973). The resistance is expressed as a restriction of N- and B-tropic leukemia viruses by cells with the respective Fv-1^{bb} and Fv-1^{nn} alleles. The F_1 hybrids (Fv-1^{nb}) restrict both viruses, but a class of primarily laboratory-derived virus strains, designated NB-tropic, are not restricted by this locus (Hartley et al., 1970).

Previous studies on the mechanism of the Fv-1 restriction have shown that the inhibition is intracellular (Eckner, 1973; Huang et al., 1973; Krontiris et al., 1973). We analyzed the fate of virus in heterokarya formed by the fusion of permissive and nonpermissive cells and found that both N- and B-tropic viruses were restricted in heterokarya but not in synkarya of permissive cells (Tennant et al., 1974a). We then attempted to determine the latest relative step in virus replication restricted by nonpermissive cells. The Fv-1^{nn} cells that had been labeled with [^{3}H]thymidine were fused with Fv-1^{bb} cells at 2, 6, and 12 hr after infection with N-tropic virus. At 60 hr after infection, the cultures were analyzed for virus protein synthesis in heterokaryons by simultaneous autoradiography and fluorescent antibody staining. As shown in Fig. 1a, virus infection was restricted in heterokarya formed within 6 hr after infection, but the number of permissive heterokarya approximately doubled in the group fused 12 hr after infection. In a reciprocal experiment

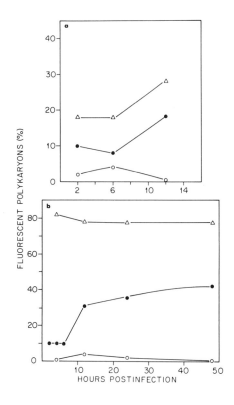

FIG. 1. *Top,* Fate of N-tropic virus in heterokarya formed after infection. The N-type cells were infected with N-tropic virus and then fused with ³H-labeled B-type cells at the indicated intervals. All cultures were collected at 60 hr after infection. At least two coverslips per group and five to ten fields per coverslip were counted, and the standard error of each value was within ±6%. The ordinate indicates the proportion of specific polykarya in the culture that were fluorescent. B/B cell synkaryons (non-permissive) (O—O), N/N cell synkarya (permissive) (△—△), N/B heterokaryons (●—●). *Bottom,* Fate of B-tropic virus in heterokarya formed after infection. The B-type cells were infected with B-tropic virus and then fused with N-type cells, as described above. N/N cell (non-permissive) synkarya (O—O), B/B cell synkarya (permissive) (△—△), N/B heterokarya (●—●). [By permission from Tennant et al. (1974): *Intl. J. Cancer,* 14:509].

with B-tropic virus (Fig. 1b), the number of permissive heterokarya approximately tripled between 6 and 12 hr. The results therefore suggested that the Fv-1 restriction functions primarily at some event in virus replication occurring within 6 hr after infection.

Inhibition of Infection by Extracts of Nonpermissive Cells

In subsequent experiments, we tested the effect of extracts of mouse cells with the Fv-1 gene locus on infection of permissive cells by N- and B-tropic host-range types of leukemia virus. The extracts of sonic-disrupted or Dounce-homogenized cells were applied to DEAE-dextran–treated cells prior to infection. As shown in Table 4, extracts from cells with the Fv-1^{nn} allele significantly inhibited only B-tropic virus, and Fv-1^{bb} allele cell extracts inhibited only N-tropic virus. Heterozygous Fv-1^{nb} cell extracts inhibited both N- and B-tropic viruses, but none of the extracts inhibited NB-tropic virus, which is not restricted by the Fv-1 locus. The extract from SC-1 mouse cells, which lack the Fv-1 gene (Janet Hartley, *personal communication*), did not inhibit the three viruses, but extracts of the other cells were inhibitory when tested against the appropriate viruses in SC-1 cells (Tennant et al., 1974b).

The inhibitor(s) in the crude extracts were very unstable (2 hr at 37°C or

TABLE 4. Percent of virus-infected cells in Fv-1$^{-/-}$ cultures treated with cell extracts[a]

Virus	Fv-1^{bb}	Fv-1^{nn}	Fv-1^{nb}	Fv-1$^{-/-}$	No extract
B-tropic	34 ± 4 (10.5)	22 ± 5 (42.1)	18 ± 3 (52.6)	36 ± 4 (5.3)	36 ± 3
N-tropic	14 ± 2 (46.2)	35 ± 5 (0)	16 ± 3 (38.5)	28 ± 5 (0)	26 ± 3
NB-tropic	79 ± 2 (0)	79 ± 4 (0)	78 ± 3 (0)	74 ± 3 (3.9)	77

[a] Fv-1$^{-/-}$ cells were pretreated with DEAE-dextran for 1 hr at 37°C and then washed and incubated with extract for 2 hr. Next, the cells were washed prior to viral infection, washed again 2 hr after virus addition, and medium was added. Coverslip cultures were collected 28 hr after infection, and the number of infected cells was determined by immunofluorescent cell counts on at least 1,000 cells/group. Numbers in parentheses represent percent inhibition. (By permission, from Tennant et al. (1974): Proc. Natl. Acad. Sci. USA, 71:4243.)

4 hr at 4°C). The inhibitor did not react directly with virus, inhibit the attachment of radioactively labeled N-tropic virus, or have cytotoxic effects on cells. The degree of inhibition measured by fluorescent antibody or plaque (XC) assay was only 50 to 80% but could be the result of the lability of the crude inhibitor or the effect of the high virus concentrations used. The restriction by the Fv-1 gene in cells, however, also is not absolute, and is expressed as a 10- to 1,000-fold reduction of infection and a multi-hit titration pattern (Lilly and Pincus, 1973). These results therefore suggested that a product of cells with the Fv-1 locus could specifically restrict virus infection.

Genetic Specificity of the Inhibitor

Although the previous studies indicated that the inhibition could be due to a specific gene product, additional studies were performed to test this assumption. Additional strains of mice with known Fv-1 alleles were tested by preparing embryo cell cultures from which extracts were made and assayed against N- and B-tropic leukemia viruses. Significant inhibition of B-tropic virus was seen only with extracts of homozygous Fv-1^{nn} (strains NIH Swiss, C3H, AKR, C57L, DBA/2, and RF) and heterozygous Fv-1^{nb} (strains B6C3F$_1$ and CD2F$_1$) cell extracts; N-tropic virus infection was restricted only by extracts of cells with the Fv-1^{bb} (BALB/c and C57BL/6) and Fv-1^{nb} alleles. There was no significant restriction of NB-tropic virus by any cell extracts. In some cases, there was a partial inhibition of virus that was not sensitive to the Fv-1 gene, but this was three to six times less than the restriction of the sensitive virus.

Although the above results suggest that the inhibitor is specifically related to the Fv-1 locus, a direct correlation was established by simultaneously testing individual mice for Fv-1 genotype and specific inhibitory activity. These B6C3F$_1$ mice (C57BL6 × C3H; Fv-1^{nb}) were mated, and the individual embryos, which should segregate the Fv-1 alleles in an approximate 1:2:1 ratio, were cultured. The individual embryo cultures were divided in the second passage, and each group was randomly coded. The Fv-1 genotype was determined for one-half of each of the cultures by titration of N- and B-tropic

TABLE 5. *Distribution of the Fv-1 gene in B6C3F$_2$ mouse embryos*

Embryo	Virus susceptibility (log$_{10}$ PFU^a/ml difference between N- and B-tropic virus)	Fv-1 genotype^b	Extract effect (% inhibition) on		Inhibitor specificity
			N-tropic virus	B-tropic virus	
D-1	0.1	nb	67	47	nb
D-2	0.3	nb	61	68	nb
D-3	0.8	nb	64	61	nb
D-4	~3.1	nn	14	66	nn
D-5	0.8	nb	31	34	nb
D-6	0.7	nb	56	58	nb
D-7	2.6	nn	0	58	nn
D-8	3.5	bb	67	0	bb
D-9	0	nb	72	77	nb
D-10	0.3	nb	61	64	nb
E-1	1.4	nb	61	69	nb
E-2	3.1	bb	67	5	bb
E-3	3.0	bb	61	8	bb
E-4	3.5	bb	44	3	bb
E-5	0.4	nb	53	39	nb
E-6	0.6	nb	53	21	nb
E-7	0	nb	69	77	nb
E-8	3.2	nn	0	69	nn
E-9	0.2	nb	44	71	nb

^{a} Plaque-forming units.
^{b} Distribution: nn, 3; nb, 12; bb, 4.

virus. The genotype was indicated by a two- to fourfold log$_{10}$ difference between the N- and B-tropic virus titers; the restricted virus demonstrated the genotype. The second one-half of the individual embryo culture was extracted, and the effect of the extract was tested against the two virus host-range types. The results of testing the progeny of two matings are shown in Table 5 and indicate a clear correlation between Fv-1 genotype and extract specificity. The extract specificity of the same embryo culture was indicated by the percent inhibition values for which nonspecific inhibition is considered to be $\leq 20\%$. The distribution of the genotypes was 3:12:4, and these frequencies were not significantly different at the chi square 5% level from those expected of a 1:2:1 ratio. The embryos of additional F$_1$ matings are now being tested to confirm these results.

DISCUSSION

The results of the two studies presented above relate to two classes of cellular functions that are important in viral oncogenesis. The studies utilized model cell-culture systems but also have important implications for understanding the mechanisms of virus-radiation oncogenesis *in vivo;* they relate to viral–chemical cocarcinogenesis and to circumstances under which the virus alone induces neoplasia. The first system was used to demonstrate that irradiation can activate endogenous leukemia virus in cultured cells. The efficiency of radiation activation cannot be compared directly with chemical activation because it is not possible to relate the doses of each activator. But, we have presented evidence that some event(s) associated with cell division are required for radiation activation—as has been demonstrated for virus activation by halogenated pyrimidines. Future studies will be directed at determining the specific nature of these cell functions, particularly if some function common to both radiation and chemicals is involved. In the case of chemical activation, two discrete cell divisions appear to be required. First, cell division must occur during exposure to IdUrd or BrUrd for the compounds to be incorporated into cellular or proviral DNA (Teich et al., 1973; Ihle et al., 1974). But, if dividing cells are exposed to the compounds, virus expression does not appear unless cell division is allowed to continue (Ihle et al., 1974). The nature of the functions required in the second cell division are not apparent but may be related to the cell division function(s) required for exogenous infection by avian and murine oncornaviruses (Temin, 1967; Yoshikura, 1970).

As a working hypothesis, it may be assumed that cells normally synthesize some type of repressor that restricts endogenous provirus transcription. Incorporation of the halogenated pyrimidines, or the direct action of radiation, may serve to decrease the affinity of such a repressor for the provirus, which could allow subsequent transcription. In addition, some function(s) associated with cell division may be required for the initiation of transcription of the "activated" endogenous provirus or of the provirus formed by the viral reverse transcriptase in exogenous infection. This second function, therefore, may be the element common to the expression of the provirus in both the endogenous and the exogenous state. Such a hypothesis, however, fails to account for many aspects of virus expression, and particularly why the exogenous provirus does not appear to come under the control of the putative repressor. Obviously, it is important to define the specific nature of the cellular functions involved in virus activation, and the radiation-activation system we have described (Otten et al., 1975) may provide an important model in these studies.

The second aspect of our studies also relates to cellular control of virus expression. Since it has been shown that an N-tropic virus can be activated from cells with the $Fv-1^{bb}$ allele, but that the activated virus fails to perpetuate in the cells, it has been proposed that the Fv-1 locus does not restrict virus activation but rather some function associated with exogenous virus replication. It is possible, however, that in addition to activating the endogenous virus, the halogenated pyrimidines may also interfere with the Fv-1 locus on virus activation. The gene is an important component in the complex problem of viral carcinogenesis, and an understanding of the mechanism of the restriction is important for future progress.

The results we have presented show that a product from cells with the Fv-1 locus can transfer resistance to specific virus host-range types. This observation suggests that the Fv-1 locus specifies a unique mechanism of resistance to oncornaviruses—a mechanism that involves a gene product that functions intracellularly. It is not clear whether the inhibitor acts directly or induces some product(s), which interact with specific viral functions. Studies are in progress to determine the biochemical nature and mechanism of action of the inhibitor.

ACKNOWLEDGMENTS

This research was sponsored jointly by the Virus Cancer Program of the National Cancer Institute, and by the Energy Research and Development Administration under contract with the Union Carbide Corporation. John M. Quarles is a postdoctoral investigator supported by Public Health Service Research Grant No. CA00157 from the National Cancer Institute.

REFERENCES

Crittenden, L. B. (1968): Observations on the nature of genetic cellular resistance to avian tumor viruses. *J. Natl. Cancer Inst.,* 41:145–153.

Declève, A., Niwa, O., Gelmann, E., and Kaplan, H. W. (1976): Radiation activation of endogenous leukemia viruses in cell culture: Acute X-ray irradiation. In: *The Biology of Radiation Carcinogenesis,* edited by J. M. Yuhas, R. W. Tennant, and J. D. Regan, pp. 217–226.

Eckner, R. J. (1973): Helper-dependent properties of Friend spleen focus-forming virus: Effect of the Fv-1 gene on the late stages in virus synthesis. *J. Virol.,* 12:523–533.

Gross, L. (1958): Attempt to recover a filterable agent from X-ray-induced leukemia. *Acta Hemat.,* 19:353–361.

Hartley, J. W., Rowe, W. P., and Huebner, R. J. (1970): Host range restrictions of murine leukemia viruses in mouse embryo cell cultures. *J. Virol.,* 5:221–225.

Huang, A. S., Besner, P., Chu, L., and Baltimore, D. (1973): Growth of pseudotypes of vesicular stomatitis virus with N-tropic murine leukemia virus coats in cells resistant to N-tropic viruses. *J. Virol.,* 12:659–662.

Ihle, J. N., Kenney, F. T., and Tennant, R. W. (1974): Evidence for a stable intermediate in leukemia virus activation in AKR mouse embryo cells. *J. Virol.,* 14:451–456.

Kaplan, H. S. (1957): The pathogenesis of experimental lymphoid tumors in mice. In: *Proceedings of the Second Canadian Cancer Conference,* Vol. II, edited by R. W. Begg, Academic Press, New York, pp. 127–141.

Krontiris, T. G., Soeiro, R., and Fields, B. N. (1973): Host restriction of Friend leukemia virus. Role of the viral outer coat. *Proc. Natl. Acad. Sci. USA,* 70:2549–2553.

Lilly, F., and Pincus, T. (1973): Genetic control of murine viral leukemogenesis. *Adv. Cancer Res.,* 17:231–277.

Otten, J. A., Quarles, J. M., and Tennant, R. W. (1975): Activation of murine leukemia virus in cell culture by gamma irradiation. *Virology (In press).*

Rowe, W. P. (1973): Genetic factors in the natural history of murine leukemia virus infection. *Cancer Res.,* 33:3061–3068.

Rowe, W. P., Hartley, J. W., Lander, M. R., Pugh, W. E., and Teich, N. (1971): Noninfectious AKR mouse embryo cell lines in which each cell has the capacity to be activated to produce infectious murine leukemia virus. *Virology,* 46:866–876.

Rowe, W. P., Pugh, W. E., and Hartley, J. W. (1970): Plaque assay techniques for murine leukemia viruses. *Virology,* 42:1136–1139.

Teich, N., Lowy, D. R., Hartley, J. W., and Rowe, W. P. (1973): Studies on the mechanism of induction of infectious murine leukemia virus from AKR mouse embryo cell lines by 5-iododeoxyuridine and 5-bromodeoxyuridine. *Virology,* 51: 163–173.

Temin, H. M. (1967): Studies on carcinogenesis by avian sarcoma viruses. V. Requirement for new DNA synthesis and for cell division. *J. Cell Physiol.,* 69:53–64.

Tennant, R. W., Myer, F. E., and McGrath, L. (1974a): Effect of the Fv-1 gene on leukemia virus in mouse cell heterokaryons. *Int. J. Cancer,* 14:504–513.

Tennant, R. W., Schluter, B., Yang, W. K., and Brown, A. (1974b): Reciprocal inhibition of mouse leukemia virus infection by Fv-1 allele cell extracts. *Proc. Natl. Acad. Sci. USA,* 71:4241–4245.

Upton, A. C. (1962): Leukemogenesis—Role of viruses and cytological aspects. In: *Cellular Basis and Etiology of Late Somatic Effects of Ionizing Radiation,* Academic Press, New York, pp. 67–82.

Yoshikura, H. (1970): Dependence of murine sarcoma virus infection on the cell cycle. *J. Gen. Virol.,* 6:183–185.

Biology of Radiation Carcinogenesis, edited by
J. M. Yuhas, R. W. Tennant, and J. D. Regan.
Raven Press, New York © 1976.

Anomalous Viral Expression in Radiogenic Lymphomas of C57BL/Ka Mice

M. Lieberman, H. S. Kaplan, and A. Declève

Department of Radiology, Stanford University School of Medicine, Stanford, California 94305

Fractionated, whole-body X-irradiation of C57BL/Ka mice leads to the development of thymus-dependent lymphomas, with onset after about three months and final incidence above 90% (Kaplan and Brown, 1952). From these lymphomas, we recovered a subcellular agent that induced similar neo-plasms in unirradiated mice of the same strain (Lieberman and Kaplan, 1959). The agent was identified as a murine leukemia virus and was desig-nated the radiation leukemia virus (RadLV). After inoculation, RadLV replicates preferentially in the thymus and can be detected within a few days by the intrathymic appearance of virus-related intracellular antigens (Declève et al., 1974*b*). The virus can also be adapted to growth in cultures of C57BL/Ka embryo fibroblasts (Lieberman et al., 1973). Its growth kinetics in cells from strains of mice differing at the Fv-1 gene locus identify it as a B-tropic virus (Declève et al., 1975), according to the nomenclature of Pincus et al. (1971).

In this chapter we present a preliminary report of an investigation designed to determine the time course of appearance and the localization of RadLV in the tissues of C57BL/Ka mice following a leukemogenic course of X-irradia-tion. The presence of virus was monitored by visualization of viral antigens in lymphoid cells of various organs by means of immunofluorescence.

C57BL/Ka mice were exposed beginning at 5 to 6 weeks of age to four weekly, whole-body X-irradiations of 168 R each. At intervals after the last exposure, groups of mice were sacrificed, and the thymus, spleen, bone mar-row, and lymph nodes were processed for immunofluorescence microscopy, as previously described (Declève et al., 1974*a;* Declève et al., 1947*b*). Begin-ning 1 month after the last irradiation, the presence of transformed cells in the thymus was ascertained by examination of stained sections.

As has been described earlier (Kaplan, 1960; Siegler et al., 1966), the first clusters of recognizably transformed cells appeared in the thymic cortex at about 6 weeks after the last X-ray exposure and gradually enlarged and coalesced thereafter.

The immunofluorescence findings, however, were unexpected. Whereas over 80% of C57BL/Ka thymocytes show the presence of viral antigens by three weeks after inoculation of RadLV, the thymocytes of X-irradiated

C57BL/Ka mice remained essentially negative throughout the course of lymphoma development. At 4 months, only 3 of 16 thymic lymphomas contained antigen-positive cells at barely detectable levels (0.02 to 0.07%). Of the other tissues tested, bone marrow was the most consistently positive. Beginning at two weeks after termination of treatment, positive cells became visible in the marrow at frequencies ranging from 0.1 to 1.5%, increasing thereafter in occasional mice to levels as high as 4% (Table 1). Findings for the spleen were much the same as those for the bone marrow, except that the proportion of mice showing positive cells was much lower. The lymph nodes did not become positive until approximately 3 months after irradiation, at a time when the positive cells could well have represented dissemination of thymic lymphoma cells, and the fraction of positive cells they contained did not exceed 1%.

When RadLV was first recovered from radiation-induced lymphomas of C57BL/Ka mice, its leukemogenic potential was very low, and it was only after repeated serial passage that it acquired its present high level of activity (Lieberman and Kaplan, 1959; Kaplan, 1967). In an attempt to reproduce this amplification, thymic cells from individual leukemic mice were serially transplanted by intrathymic injection in weanling recipients. At 3-week intervals, the resultant thymic tumors were passed again and were also processed for immunofluorescence. The results are shown in Table 2. It appears that after one or more passages, viral antigen-positive cells appear in the thymic tumors, in low numbers at first and increasing thereafter. Experiments are in progress to answer the question: Do the cells in radiation-induced lymphomas appear devoid of viral antigen because viral expression is incomplete or because the quantity of viral antigen per cell is so low as to escape detection by the immunofluorescence method? Cell-free extracts from lymphoid tissues of leukemic mice have been inoculated intrathymically into weanling C57BL/Ka mice to determine their leukemogenic potential. No lymphomas have developed in the recipients after 8 to 9 months, but a long latent period is not unusual in the case of first-passage virus preparations.

In order to acquire additional information about the "cryptic" virus in radiation lymphomas, its replication characteristics *in vitro* were investigated. In a first experiment, thymus and marrow cells from the second passage of donor No. 1 (see Table 2) were inoculated onto monolayers of C57BL/Ka, BALB/c, and NIH-Swiss fibroblasts. When the monolayer became confluent, the lymphoid cells were washed off, and the fibroblasts were trypsinized and subcultured. An aliquot was processed for immunofluorescence, as were the washed-off lymphoid cells; all were negative (Table 3). At the second subculture, the fibroblasts that had been co-cultivated with leukemic thymocytes were still negative, but of those which had been cocultivated with leukemic marrow cells, 10% in the C57BL/Ka cultures and 5% in the BALB/c cultures were antigen-positive. The NIH-Swiss cells remained negative. Unfortunately, bacterial contamination necessitated termination of the experiment at the next passage.

TABLE 1. Viral antigen-positive cells in thymus, spleen, bone marrow, and lymph nodes of C57BL/Ka mice at intervals after X-irradiation

Tissue	Time after last x-ray exposure							
	3 days	1 week	2 weeks	1 month	1½ months	2 months	3 months	4 months
Thymus	0/14	0/8	0/14	1/12 (0.2)	0/12	1/16	1/6 (0.1)	3/16 (0.02–0.07)
Spleen	0/14	0/8	3/14[a] (0.2–0.5)[b]	7/12 (0.5–5.0)	5/11 (0.1–1.3)	6/15 (0.2–0.6)	3/6 (0.1–0.3)	3/15 (0.1 –0.8)
Marrow	0/14	0/8	6/14 (0.1–1.5)	11/12 (0.6–2.0)	11/12 (0.4–3.5)	13/15 (0.03–0.9)	6/6 (0.8–4.0)	5/13 (0.02–3.6)
Nodes	0/14	0/8	0/14	0/6	0/12	0/8	6/6 (0.2–1.0)	4/10 (0.02–0.8)

[a] Number of mice with antigen-positive cells/total number of mice.
[b] Percent fluorescing cells in positive mice, range.

TABLE 2. *Serial syngeneic passage of leukemic cells from radiation-induced lymphomas of C57BL mice*

	Viral antigen in thymic tumors passage generation							
	1		2		3		4	
Donor	No. positive mice/total	% fluorescing cells	No. positive mice/total	% fluorescing cells	No. positive mice/total	% fluorescing cells	No. positive mice/total	% fluorescing cells
1	0/3	—	0/3	—				
2	1/4	7	3/3	11,17,20	3/3	11,11,18	3/3	40,50,60
3	2/2	10,12	Terminated		Terminated		Terminated	
4	0/2	—	0/2	—	2/2	6,17	2/2	10,20[a]
5	0/2	—	0/2	—	0/2	—	Terminated	

[a] Diminished intensity of fluorescence.

TABLE 3. In vitro passage of virus from radiation-induced lymphomas of C57BL/Ka mice

| | IF-positive cells in C57BL/Ka, BALB/c, and NIH-Swiss fibroblasts (%) | | | | | | | | | | | |
| | Passages 1 and 2 | | | Passage 3 | | | Passage 4 | | | Passage 6 | | |
Inoculum	C57BL	BALB/c	NIH-SW	C57BL	BALB/c	NIH-SW	C57BL	BALB/c	NIH-SW	C57BL	BALB/c	NIH-SW
Donor No. 1, passage 2 cells	0	0	0	10	5	0	Terminated					
Leukemic donor												
Thymus extract	0	N.D.[a]	0	0	N.D.	0	0	N.D.	0			
Spleen extract	0	N.D.	0	0	N.D.	12	0	N.D.	25	Terminated		
Marrow extract	0	N.D.	0	0	N.D.	12	0	N.D.	60			
Leukemic donors												
Thymus extract	0	N.D.	0	0	N.D.	0	0	N.D.	26	0	N.D.	70
Spleen extract	0	N.D.	0	0	N.D.	0	0	N.D.	0	0	N.D.	0
Marrow extract	0	N.D.	0	0	N.D.	0	0	N.D.	0	0	N.D.	0

[a] N.D., Not done.

In a second experiment, cell-free extracts from the thymus, spleen, and marrow of a mouse with radiogenic lymphoma were inoculated onto monolayers of C57BL/Ka, NIH-Swiss, and SIRC fibroblasts. The cells were subcultured when they became confluent, and at each passage, an aliquot was processed for immunofluorescence. The results are shown in Table 3. Through four subcultures, the thymus extract-infected fibroblasts remained negative. However, positive cells appeared in the third subculture of the NIH-Swiss cells that had received an inoculum of either spleen or marrow extract, and their number increased on passage. The C57BL/Ka and SIRC fibroblasts remained negative.

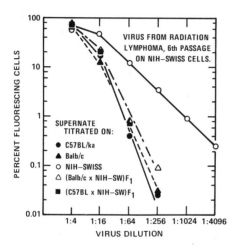

FIG. 1. Percent of target cells that fluoresce following the addition of varying dilutions of the supernatant obtained from the sixth passage of a radiation-induced C57BL/Ka lymphoma on NIH-SWISS cells.

In a third experiment, two thymus extracts and one spleen extract from individual donors were used. Cell cultures were as above, except that NRK cells were used instead of SIRC. Through six subcultures, only one of the thymus extracts eventually yielded virus, and this again only on NIH-Swiss cells (Table 3). The virus-containing supernatant of the sixth-passage NIH-Swiss cells was used to determine virus tropism. Serial dilutions were titrated on the following cell cultures: C57BL/Ka, NIH-Swiss, BALB/c, (BALB/c × NIH-Swiss) F_1, and (C57BL/Ka × NIH-Swiss) F_1. The extent of viral replication was assessed by monitoring the fraction of cells showing viral antigen by immunofluorescence. The results are shown in Figure 1, in which the percentage of antigen-positive cells is plotted against virus dilution for each cell type. It is apparent that two types of kinetics were obtained in this experiment: a one-hit response (45° slope), in the case of virus replicating in NIH-Swiss cells, and two-hit kinetics (~ 63° slope) for the other four cell types. To our knowledge, this is the first evidence for the existence of N-tropic MuLV in strain C57BL.

Two major conclusions are suggested by the present experiments.

1. The radiation-induced lymphomas of C57BL/Ka mice differ strikingly from those induced by the passaged virus originally obtained from them in that viral antigen is either absent or only minimally detectable in the thymic lymphoma cells by the immunofluorescence procedure employed. The status of the virus in these mice is not presently known. As a working hypothesis, we postulate that irradiation of the animal leads to a derepression or activation of a latent viral genome and that thereafter only partial virus expression is required to initiate transformation in susceptible cell types. A very small fraction of the virus population may proceed to complete expression of all virus-associated properties, including antigenicity and infectivity. Although this fraction is too small to be detected initially by the methods used, it is sufficient to infect and transform susceptible host cells after inoculation, although with low efficiency. Serial, *in vivo* viral passage thereafter leads to marked and fairly rapid increases in both antigenic expression and infectivity, but the mechanisms through which these changes are effected are not known.

2. An interesting feature, manifested after infection of fibroblasts *in vitro* with subcellular extracts from radiogenic lymphomas, is that the emergent virus may exhibit N-tropism, with single-hit kinetics on Fv-1^n cells, whereas passaged RadLV is distinctly B-tropic when adapted to growth *in vitro* (Lieberman et al., 1973; Declève et al., 1975). This N-tropism has not been observed after *in vivo* passage of viable or radiation-killed leukemic cells from C57BL/Ka mice with radiogenic lymphomas; after one or more passages, such cells yield detectable virus in C57BL/Ka mice, but detectable virus has not been observed to date in NIH-Swiss mice, the prototype of the Fv-1^n allotype. What is the relationship between RadLV and the N-tropic virus? Which of these viruses mediates leukemogenesis in irradiated mice, if only one is involved? How do they interact, if both are involved? Does the xenotropic virus of C57BL mice also have a role in the disease process? To what extent is viral expression needed for neoplastic transformation? These are some of the questions that are raised by these experimental results; much additional work will be needed before they can be answered.

ACKNOWLEDGMENTS

The excellent technical assistance of Nancy Ginzton, Joan Kojola, and Barbara Franks is gratefully acknowledged. Supported by grants CA 03352 and CA 10372 from the National Cancer Institute, National Institutes of Health, Bethesda, Maryland.

N.B. After submission of this manuscript it came to our attention that evidence for the presence of N-tropic MuLV in the spleen of C57BL mice was recently presented by T. Okada (1975): *J. Virol.* 15:332.

REFERENCES

Declève, A., Niwa, O., Gelmann, E., and Kaplan, H. S. (1975): Replication kinetics of N- and B-tropic murine leukemia viruses on permissive and nonpermissive cells *in vitro. Virology,* 65:320.

Declève, A., Niwa, O., Hilgers, J., and Kaplan, H. S. (1974*a*): An improved murine leukemia virus immunofluorescence assay. *Virology,* 57:491.

Declève, A., Sato, C., Lieberman, M., and Kaplan, H. S. (1974*b*): Selective thymic localization of murine leukemia virus-related antigens in C57BL/Ka mice after inoculation with radiation leukemia virus. *Proc. Natl. Acad. Sci. USA,* 71:3124.

Kaplan, H. S. (1960): Early microscopic diagnosis of lymphosarcoma *in situ* in thymus of irradiated mice. *Fed. Proc.,* 19:399 (abstr.).

Kaplan, H. S., and Brown, M. B. (1952): A quantitative dose-response study of lymphoid tumor development in irradiated C57 black mice. *J. Natl. Cancer Inst.,* 13: 185.

Lieberman, M., and Kaplan, H. S. (1959): Leukemogenic activity of filtrates from radiation-induced lymphoid tumors of mice. *Science,* 130:387.

Lieberman, M., Niwa, Declève, A., and Kaplan, H. S. (1973): Continuous propagation of radiation leukemia virus on a C57BL mouse embryo fibroblast line, with attenuation of leukemogenic activity. *Proc. Natl. Acad. Sci. USA,* 70:1250.

Pincus, T., Hartley, J. W., and Rowe, W. P. (1971): A major genetic locus affecting resistance to infection with murine leukemia viruses. I. Tissue culture studies of naturally occurring viruses. *J. Exp. Med.,* 133:1219.

Siegler, R., Harrell, W., and Rich, M. A. (1966): Pathogenesis of radiation-induced thymic lymphoma in mice. *J. Natl. Cancer Inst.,* 37:105.

Biology of Radiation Carcinogenesis, edited by
J. M. Yuhas, R. W. Tennant, and J. D. Regan.
Raven Press, New York © 1976.

Pathways in Murine Radiation Leukemogenesis—Coleukemogenesis

Nechama Haran-Ghera

Department of Chemical Immunology, The Weizmann Institute of Science, Rehovot, Israel

The experimental systems used in the present studies involve lymphatic leukemia induction in C57BL/6 mice by exposure to fractionated whole-body irradiation or by inoculation of the radiation leukemia virus.

The C57BL strain of mice, which exhibits a very low spontaneous lymphatic leukemia incidence, is extremely susceptible to the induction of lymphatic leukemia by exposure to X-rays. This strain was, therefore, extensively investigated in relation to murine radiation leukemogenesis. Different studies have indicated the optimal conditions for leukemia induction and prevention (Kaplan, 1964). Susceptibility to radiation was found to be age dependent, namely, with increasing age a significant decrease in leukemia incidence was observed (Kaplan, 1948). The optimal leukemia incidence was obtained when a dose of X-rays was divided into repeated exposures within a few days interval (i.e., four whole-body exposures of 150 to 170 r at weekly intervals) rather than as a single exposure; a delay in the time intervals between the repeated radiation exposures (14 to 21 days) markedly reduced leukemia incidence (Kaplan and Brown, 1952). Although most of the lymphatic leukemias induced by irradiation in the C57BL strain of mice originated in the thymus, radiation of the thymic area did not cause leukemia (Kaplan, 1949). Prevention of radiation leukemogenesis was afforded by shielding the spleen (Lorenz et al., 1953) or bone marrow (Kaplan and Brown, 1951) during exposure of the rest of the body to X-rays, or by injecting isologous bone marrow cells into irradiated hosts shortly after termination of the radiation treatment (Kaplan et al., 1953). The demonstration that thymic grafts restored the incidence of lymphomas in thymectomized irradiated C57BL mice indicated the existence of an indirect induction mechanism (Kaplan et al., 1956). These findings led to a search for leukemogenic viruses in radiation-induced lymphomas. It was shown that cell-free preparations from either primary or transplanted radiation-induced leukemias in the C57BL/6 strain of mice (Lieberman and Kaplan, 1959) or from irradiated non-leukemic bone marrow (Haran-Ghera, 1966a) contained an agent with leukemogenic activity. The leukemogenic activity of this isolated agent was first demonstrated by its tumorigenic effect upon injection into isologous newborn mice. A more sensitive technique for demonstrating the leukemogenic activity of the agent involved injection of the leukemogenic agent directly into the intact thymus of an adult mouse (Haran-Ghera, 1969a). Although the virus exerted its leukemogenic effect locally and directly on the thymus (Haran-Ghera et al., 1966b), host treatment (X-rays, antithymocyte serum) markedly increased tumor incidence, provided it was administered within several days after virus inoculation (Haran-Ghera, 1971).

Usually in experimental leukemogenesis, several months elapse between the termination of the leukemogenic treatment and the occurrence of overt disease. Exposure of C57BL/6 mice, for example, to fractionated irradiation induces a high incidence of lymphatic leukemia (70 to 90%) at an average latent period of 200 days. Is this long latent period related to delayed neoplastic transformation or with the proliferation of leukemic cells affected by host factors? The mode of action of radiation as a leukemogenic and coleukemogenic factor relative to the onset of neoplastic transformation and its effects on specific lymphoid cell populations and virus-lymphoid cell interaction are analyzed in the studies presented here.

DETECTION OF PRELEUKEMIC CELLS DURING THE LATENT PERIOD OF LEUKEMIA DEVELOPMENT

A method to establish the presence of preleukemic cells in mice at a stage when they do not show clinical manifestations of the disease (Haran-Ghera, 1973), has been used in the present studies. This method involved intravenous injection of bone marrow cells from donor mice treated with fractionated irradiation (collected at different time intervals following termination of the leukemogenic treatment) into irradiated syngeneic C57BL/6 or hybrid (BALB/c × C57BL/6)F_1 mice. The transfer was always performed from one donor to one recipient to avoid possible contamination of the pool by one single preleukemic mouse. The use of hybrid mice in this analysis enabled the identification of the preleukemic cell genotype, whether of donor or recipient origin (by transplanting the tumor cells developing in F_1 hybrid mice into F_1 and parental strains). The origin of leukemic cells from the parental C57BL/6 donor strain would indicate the actual transfer of established preleukemic or leukemic cells among the transferred bone marrow cells, whereas leukemias of F_1 host origin would indicate the presence of a leukemogenic non-cellular agent among the transferred cells that caused neoplastic transformation in the thymus or other lymphoid organs of the host. Exposure of 6 to 8 week-old female C57BL/6 mice to four weekly doses of 170 r wholebody irradiation induced 72% lymphatic leukemia at an average latent period of 210 days. Transplantation of 3×10^7 normal syngeneic bone marrow cells into the irradiated mice (intravenously), within 1 to 3 hr after the last radiation exposure, reduced the leukemia incidence to 25%, whereas thymus removal, before the radiation treatment, abolished overt leukemia development completely (Table 1). Transfer experiments demonstrated the "release" phe-

TABLE 1. Leukemia induction following transfer of bone marrow cells from radiation treated young C57BL/6 mice

Donor strain[a]	Donor treatment (r × 4)	Time of transfer after treatment (days)	Bone marrow recipient strain[b]	Pretreatment of recipient (r)	Leukemia incidence and ALP[c] (days)	Leukemia origin	
						Donor	Recipient
C57BL/6	170				13/18-72% (210)	—	—
C57BL/6	170 (+BM)				5/20-25% (185)	—	—
Thx[d] C57BL/6	170				0/20 —	—	—
C57BL/6	170	7	C57BL/6	400	5/12-40% (190)	—	—
C57BL/6	170	30	C57BL/6	400	16/20-80% (185)	—	—
C57BL/6	None	—	C57BL/6	400	1/20- 5% (230)	—	—
C57BL/6	170	7	(BALB/c × C57BL/6)F$_1$	400	6/20-30% (202)	—	5/5
C57BL/6	170	30	(BALB/c × C57BL/6)F$_1$	400	10/18-55% (163)	6/8	2/8
C57BL/6	None	—	(BALB/c × C57BL/6)F$_1$	400	0/15 —	—	—
C57BL/6	170 (+BM)	7	C57BL/6	400	4/12-33% (190)	—	—
C57BL/6	170 (+BM)	7	(BALB/c × C57BL/6)F$_1$	400	4/24-16% (180)	—	3/3
C57BL/6	170 (+BM)	30	C57BL/6	400	10/18-55% (185)	—	—
C57BL/6	170 (+BM)	30	(BALB/c × C57BL/6)F$_1$	400	18/23-78% (211)	14/15	1/15
Thx[d] C57BL/6	170	7	C57BL/6	400	3/10-30% (200)	—	—
Thx[d] C57BL/6	170	7	(BALB/c × C57BL/6)F$_1$	400	9/20-45% (236)	—	6/6
Thx[d] C57BL/6	170	30	C57BL/6	400	11/16-70% (194)	—	—
Thx[d] C57BL/6	170	30	(BALB/c × C57BL/6)F$_1$	400	16/20-80% (185)	14/14	—

[a] Female C57BL/6 were thymectomized at the age of 6 weeks; at the age of 8 weeks these thymectomized mice, as well as intact mice, were exposed to four weekly doses of 170 r whole body irradiation, and 3 × 10^7 normal bone marrow was injected intravenously 1 to 3 hr after the last fractionated irradiation: +BM, plus bone marrow.

[b] Six- to 8-week-old female C57BL/6 or (BALB/c × C57BL/6)F$_1$ hybrid mice were exposed to 400 r whole-body irradiation, and 10^7 to 3 × 10^7 bone marrow cells, collected from irradiated (170 r × 4) donors (transfer from one donor to one recipient) were injected intravenously 1 to 3 hr after exposure to X-rays.

[c] Average latent period from time of cell transfer.

[d] Thymectomized.

nomenon of a leukemogenic agent in the bone marrow within several days of termination of the radiation treatment. Bone marrow cells, collected 7 days after the last radiation exposure from intact, thymectomized or intact mice reconstituted with normal bone marrow cells, when transferred into irradiated recipients caused leukemia development in 30 to 40% of the treated mice. The genotype analysis of these leukemias (induced in F_1 hybrids) indicated that they were all of recipient F_1 origin probably due to a non-cellular leukemogenic agent present among the transferred C57BL/6 irradiated bone marrow cells (Table 1). It is interesting to point out that thymectomy or bone marrow injection following the radiation treatment did not prevent the "release" of the leukemogenic agent within several days after last radiation exposure. Preleukemic-leukemic cells were observed in the bone marrow of irradiated mice within 30 days following termination of the radiation treatment (Table 1), as the genotype analysis indicated that most of the developing leukemias were of donor C57BL/6 origin. The methods known to reduce (bone marrow transplantation shortly after radiation) or prevent (by thymectomy before or immediately after irradiation) radiation leukemogenesis did not abolish or decrease the occurrence of preleukemic cells in the bone marrow within 30 days after radiation treatment (all the leukemias developing in the different experimental groups being of donor origin, Table 1). These results indicated the presence of preleukemic cells within four weeks following radiation treatment (although the acute disease occurred at about 200 days), irrespective of the ultimate susceptibility of the treated mice to the development of overt leukemia.

RADIATION-INDUCED HOST EFFECTS

Different tests were carried out to evaluate the possible contribution of host immune impairment, following fractionated irradiation, to leukemia development. A marked depression in plaque-forming capacity of the 19 S type to sheep red blood cells (SRBC) was observed in the irradiated mice for several months (tested up to 140 days after last X-ray exposure). This impairment could be associated with the suppressive effect of the radiation leukemia virus (Peled and Haran-Ghera, 1971a) "released" following bone marrow injury by irradiation (Haran-Ghera, 1966a). The possible correlation between this impairment and the incidence or latent period of tumor development was estimated in the following way: After spleen removal, for the evaluation of plaque formation, the mice were kept alive for further follow-up of leukemia development. The level of plaque-forming capacity did not correlate with leukemia development. Leukemia appeared in mice exhibiting either a low or high response to SRBC, and the latency was also found to be unrelated to the degree of immunosuppression induced by radiation.

The capacity to cause a graft-versus-host (GVH) response after radiation treatment was tested by injecting 10^7 spleen cells from irradiated mice (7, 14,

28, and 62 days after the last X-ray exposure; 10 spleens per age group were tested) into 10-day-old (BALB/c × C57BL/6)F$_1$ hybrid mice, and spleen indices were determined 9 days later. Spleen cells from normal age-matched C57BL/6 mice served as controls. Significant reduced GVH capacity was observed up to 1 month following radiation (control values being 3.0 ± 0.14 versus 1.6 ± 0.10 after 7 days; 1.7 ± 0.11 after 14 days; and 2.1 ± 0.12 after 28 days; the P value in all these groups being <<0.001). Skin graft survival (grafting C3H/eb skin) was not prolonged in irradiated mice, nor could such mice accept an allogeneic tumor graft (3:4-benzopyrene-induced fibrosarcoma in C3H/Jax mice). The possible contribution of immune impairment caused by fractionated irradiation to radiation leukemogenesis seemed, therefore, quite doubtful.

In recent studies (Haran-Ghera et al., 1974), we have shown that the majority of radiation and radiation leukemia virus induced lymphatic leukemias consisted of T lymphocytes bearing high levels of surface H-2 alloantigens. Could irradiation induce changes in the pattern and distribution of lymphoid cells involved in the neoplastic transformation and/or leukemic cell proliferation? As the target organ for overt lymphatic leukemia expression is the thymus, the possibility that a specific lymphoid thymus subpopulation could be a prerequisite for leukemic development was studied further. Thymus subpopulations can be classified on the basis of cell surface antigens and biologic properties. Approximately 85% of T cells within the thymus (considered to be steroid- and radiation-sensitive cells) are characterized by a low level of surface H-2 alloantigens and high level of surface θ antigen. The remaining 15% of thymus lymphocytes have the surface characteristics of T lymphocytes in the peripheral tissues, namely, high levels of H-2 (assumed to be corticoid and radiation resistant) and lower levels of θ (Cerottini and Brunner, 1967; Raff, 1970). Tests were carried out to find out whether fractionated radiation could change the pattern of the normal thymus subpopulations and whether further treatment with bone marrow would alter the radiation-induced thymus population pattern. The presence of θ antigen and high levels of H-2 alloantigen on thymocytes after each radiation exposure and after bone marrow reconstitution following the last radiation treatment was determined using a cytotoxic test (trypan blue dye exclusion test). Anti-θ C3H serum (prepared by six weekly injections of 10^7 C3H thymus cells into AKR mice) or H-2 alloantiserum, shown to be cytotoxic only to thymocytes having high levels of H-2 antigen (obtained following six weekly injections of 10^8 C57BL/6 spleen cells into C3H mice), were used in this analysis. The results obtained are summarized in Fig. 1. Fractionated irradiation did indeed change, for several weeks, the pattern of the normal thymus population, namely, an abundance of high H-2 thymus-derived lymphocytes were present in the thymus (60 to 80%), after the last exposure, in spite of the fact that the thymus had already regenerated and almost regained its initial normal weight (Fig. 1). Bone marrow administration after the last radiation exposure

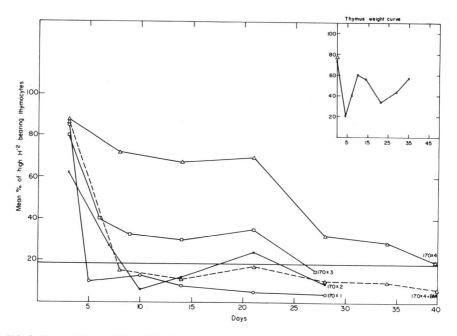

FIG. 1. Mean incidence of high H-2^b alloantigen-bearing thymocytes in C57BL/6 female mice following each fractionated radiation exposure; level in normal unirradiated thymus, baseline. The analysis was started 5 days following the first, second, third, or fourth exposure to X-rays. The radiation dose was 170 r whole-body irradiation in 6- to 8-week-old female C57BL/6 mice; the interval between exposures was 7 days. Eight-week-old female mouse 3 × 10^7 syngeneic bone marrow cells were injected intravenously within 1 to 3 hr after the last radiation exposure. *Inset*, Thymus weight curve (mg) following four weekly exposures to X-rays.

reduced drastically the radiation-induced, elevated high H-2 population pattern. The absence of this thymus subpopulation following radiation and bone marrow treatment could, perhaps, be considered as a factor in preventing leukemic cell proliferation. The fact that one single administration of bone marrow cells after the last radiation exposure is as effective in preventing leukemia development as repeated bone marrow injections after each radiation exposure coincides with the present findings that the susceptible high H-2 thymus subpopulation is present in abundance only after the last radiation exposure.

The length of the interval between the repeated exposures was shown to affect leukemia incidence (Kaplan and Brown, 1952). A comparative follow-up analysis of thymus subpopulations after exposing six- to eight-week-old mice to four doses of 170 r whole-body irradiation with a 7- or 14-day interval between the repeated exposures indicated a marked reduction in the availability of the high H-2 population when the 14-day interval (which resulted in a reduced leukemia incidence, 35% versus 75% at the 7-day interval) was introduced (Fig. 2).

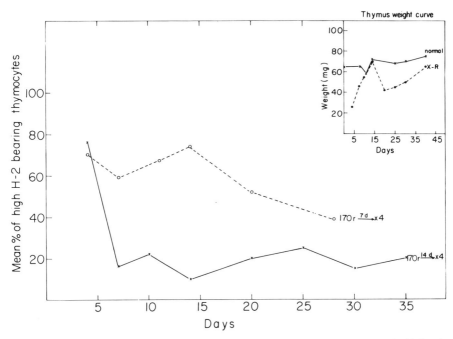

FIG. 2. The mean incidence of high H-2^b alloantigen-bearing thymocytes in 6- to 8-week-old female C57BL/6 mice within 35 days following last exposure to fractionated irradiation. The mice received four doses of 170 r each whole-body irradiation at weekly or fortnightly intervals. *Inset,* Thymus weight curve (mg).

The majority of leukemias developing in the thymus were shown to originate from the minor high H-2 thymus subpopulation (Haran-Ghera et al., 1974), and because there is a correlation between radiation treatment yielding high leukemia incidence and a transient thymus pattern consisting mainly of thymocytes bearing high levels of H-2 alloantigens, it might be assumed that a certain level of this population is a prerequisite for overt leukemia development.

AGE-DEPENDENT SUSCEPTIBILITY TO RADIATION LEUKEMOGENESIS

The susceptibility of C57BL/6 mice to radiation leukemogenesis is age dependent, namely, older mice are less susceptible to lymphatic leukemia induction following exposure to X-rays (Kaplan, 1948). The target organ for leukemia development is the thymus, and it could be assumed that the alteration of susceptibility with age is related to thymus involution or lack of target cells in the thymus of older mice. The age-related susceptibility could also be affected by other host factors. As the radiation leukemia virus is present during postnatal life in non-irradiated C57BL mice, and its titer increases with aging (Haran-Ghera and Peled, 1967), it could be proposed that reduction in susceptibility to radiation leukemogenesis with age increase might be attributed to a natural build-up of immunity in older mice. Findings concerning resistance against isotransplantation of leukemic cells in normal five- to eight-month-old C57BL/6 mice and the presence of neutralizing antibodies against the radiation leukemia virus in 5- 12-month-old normal C57BL/6 mice (Haran-Ghera, 1972) did, indeed, suggest that some natural immunization by the radiation leukemia virus, present in non-irradiated C57BL/6 mice, might occur with increase in age. The possible role of age-related changes in the thymus in radiation leukemogenesis was further evaluated in the following experiment. Female C57BL/6 mice aged 1, 5, and 8 months were thymectomized and 7 days later they were grafted with a newborn isologous thymus under the kidney capsule. Thus, mice of variable ages were carrying a similar young thymus graft of the same age. The thymus graft developed well in the three age groups (weighing 40 to 60 mg in the different age groups tested within 4 weeks after grafting). When the thymus graft was 30 days old, these animals, as well as control intact mice of the same age groups, were exposed to four weekly doses of 170 r each whole-body irradiation, and leukemia incidence in the irradiated mice was recorded (each experimental group consisted of 20 to 30 mice). The age-dependent susceptibility to radiation leukemogenesis was obvious: 2-month-old intact irradiated mice had an 80% incidence (203 days) versus 50% (184 days) in 6-month-old mice and only 30% (265 days) in the 9-month-old intact C57BL/6 mice. This age-dependent susceptibility was also seen in the thymectomized, thymus intrarenal grafted irradiated mice. The leukemia incidence in the 2-month-old grafted mice was 65% (165 days) (thereby demonstrating the susceptibility of the thymus whether *in situ* or grafted at another site to become leukemic), 35% (220 days) in the six-month-old ones, and 18% (255 days) in the 9-month-old mice. Hence, an age-dependent decrease in leukemia incidence was observed, although the thymus in these tested mice was of the same age, and the variable factor was the host's age.

The capacity of radiation to affect the "release" of a leukemogenic factor and leukemic cell transformation in older C57BL/6 mice was further tested using the bone marrow transfer method previously described. Female C57BL/6 mice aged 6 and 9 months were exposed to fractionated irradiation (four weekly exposures of 170 r whole-body irradiation) and the bone marrow was harvested 7 and 30 days after radiation treatment and transplanted into (BALB/c × C57BL/6)F_1 (8 to 10-week-old) mice previously exposed to 400 r. The results obtained are summarized in Table 2. Leukemic cells were found among the irradiated bone marrow cells in both age groups tested. In 6-month-old irradiated mice the findings were similar to those described previously in the young 6- to 8-week-old irradiated mice (the "release" of a leukemogenic agent present among bone marrow cells within several days after last radiation treatment and preleukemic-leukemic cells mostly of donor origin within 30 days following irradiation). In the 9-month-old irradiated

TABLE 2. Leukemia induction following transfer of marrow cells from six- and nine-month-old, radiation-treated C57BL/6 mice

Age (months)	Donor strain[a]	Donor treatment (r × 4)	Time of bone marrow transfer after treatment	Bone marrow recipient strain[b]	Pretreatment of recipient	Leukemia incidence and ALP[c] (days)	Leukemia origin	
							Donor	Recipient
6	C57BL/6	170				8/20–40% (270)	—	—
9	C57BL/6	170				5/18–27% (295)	—	—
6	C57BL/6	170	7	(BALB/c × C57BL/6)F₁	400	7/20–35% (165)	—	7/7
6	C57BL/6	170	30	(BALB/c × C57BL/6)F₁	400	13/20–65% (240)	10/12	2/12
6	C57BL/6	None		(BALB/c × C57BL/6)F₁	400	0/20 —	—	—
9	C57BL/6	170	7	(BALB/c × C57BL/6)F₁	400	17/20–85% (124)	14/17[d]	—
9	C57BL/6	170	30	(BALB/c × C57BL/6)F₁	400	12/14–84% (135)	8/10[d]	—

[a] Female C57BL/6 mice at the age of six and nine months were exposed to four weekly doses of 170 r whole body irradiation.
[b] Six- to eight-week-old (BALB/c × C57BL/6)F₁ mice were exposed to 400 r whole body irradiation and 1 to 3 hr later they received an intravenous injection (10^7 to 3×10^7) of bone marrow cells collected from an irradiated C57BL/6 donor; the cells were transferred from one donor to one recipient. The genotype analysis of the leukemias occurring in the F₁ hybrid mice was done by transplanting the leukemic cells into the parental strains and the hybrid mice.
[c] Average latent period from time of cell transfer.
[d] The mice developed mostly reticulum cell neoplasm type A; three transplanted tumors in each test group did not grow.

mice, leukemic cells of donor origin were detected in the bone marrow within 7 days after termination of the radiation treatment. It is interesting to stress the unique occurrence of reticulum cell neoplasms type A following transplantation of bone marrow cells taken from 9-month-old irradiated mice. These findings perhaps indicate a direct action of X-rays on bone marrow stem cells. In young mice, these "transformed" stem cells would eventually migrate and reach the thymus and become T leukemic cells (and thereafter sequestrate back to bone marrow as T cells). In older mice, the thymus function to affect bone marrow stem cell differentiation might already be defective and, therefore, these transformed cells would remain in the more primitive undifferentiated reticulum cell form and ultimately develop into reticulum cell neoplasms. The results obtained clearly indicated that age increase did not affect the susceptibility of lymphoid cells to neoplastic transformation.

The thymus subpopulation patterns in relation to age were also evaluated. Female C57BL/6 mice aged 6 weeks, 5 months, and 8 months were exposed to fractionated irradiation, and after the radiation treatment, the mean percent of the high H-2^b bearing thymocytes was tested. A marked decrease in this specific thymus subpopulation was observed in the 5- and 8-month-old irradiated mice (65 to 55% within 10 to 25 days after radiation of 6-week-old

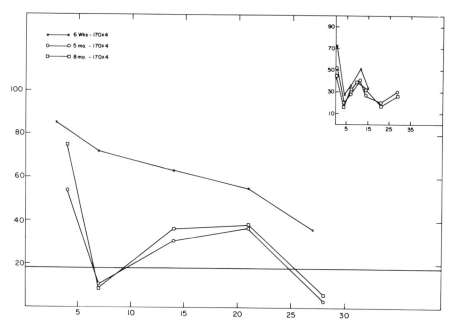

FIG. 3. Comparative incidence of high H-2^b thymus subpopulation in C57BL/6 mice following exposure to four weekly doses of 170 r whole-body irradiation at the age of 6 weeks, 5 months, or 8 months. The baseline expresses the normal level of this thymus subpopulation in 1- to 12-month-old C57BL/6 mice. *Inset,* Thymus regeneration weight curve (mg) of the different age groups following X-ray treatment.

mice versus 20 to 35% at similar time intervals in the older tested mice) (Fig. 3). The relative, age-dependent decreased incidence of the high H-2 thymus subpopulation in irradiated mice could affect the ultimate leukemia development in older mice.

RADIATION COLEUKEMOGENIC ACTIVITY

The conventional procdure to test the leukemogenic activity of the radiation leukemia virus (RLV) is by inoculation into newborn C57BL mice. In previous studies, we have shown that inoculation of RLV directly into the thymus of adult C57BL/6 mice further exposed to a low dose (300 to 400 r) of X-rays caused leukemia development in a more effective way (Haran-Ghera, 1969a). It was also shown that inoculation of the virus directly into the thymus of adult mice, without further exposure to radiation, induced a low leukemia incidence and actually rendered these injected mice resistant to further leukemic cell challenge (Haran-Ghera, 1969b). Sera from such immunized mice nullified the leukemogenic activity of the radiation leukemia virus, and lymphoid cells from these immunized mice when added to leukemic cell challenge prevented the proliferation of leukemic cells (Peled and Haran-Ghera, 1971b). The fact that bone marrow administration (10^6 to 10^7 cells) following exposure to X-rays (several days after virus inoculation intrathymically) did not reduce leukemia incidence could propose that the coleukemogenic action of radiation might affect host factors other than host immune impairment.

Many leukemogenic viruses, including the radiation leukemia virus, were found to cause immune impairment, namely, virus-inoculated mice had a reduced capacity to produce antibodies to SRBC (Peled and Haran-Ghera 1971a). The mechanism by which the virus suppresses the immune response is not yet clear. Several investigations have proposed that virus and antigen compete for a stem cell that has immunoproliferative potential (Siegel and Morton, 1966; Ceglowski and Friedman, 1967). The radiation leukemia virus used in the present studies was originally obtained from bone marrow of irradiated C57BL/6 mice (Haran-Ghera, 1966a) and kept by serial passage lines of the virus in thymic tissue of C57BL/6 mice. In general, such serial passage lines of virus, when injected directly into adult C57BL/6 thymus, induce a low leukemia incidence (0 to 20%). The incidence can be increased to 80 to 100% by further exposure (within a few days after virus inoculation) of the injected mice to X-rays. This type of virus passage is designated in the present study as RLV "passage 127." Sometimes, however, a serial passage line of the virus when injected intrathymically into normal C57BL/6 mice would yield a high leukemia incidence (70 to 100%) without any further exposure to X-rays. Yet, when this virus preparation is injected into the thymus of (BALB/c × C57BL/6)F_1 mice, its high leukemogenic activity depends on further exposure of the inoculated mice to radiation (it acts similarly to passage 127 in C57BL/6 mice). Such a virus preparation tested in the present analysis was designated as "passage 136." It seemed of interest to determine whether the immunosuppressive effect of these two different virus preparations (passage 127 and passage 136) (injected in C57BL/6 and F_1 mice) would be similarly attributed to either a thymus- or bone marrow-derived population of immunocytes, or both, and whether radiation exposure following virus inoculation (testing X-ray treatment shortly after virus inoculation, which would increase leukemia incidence, or delaying radiation exposure and thereby decrease its coleukemogenic activity) would alter this virus-lymphoid cell interaction and thereby introduce the suitable interaction leading to leukemia development. The cell transfer technique of Mitchell and Miller (1968), which demonstrated either the presence or absence of specific antigen-sensitive or antibody-forming cells, or both, was chosen to study whether the two different virus passages interfered with the function of T and/or B cells. Here, C57BL/6 and (BALB/c × C57BL/6)F_1 mice were injected with virus passage 127 or passage 136 (with or without further exposure to X-rays), and 1 month later, suspensions of thymus and bone marrow cells collected from the virus-inoculated hosts were suspended in Tyrode solution. Aliquots of 5×10^7 thymocytes were mixed with 2×10^7 bone marrow cells, and 0.5 ml of 10% SRBC was added to the mixed cell suspension; the total of 1 ml volume was injected intravenously into syngeneic recipients that had been exposed to 700 r whole body irradiation a few hours earlier. The following cell combinations were tested: (1) normal thymus and normal bone marrow cells; (2) thymus cells from normal donors with bone marrow cells from virus-injected mice; (3) thymocytes from virus-injected donors with normal bone marrow cells; (4) thymocytes and bone marrow cells from virus-injected mice. The spleens from the different treated groups were removed 8 days after the cell transfer, and the number of plaque-forming cells (PFC) per spleen was evaluated. The results are summarized in Table 3. Results of the transfer experiments testing thymus and bone marrow cell combinations from donor mice injected with passage 127 (causing a low leukemia incidence when inoculated into adult C57BL/6 thymus) indicated that this virus preparation affected the marrow cell population of immunocytes (thymus cells from passage 127-inoculated donors with normal bone marrow cells yielded 620 ± 139 PFC/spleen versus 120 ± 98 PFC/spleen when bone marrow cells originated from virus-injected mice). The route of virus administration whether injected intraperitoneally or intrathymically (Table 3) did not affect the virus T–B cell interaction ratio. Exposure to 400 r within 2 days after passage 127 intrathymic injection, a procedure that markedly increased leukemia incidence, was found to cause a change in virus-immunocompetent cell interaction, namely, both thymus and bone marrow cells became functionally impaired (Table 3). Delaying the radiation exposure to 15 or 30 days after intrathymic virus injection (thereby reducing leukemia incidence to 32% and 15%, respectively) did not affect the immunocompe-

TABLE 3. The effect of radiation leukemia virus passages on thymus and bone marrow cells in response to SRBC

Donor treatment (test done 30 days after termination of treatment)	Leukemogenic activity		Direct PFC/spleen (± SE) in the following cell combinations[a]			
	incidence (%)	Latent period (days)	Nor Thy + Nor BM	Nor Thy + virus BM	Virus Thy + Nor BM	Virus Thy + virus BM
Passage 127 in C57BL/6 (intraperitoneal)	0		1386 ± 320	260 ± 102	1400 ± 398	210 ± 86
Passage 127 in C57BL/6 Thy	10	108	748 ± 198	120 ± 98	620 ± 139	108 ± 94
Passage 127 in C57BL/6 Thy 2 d[b] 400 r	95	85	800 ± 132	194 ± 68	170 ± 93	130 ± 78
Passage 127 in C57BL 6 Thy 15 d[b] 400 r	32	120	900 ± 124	284 ± 75	662 ± 102	230 ± 104
Passage 127 in C57BL/6 Thy 30 d[b] 400 r	15	98	840 ± 114	150 ± 87	555 ± 165	170 ± 65
Passage 136 in C57BL/6 Thy	90	96	900 ± 165	751 ± 102	212 ± 68	180 ± 80
Passage 136 in (BALB/c × C57BL/6)F$_1$ Thy	8	124	920 ± 120	226 ± 55	780 ± 155	220 ± 66
Passage 136 in (BALB/c × C57BL/6)F$_1$ Thy 2 d[b] 400 r	82	102	940 ± 137	210 ± 83	279 ± 113	196 ± 58

[a] Normal (Nor) thymus and bone marrow cells were taken from eight-week-old female mice, and 5×10^7 thymus cells (Thy) with 2×10^7 bone marrow cells (BM) were mixed with 0.5 ml of 10% SRBC and injected intravenously into isogeneic 750 r irradiated, 12-week-old hosts. The direct PFC of the spleens were tested eight days after cell transfer. Fifteen mice were used in each group, and ten mice from each group were kept aside for follow-up of leukemia incidence.
[b] Days.

tence of thymus cells collected from virus (passage 127)-injected donors (contrary to the results obtained with radiation within 2 days of virus treatment). In contrast, a reduced response to SRBC (212 ± 68 PFC/spleen) was obtained when thymus cells from virus passage 136-inoculated donors were mixed with normal bone marrow cells. Whereas bone marrow cells from virus passage 136-inoculated donors, when mixed with thymus cells from normal PBS-injected donors, showed a normal response (751 ± 102 PFC/spleen) similar to that obtained following the injection of normal thymus and normal bone marrow cells (900 ± 165 PFC/spleen). These results suggest that the thymus-derived cells per se were affected by the radiation leukemia virus passage 136 (which is highly leukemogenic when injected into adult thymus without any further host treatment), since their immunocompetent function was impaired. The virus passage 136 preparation when injected into (BALB/c × C57BL/6)F_1 mice (inducing low leukemia incidence, contrary to its high leukemogenic activity when injected into C57BL/6 adult thymus) rendered the bone marrow cells functionally impaired. Further exposure of these F_1 (passage 136)-inoculated mice to 400 r affected the function of thymus cells, which become functionally impaired. These results could suggest that unless the virus interacts with the thymus population (to such a level that thymocyte function is impaired), which is the susceptible population to neoplastic proliferation, no leukemias would develop in spite of virus introduction and its persistant presence in the thymus. Radiation treatment has actually introduced a change in virus-lymphoid cell interaction and thereby, perhaps, acted as a coleukemogenic factor.

CONCLUSIONS

These studies indicate that within 4 weeks after termination of radiation treatment, preleukemic cells were present in the bone marrow of irradiated mice, although these mice were clinically normal for several months before overt disease was observed. The methods known to reduce or prevent radiation leukemogenesis did not affect the degree of leukemogenic agent "release" demonstrated in irradiated bone marrow, nor did these treatments decrease the level of neoplastic transformation among the irradiated bone marrow cells, irrespective of the ultimate susceptibility of the treated mice to the development of overt leukemia. Although the susceptibility of C57BL/6 mice to radiation leukemogenesis is age dependent (older mice are less susceptible to development of the overt disease), the increased age (tested in 9-month-old mice) did not affect the susceptibility of lymphoid cells to neoplastic transformation. Overt leukemia development could be related to the ultimate capacity of preleukemic cells to escape immune system control, dependent on changes in cell-mediated immunity and the function of humoral immune responses during the long latent period. Another plausible assumption could be that, within the long latent period, these preleukemic-early occurring cells could acquire new properties to allow their uncontrolled proliferation. The transient immune impairment induced by fractionated whole body irradiation did not seem to contribute to the proliferation of preleukemic cells detected shortly after termination of the leukemogenic treatment.

Fractioned radiation was shown to affect and change the normal pattern of thymus subpopulation, namely increase markedly the incidence of thymocytes bearing high levels of H-2 alloantigens. Transplantation of bone marrow cells after the radiation treatment, the lengthening of the time intervals between the repeated radiation exposures, or exposure of older mice to radiation treatment, procedures known to reduce the incidence of radiation-induced leukemias, were all shown to interfere with and reduce the radiation effect on thymus high H-2 populations. It thus could be proposed that the transient availability of this high H-2 thymus subpopulation, following radiation damage, in abundance (beyond 15 days after the last radiation exposure) might be a prerequisite for the development of overt leukemia.

Concerning the effect of radiation in promoting leukemia induction by the radiation leukemia virus, we found that the initial direct virus-thymus cell interaction would lead to high leukemia induction potency without need for further host treatment, whereas virus-bone marrow interaction (the general pattern) would yield a low leukemia incidence unless a change in this virus-lymphoid cell relationship were introduced. Radiation might act as a co-leukemogenic agent due to its capacity to change the virus-T and B cell interaction.

ACKNOWLEDGMENT

This investigation was supported in part by USPHS Research Contract No. 1-CB-43930.

REFERENCES

Ceglowski, W. S., and Friedman, H. (1967): Suppression of the primary antibody plaque response of mice following injection with Friend virus. *Proc. Soc. Exp. Biol. Med.*, 126:662–667.

Cerottini, J. C., and Brunner, K. T. (1967): Localization of mouse isoantigens on the cell surface as revealed by immunofluorescence. *Immunology*, 13:395–403.

Haran-Ghera, N. (1966a): Leukemogenic activity of centrifugates from irradiated mouse thymus and bone marrow. *Int. J. Cancer*, 1:81–87.

Haran-Ghera, N., Lieberman, M., and Kaplan, H. S. (1966b): Direct action of a leukemogenic virus on the thymus. *Cancer Res.*, 26:438–441.

Haran-Ghera, N., and Peled, A. (1967): The mechanism of radiation action in leukemogenesis. Isolation of a leukemogenic filtrable agent from tissues of irradiated and normal C57BL mice. *Br. J. Cancer*, 21:730–738.

Haran-Ghera, N. (1969a): The role of immune impairment in viral leukemogenesis. In: *Immunity and Tolerance in Oncogenesis*, edited by L. Severi, pp. 585–597.

Haran-Ghera, N. (1969b): Host resistance against isotransplantation of lymphomas induced by the radiation leukemia virus. *Nature*, 222:992–993.

Haran-Ghera, N. (1971): Influence of host factors on leukemogenesis by the radiation leukemia virus. *Israel J. Med. Sci.*, 7:17–25.

Haran-Ghera, N. (1972): The role of immunity in radiation leukemogenesis. In: *Unifying Concepts of Leukemia,* edited by R. M. Dutcher and L. Chieco-Bianchi, pp. 671–676. Karger, Basel.

Haran-Ghera, N. (1973): Relationship between tumor cell and host in chemical leukemogenesis. *Nature [New Biol.],* 246:84–86.

Haran-Ghera, N., Ben-Yaakov, M., Chazan, R., and Peled, A. (1974): Pathways in thymus and bone marrow derived lymphatic leukemia in mice. In: *Comparative Leukemia Research, 1973,* edited by Y. Ito and R. M. Dutcher, pp. 133–141. Univ. of Tokyo Press, Tokyo and Karger, Basel.

Kaplan, H. S. (1948): Influence of age on susceptibility of mice to the development of lymphoid tumors after irradiation. *J. Natl. Cancer Inst.,* 9:55–56.

Kaplan, H. S. (1949): Preliminary studies of the effectiveness of local irradiation in the induction of lymphoid tumors in mice. *J. Natl. Cancer Inst.,* 10:267–270.

Kaplan, H. S., and Brown, M. B. (1951): Further observations on inhibition of lymphoid tumor development by shielding and partial body irradiation of mice. *J. Natl. Cancer Inst.,* 12:427–436.

Kaplan, H. S., and Brown, M. B. (1952): A quantitative dose response study of lymphoid tumor development in irradiated C57BL mice. *J. Natl. Cancer Inst.,* 13:185–208.

Kaplan, H. S., Brown, M. B., and Paull, J. (1953): Influence of bone marrow injections on involution and neoplasia of mouse thymus after systemic irradiation. *J. Natl. Cancer Inst.,* 14:303–316.

Kaplan, H. S., Carnes, W. H., Brown, M. B., and Hirsch, B. B. (1956): Indirect induction of lymphomas in irradiated mice. I. Tumor incidence and morphology in mice bearing non irradiated thymic grafts. *Cancer Res.,* 16:422–425.

Kaplan, H. S. (1964): The role of radiation in experimental leukemogenesis. *J. Natl. Cancer Inst. Monogr.,* 14:207–217.

Lieberman, M., and Kaplan, H. S. (1959): Leukemogenic activity of filtrates from radiation-induced lymphoid tumors in mice. *Science,* 130:387–388.

Lorenz, E., Congdon, C. C., and Uphoff, D. (1953): Prevention of irradiation-induced lymphoid tumors in C57BL mice by spleen protection. *J. Natl. Cancer Inst.,* 14:291–301.

Mitchell, G. F., and Miller, J. F. A. P. (1968): Immunological activity of thymus and thoracic duct lymphocytes. *Proc. Natl. Acad. Sci. USA,* 59:296–305.

Peled, A., and Haran-Ghera, N. (1971a): Immunosuppression by the radiation leukemia virus and its relation to lymphatic leukemia development. *Int. J. Cancer,* 8:97–106.

Peled, A., and Haran-Ghera, N. (1971b): Immunological studies on the radiation leukemia virus in C57BL mice. *Nature [New Biol.],* 232:244–245.

Raff, M. C. (1970): Two distinct populations of peripheral lymphocytes in mice distinguishable by immunofluorescence. *Immunology,* 19:637–650.

Siegel, B. V., and Morton, J. I. (1966): Serum agglutination levels to sheep red blood cells in mice injected with Rauscher virus. *Proc. Soc. Exp. Biol. Med.,* 123:467–470.

Biology of Radiation Carcinogenesis, edited by
J. M. Yuhas, R. W. Tennant, and J. D. Regan.
Raven Press, New York © 1976.

Characterization of Natural Antibodies in Mice to Endogenous Leukemia Virus

J. N. Ihle, J. C. Lee, and M. G. Hanna, Jr.

Basic Research Program, NCI–Frederick Cancer Research Center, Frederick, Maryland 21701

The immunosuppressive and carcinogenic effects of ionizing radiation have been well documented. However, the relationship between these effects and their relative contribution to the induction and propagation of neoplasia have been largely speculative. Immunosuppression may be the single factor in radiation carcinogenesis, or it may be completely independent of the carcinogenic event. The induction of neoplasia is probably due to both a carcinogenic effect and an immunosuppressive effect. Our inability to define the relationship between these two effects of radiation and measure their relative significance has largely been due to the inability to quantitatively evaluate the contribution of immune surveillance to the regulation of neoplasia and to quantitatively evaluate changes in presumptive oncogenic events induced by radiation.

The spectrum of radiation-induced malignancy is extremely broad, and the absolute relationship between the immunosuppressive and carcinogenic effects of radiation-induced malignancies probably vary. There are now some systems available, however, that are amenable to the quantitative approach necessary to understand the comprehensive changes occurring during radiation that lead to cancer. Perhaps the most amenable system available is radiation-induced lymphomas in mice.

The predominant lympho-proliferative disease occurring in mice is thymic lymphoma. These tumors occur naturally in the majority of mouse strains, constitute the predominant tumor in some strains of mice, such as AKR, and are readily induced in several strains of mice by radiation (Kaplan, 1967). The etiologic agent of thymic lymphoma in mice is an RNA tumor virus, and similar, if not identical, viruses are associated with radiation-induced leukemias (Kaplan, 1967). These viruses are endogenous to the host. They are spontaneously activated throughout life, and can be chemically activated from virus-negative mouse embryo fibroblast cell lines (Rowe et al., 1971). Two genetically distinct oncornaviruses have been isolated and are distinguishable on the basis of host range (Aaronson and Stephenson, 1973). The ecotropic murine leukemia virus is capable of replicating in mouse cells and is the etiologic agent of the majority of thymic lymphomas. A second virus, termed xenotropic, does not replicate in mouse cells but will replicate in cells of other species; the relationship of this virus to spontaneous neoplasia is unknown.

The ability of radiation to induce thymic lymphomas in susceptible mice is presumably related to its ability either to induce or activate expression of the endogenous leukemia virus or its ability to immunosuppress the host sufficiently to allow escape of the virus from host regulation, or both. Techniques to quantitatively measure changes in virus expression induced by radiation now exist. For example, in tissue culture, it has been demonstrated that radiation can induce at low but significant frequencies spontaneous expression of the virus (Rowe et al., 1971). This suggests that a similar induction by radiation can be achieved *in vivo*. The relative role of the immunosuppressive effects of radiation must also be examined. We have previously shown that the spontaneous expression of endogenous leukemia viruses induces a chronic humoral response to the virus, which may contribute to the regulation of the pathologic expression of the virus (Ihle et al., 1973). Here we will review our techniques and findings on this autogenous immune response as it relates to the immunosuppressive effects of radiation in the induction of thymic lymphomas in mice.

MATERIALS AND METHODS

Animals. Male, 1-year-old mice of various strains were used. All mice were specific-pathogen-free (SPF).

Test sera. Blood was collected from mice by cardiac puncture. Sera were separated by centrifugation at 400 × *g* for 15 min and were stored at −70°C prior to use. Hyperimmune serum from rabbits immunized against p15 or gp71 isolated from Friend MuLV, was kindly provided by Dr. W. Schäfer, Max Planck Institute, Tubingen, Germany.

Viruses. Viruses used included AKR virus, isolated from an established line of AKR mouse embryo cells [FIC2(16a)] (obtained initially from Dr. W. P. Rowe, National Institutes of Health), which had spontaneously initiated virus synthesis. Moloney leukemia virus was isolated from a chronically infected continuous-passage Swiss mouse embryo cell line (SME). Rauscher MuLV was purified from the JLS-V5 cell line. A chemically induced endogenous virus of BALB/c mouse cells, BALB:virus-2 (kindly provided by Dr. S. A. Aaronson, National Cancer Institute) was routinely carried in normal rat kidney cells (NRK). The RD-114 virus was isolated from the RD cell line. Rat leukemia virus was isolated from a W/Fu rat cell line productively infected with rat leukemia virus.

Preparation of radioactive-labeled virus. [³H]leucine-labeled virus was prepared as previously described (Ihle et al., 1973) except 10^{-6} M hydrocortisone was incorporated in the culture medium to enhance virus yield. All viruses were purified through a final step of isopycnic banding in a 15 to 50%

linear sucrose gradient. In some cases, an additional step of sedimentation centrifugation was necessary to obtain homogeneous virus preparations.

The viruses were prepared under identical conditions and had similar radiospecific activities of 1 to 3 $\times$ 10^7 cpm/mg protein. Purified virus pools with acceptable specific activity were stored at $-70°C$, then used immediately upon thawing.

Preparation of unlabeled AKR virus. Nonradioactive AKR leukemia virus was purified as above from 12-hr harvests of culture medium from AKR cells grown in roller bottles. Protein concentrations were determined by the method of Lowry (1951).

Radioimmune precipitation assays against intact virus. The radioimmune precipitation assay against intact radioactive-labeled AKR virus has been described in detail elsewhere (Ihle et al., 1973). Briefly, 0.1 ml of the test serum, or serum fraction, was serially diluted twofold in TNE buffer (0.05 M Tris-hydrochloride, pH 7.5, 0.1 M NaCl, 1mM EDTA), 0.1 ml (6,000 cpm) of labeled virus was added, and the mixture was incubated 1 hr at 37°C to allow the formation of immune complexes. Subsequently, a volume of 0.1 ml of anti-γ-globulin (Cappel anti-mouse γ-globulin) diluted 1:2 in TNE was added, the mixture incubated again at 37°C for 1 hr, and finally incubated at 4°C for 2 hr. The precipitates were collected by centrifugation at 1200 $\times$ g for 15 min, and the supernatant was removed for determination of radioactivity. The precipitates were washed three times with TNE, resuspended in 0.4 ml TNE, and prepared for counting. All samples were counted in 10-ml Aquasol (New England Nuclear, Boston, Mass.) in a Packard Tricarb scintillation counter. The percent precipitation was expressed as the percentage of counts in the precipitate relative to the combined counts in the precipitate and in the first supernatant. A number of parameters of the radioimmune precipitation assay were found to affect the results, as described in a previous report (Ihle et al., 1973).

To prepare immune precipitates for SDS-polyacrylamide gel electrophoresis, 25 to 50 μl of serum were allowed to react with 2 $\times$ 10^5 cpm of Triton-disrupted virus and subsequently precipitated with anti-γ-globulin as described by Ihle et al. (1974). The precipitates were washed four times with TNE and then sedimented through a cushion of 25% sucrose containing TNE and 0.5% deoxycholate. The precipitates were resuspended in TNE and pelleted at 1200 $\times$ g for 20 min. The pellets were carefully drained dry, resuspended in 0.5 ml of 0.01 M sodium phosphate buffer (pH 7.4) containing 1% SDS and 1% β-mercaptoethanol, and incubated at 60° for 1 hr, then at 37°C overnight.

SDS-polyacrylamide gel electrophoresis of immune precipitates. SDS-polyacrylamide gel electrophoresis was performed as described by Weber and Osborn (1969). Bromophenol blue was used as a reference standard to determine relative mobilities and was generally allowed to migrate 8 cm.

Standard protein samples were used to calibrate the system as described by Ihle et al. (1974). The gels were sectioned into 1-mm slices, which were dissolved in 30% hydrogen peroxide at 75°C overnight. The radioactivity of each gel-slice fraction was determined in a liquid scintillation counter.

RESULTS

The existence of a chronic humoral response in mice to endogenous leukemia viruses was postulated from the observation that in aged mice of certain strains, immune complexes containing this virus were detected in kidneys (Hanna et al., 1972; Oldstone et al., 1972). To further establish the existence of natural antibody to the virus and to quantitatively assess the humoral response, we developed a sensitive radioimmune precipitation assay, using [³H]leucine-labeled AKR leukemia virus purified from a cloned line of virus-producing AKR cells. Representative results of this assay are shown in Fig. 1. The specificity of the assay, previously demonstrated by Ihle et al. (1973), is provided by the observation that normal rabbit serum does not react with and precipitate labeled virus.

When age-matched sera from various strains of mice are examined for natural antibody to AKR leukemia virus, the majority are found to have significant titers (Fig. 1). But, striking variations in antibody titers are evident and appear to correlate to the incidence of spontaneous leukemias. Such strains as BALB/c, C57BL/6, and C3H have intermediate titers and are characterized by 10 to 20% incidence of spontaneous leukemias. Mouse strains with a high leukemia incidence, such as RF and AKR, have generally low and variable titers against the virus. The exception to this correlation is found in a group of strains, such as NIH, which have low levels of natural antibody and low incidences of spontaneous leukemia (Hartley et al., 1969). Another characteristic of these strains is the absence of ecotropic virus expression. The strains are thought to possess only the endogenous xenotropic virus, the expression of which is restricted to later life. Therefore, the lack of appreciable antibody titers and low rate of spontaneous leukemias in these

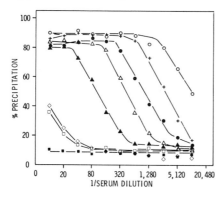

FIG. 1. Radioimmune precipitation assay of various immune sera from one-year-old mice against intact [³H]leucine-labeled AKR leukemia virus. RF (▲—▲), B6C3F₁ (+ — +), AKR (□—□), normal rabbit serum (■—■), STU (○—○), C57BL/6 (●—●), NIH (◇◇), and BALB/c (△—△).

strains may be due to limited virus expression. The above observations, in addition to the sera titration data found in other strains (Nowinski and Kaehler, 1974), suggest that a correlation exists between antibody titers, virus expression, and frequency of spontaneous leukemia. This correlation may suggest that the chronic humoral response functions in regulating virus-mediated pathogenesis.

Titer variation in various strains may be the result of either the immunologic responsiveness of the host to the virus or the extent of virus expression *in vivo* or both. First, genetic factors other than Fv-1 have been shown to be associated with resistance. In particular, the Rgv-1 gene is influential in defining resistance and may be identical to the Ir-1 gene that defines immune responsiveness to certain antigens (Lilly, 1972). Second, the relative amount of virus expression in the various mouse strains examined, particularly during early life, is similar except for such strains as AKR or RF (Hartley et al., 1969). Hence, we presently feel that the titers reflect differences in immune responsiveness either defined genetically or by some other parameter, such as the relative levels of virus expression during ontogeny of the immune response.

The relationship between the immune responsiveness of various strains and susceptibility to radiation-induced leukemia is shown in Table 1. Perhaps the most striking correlation is the observation that strains of mice highly susceptible to radiation-induced lymphomas are marginally immunologically responsive to the virus. In contrast, highly resistant strains of mice to radiation-induced leukemia have high titers of natural antibody to the virus and very low incidences of spontaneous leukemias. This correlation suggests that immunosuppressive effects of radiation may contribute significantly to radiation-induced leukemia in mice. Similarly, the immunosuppressive effects of radiation may also involve qualitative changes. To examine the antigenic specificites of the immune response, normal sera were reacted with disrupted [^{3}H]leucine-labeled virus, the immune complexes isolated, and the reactive virion proteins identified by SDS-polyacrylamide gel electrophoresis (Table 2). The results with normal B6C3F$_1$ sera are shown in Fig. 2. For comparison, the profile of the total labeled AKR virion proteins is shown in Fig. 2,A. As shown in Fig. 2,B, B6C3F$_1$ sera precipitated approximately 3 to 5% of the radioactivity from disrupted virions. Primarily three radioactive components, having molecular weights of 68,000, 43,000 and 17,000, were identified. The specificity of these techniques in detecting immune reactions is shown in Fig. 2,C, which illustrates the profile obtained when rabbit antisera to either p30 or normal rabbit serum were reacted with disrupted virions.

The specificity of the reactions detected with normal B6C3F$_1$ sera and the identity of the radioactive peaks are shown in Fig. 3. When [^{3}H]glucosamine-labeled virus was used, only the 68,000- and 43,000-molecular weight peaks were detected, suggesting that these proteins correspond to the two viral envelope glycoproteins, gp71 and gp43 (Fig. 3,A). Figure 3,B shows the

TABLE 1. Correlation of antibody titers with spontaneous and radiation-induced leukemia

Strain	Rip titer	Spontaneous leukemias (%)	Radiation leukemia (%)
AKR	0–40	80	—
RF	80–320	50	80[a]
BALB/c	160–640	20	>50[b]
C57BL/6	320–1,280	17	15–35[b]
C3H	160–640	14	3–10[b]
B6C3F$_1$	1,280–5,120	<5	—
STU	5,120–10,240	—	—
NIH	10–80	<5	—
SWR/J	10–80	<5	—

[a] Clapp and Yuhas (1973).
[b] Kirschbaum and Mixer (1947).

results of a competition assay in which rabbit antisera to gp71 were incubated with the virus prior to the addition of normal B6C3F$_1$ sera. The immune complexes were then precipitated with rabbit antisera to mouse γ-globulins and analyzed by SDS-polyacrylamide gel electrophoresis. As shown in Fig. 3,B, rabbit antisera to gp71 competes for the precipitation of the 68,000 molecular weight component, but not for the other virion proteins. Similarly, monospecific rabbit antisera to p15 compete for precipitation of the 17,000 molecular weight component (Fig. 3,C). These data taken together show that natural immune sera react individually with the virion gp71, gp43, and p15 as opposed to reacting with a complex containing gp71, gp43, or p15. Sera from other strains of mice (C3H, C57BL/6, BALB/c, STU, AKR) have shown similar reactivities.

The antibody specificity of the natural immune response is shown in Fig. 4. For these experiments, B6C3F$_1$ sera were fractionated on ammonium sulfate, and the 19S and 7S components were fractionated on G-200 Sephadex. Both fractions have radioimmune precipitation titers against intact virus (Lee et al., 1974) with the 19S fraction having a somewhat higher titer. Radioactive profiles from SDS-polyacrylamide gels of immune precipitates of 19S and 7S

TABLE 2. Experimental protocol for detecting reactive virion proteins

1. [³H]Leucine-labeled virus disrupted with 0.5% Triton (0.6 M KCl) for 1 hr at 4°C
2. Diluted 10-fold and reacted with test serum for 4 hr at 37°C
3. Antiglobulin added and reacted for 1 hr at 37°C and 2 hr at 4°C
4. a. Precipitate collected
   b. Washed four times with TNE
   c. Washed once by pelleting through 1.0 ml 25% sucrose with 0.5% DOC
   d. Washed once with TNE
5. Precipitates solubilized in SDS for polyacrylamide gel electrophoresis

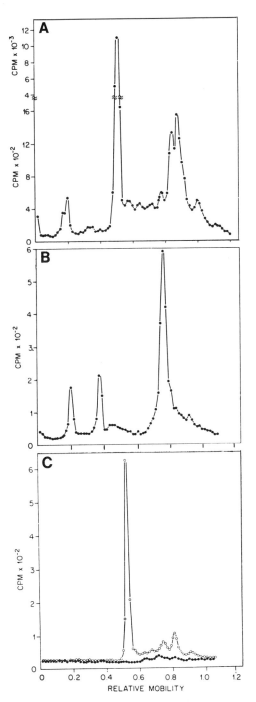

FIG. 2. SDS-polyacrylamide gel electrophoresis profiles of (A) Triton-disrupted [³H]leucine-labeled AKR MuLV; (B) immune precipitates of 1.5-year B6C3F₁ serum with Triton-disrupted, labeled AKR virus; (C) immune precipitate of normal rabbit serum (●—●) and rabbit antisera to p30 (○—○) reacted with Triton-disrupted labeled AKR virus.

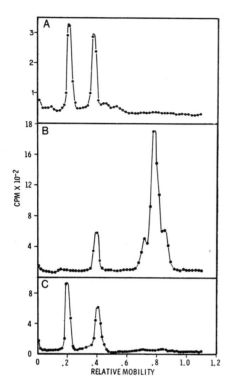

FIG. 3. SDS-polyacrylamide gel electrophoresis profiles of (A) an immune precipitate of 1.5-year B6C3F$_1$ serum reacted with Triton-disrupted, [^{3}H]glucosamine-labeled AKR MuLV; (B) an immune precipitate of 1.5-year B6C3F$_1$ serum reacted with Triton-disrupted [^{3}H]leucine-labeled AKR MuLV after reaction with rabbit antisera to gp71; (C) immune precipitates as in (B) but reacted with rabbit antisera to p15.

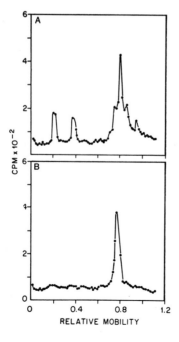

FIG. 4. SDS-polyacrylamide gel electrophoresis profiles of (A) an immune precipitate of 19S immunoglobulins from 1.5-year B6C3F$_1$ serum with Triton-disrupted, [^{3}H]leucine-labeled AKR MuLV; (B) an immune precipitate of 7S immunoglobulins from 1.5-year B6C3F$_1$ serum with Triton-disrupted, [^{3}H]leucine-labeled AKR MuLV.

fractions reacted with disrupted [³H]leucine-labeled virus are shown in Fig. 4. The 19S fraction reacted with all three viral antigens: gp71, gp43, and p15. In contrast, the 7S fraction reacted only with p15. The significance of these observations, previously noted by Lee et al. (1974), is that only the 19S fraction is capable of neutralizing xenotropic virus. These observations are of particular significance in radiation-induced leukemia, since IgM is known to have a shorter circulating half-life than IgG (Waldmann and Strober, 1969) and may, therefore, be more radiation sensitive than a chronic IgG response.

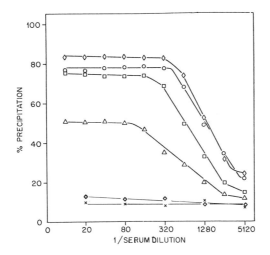

FIG. 5. Radioimmune precipitation assay of 1.5-year B6C3F₁ immune sera against different intact [³H]leucine-labeled MuLV. Titration curves of natural immune serum to AKR MuLV (□—□), Rauscher MuLV (◇—◇), Moloney MuLV (○—○), BALB:virus-2 (△—△), rat leukemia virus (◇—◇), and RD-114 (X — X).

Both gp71 and p15 have been shown previously to be virion envelope proteins (Hunsmann et al., 1974; Ihle et al., 1975). These studies and others (Strand and August, 1974) have demonstrated that heterologous antisera to gp71 cross-react with various murine viruses and weakly cross-react with C-type viruses from other species. They also detect type-specific differences between murine leukemia viruses. In contrast, heterologous antisera to p15 cross-react with all murine viruses and strongly cross-react with viruses of other species. To determine the spectrum of antigenic determinants (type, group, or interspecies) recognized by natural immune sera, we examined the ability of natural immune sera to cross-react with various C-type virus. The radioimmune precipitation curves obtained with various [³H]leucine-labeled viruses are shown in Fig. 5.

Normal B6C3F$_1$ sera had comparable titers against Rauscher, Moloney, AKR, and BALB:virus-2. In contrast, normal B6C3F$_1$ sera did not react with either rat leukemia virus or RD-114 virus, suggesting that the sera have group-specific reactivity. The inability of normal sera to distinguish between the FMR and Gross types of murine leukemia viruses is unique because heterologous antisera to these viruses detect differences. The virion proteins responsible for these serologic differences have not been characterized.

The group-specific reactivity of natural immune sera is shown in Fig. 6. For these experiments, unlabeled purified AKR virus was used as a competing antigen in radioimmune precipitation assays of limiting B6C3F$_1$ sera with Moloney, BALB:virus-2, and AKR leukemia viruses. The AKR virus was

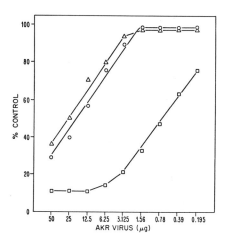

FIG. 6. Inhibition of precipitation of labeled AKR virus (□—□), labeled BALB:virus-2 (○—○), and Moloney (△—△) with 1.5-year B6C3F$_1$ serum by unlabeled AKR virus. The B6C3F$_1$ serum diluted 1:128 was incubated for 1 hr at 37°C with various concentrations of cold AKR virus. Labeled virus was then added and assayed as in the radioimmune precipitation assay.

shown to compete in a comparable manner for precipitation of all of these viruses, thus providing evidence that there are antibodies that cross-react with the various murine leukemia viruses.

The ability of natural immune sera to react equivalently with BALB: virus-2 and AKR virus was unexpected, since Aaronson and Stephenson (1974) have shown that although normal sera from several strains of mice have high titers of antibody capable of neutralizing the xenotropic BALB: virus-2, these sera only weakly neutralize the endogenous ecotropic viruses. Furthermore, neutralization resides only in the 19S antibody fraction (Lee et al., 1974) and now, as demonstrated above, appears to be dependent upon an immune response to gp71 or gp43. Heterologous antisera to gp71 are capable of virus neutralization, but antisera to p15 only weakly neutralize ecotropic viruses (Ihle et al., 1975). Therefore, the basis for the type specificity of natural immune sera in terms of neutralization is unknown, but it may depend upon the structural organization of the virus as it relates to the ability of immune complexes to neutralize it. It may also depend on infectious to non-infectious particle ratios of endogenous xenotropic viruses.

DISCUSSION

In our experiments we attempted to demonstrate a natural immune response in mice to the expression of endogenous leukemia viruses. We developed and utilized a sensitive and quantitative radioimmune precipitation assay using [³H]leucine-labeled intact virus and demonstrated that a wide variety of mouse strains have titerable antibody against C-type viruses. Perhaps the most striking observation was the diversity in titers observed among the various mouse strains. These differences may be the result of a number of factors, such as genetically defined immune responsiveness to the virus, the level of virus expression, or the initiation of virus expression relative to the ontogeny of the immune response. Experiments are in progress to determine which of these factors are responsible for these differences.

How the immune response functions in influencing the incidence of virus-induced pathogenesis has not been firmly established. We have demonstrated an inverse correlation between titers and spontaneous leukemia, but as noted above, a number of factors contribute to the titer of free antibody all of which may determine the incidence of spontaneous leukemia, i.e., the amount of virus expression. But indirect evidence for the functionality of the immune response was obtained by Hanna et al. (1972), who demonstrated that in certain strains of mice, an inverse correlation exists between the degree of glomerulonephritis (caused in part by immune complexes with C-type viruses) and the incidence of spontaneous lymphomas.

The role of the autogenous immune response in determining sensitivity to radiation-induced leukemia is not known. Our data suggest that susceptible strains have the endogenous ecotropic virus and intermediate or low titers of antibody. The involvement of an immune response, however, is indicated by a number of other observations. Clapp and Yuhas (1973) observed an inverse correlation between the degree of glomerulosclerosis and the incidence of leukemia in irradiated RF mice. From these observations, they suggest that radiation-induced leukemogenesis involves immunosuppression. Kaplan (1948) demonstrated a dramatic decrease with age in the susceptibility of C57 mice to radiation-induced lymphomas. This may be correlated with age-dependent increases in the autogenous immune response observed in several strains of mice (Ihle et al., 1973). Last, protection against the development of radiation-induced leukemia can be achieved by shielding the spleen or the marrow of the lower extremities or by injecting isologous marrow cells (Haran-Ghera, 1967). All these observations are consistent with a mechanism involving immunosuppression.

Our results also demonstrate a high degree of specificity of the autogenous immune response in terms of antigenic recognition and antibody type. Clearly, the efficacy of an immune response may depend on both antigenic and immunoglobulin differences. Heterologous antisera to virion envelope proteins have distinct differences in terms of their ability to neutralize C-type viruses.

Similarly, antibody type in other viral systems have neutralization differences —IgM being generally more effective. Therefore, any changes in specificity induced by radiation may significantly alter the efficacy of the immune response. The observation that only the 19S immunoglobulins react with gp71 is significant in terms of radiation-induced pathogenesis. The predominant reaction in normal immune sera is with gp71 (Ihle, *unpublished*) and, as shown here, is a 19S response. Furthermore, immunologic reactions with gp71 neutralize the virus, and with natural sera, neutralization of xenotropic virus is found only in the 19S fraction (Lee et al., 1974).

Based on these observations and the short circulating half-life of IgM, we predict that this reaction is the most significant in terms of the immunosuppressive effects of radiation and leukemogenesis. Furthermore, techniques now exist to more closely examine the immunosuppressive effects of radiation as they relate to induction of thymic lymphomas in mice.

ACKNOWLEDGMENTS

This research was supported by the National Cancer Institute under Contract No. NOI-CO-25423 with Litton Bionetics, Inc.

REFERENCES

Aaronson, S. A., and Stephenson, J. R. (1973): Independent segregation of loci for activation of biologically distinguishable RNA C-type virus in murine cells. *Proc. Natl. Acad. Sci. USA,* 70:2055–2058.

Aaronson, S. A., and Stephenson, J. R. (1974): Widespread natural occurrence of high titered neutralizing antibodies to a specific class of endogenous murine type-C virus. *Proc. Natl. Acad. Sci. USA,* 71:1957–1961.

Clapp, N. K., and Yuhas, J. M. (1973): Suggested correlation between radiation-induced immunosuppression and radiogenic leukemia in mice. *J. Natl. Cancer Inst.,* 51:1211–1215.

Hanna, M. G., Jr., Tennant, R. W., Yuhas, J. M., Clapp, N. K., Batzing, B., and Snodgrass, M. (1972): Autogenous immunity to endogenous RNA tumor virus in mice with a low natural incidence of lymphoma. *Cancer Res.,* 32:2226–2234.

Haran-Ghera, N. (1967): The mechanism of radiation action in leukemogenesis. The role of radiation in leukemia development. *Br. J. Cancer,* XXI:739–749.

Hartley, J. W., Rowe, W. P., Capps, W. I., and Heubner, R. J. (1969): Isolation of naturally occurring viruses of the murine leukemia virus group in tissue culture. *J. Virol.,* 3:126–132.

Hunsmann, G., Moennig, V., Pister, L., Seifert, E., and Schäfer, W. (1974): Properties of mouse leukemia viruses. VIII. The major viral glycoprotein of Friend leukemia virus. Seroimmunological, interfering and hemagglutinating capacities. *Virology,* 3:126:307–318.

Ihle, J. N., Hanna, M. G., Jr., and Roberson, L. E. (1974): Autogenous immunity to endogenous RNA tumor virus: Identification of antibody reactivity to select viral antigens. *J. Exp. Med.,* 136:1568–1581.

Ihle, J. N., Yurconic, M., Jr., and Hanna, M. G., Jr. (1973): Autogenous immunity to endogenous RNA tumor virus. Radioimmune precipitation assay of mouse serum antibody levels. *J. Exp. Med.,* 138:194–208.

Ihle, J. N., Hanna, M. G., Jr., Schäfer, W., Hunsmann, G., Bolognesi, D. P., and Hüper, G. (1975): Polypeptides of mammalian oncornaviruses. Localization of p15 and reactivity with natural antibody. *Virology,* 63:60–67.

Kaplan, H. S. (1948): Influence of age on susceptibility of mice to the development of lymphoid tumors after irradiation. *J. Natl. Cancer Inst.,* 9:55–56.

Kaplan, H. S. (1967): On the natural history of the murine leukemias: Presidential address. *Cancer Res.,* 27:1325–1340.

Kirschbaum, A., and Mixer, H. W. (1947): Induction of leukemia in eight inbred stocks of mice with varying susceptibility to spontaneous disease. *J. Lab. Clin. Med.,* 32:720–731.

Lee, J. C., Hanna, M. G., Jr., Ihle, J. N., and Aaronson, S. A. (1974): Autogenous immunity to endogenous RNA tumor virus: Differential reactivities of immunoglobulins M and G to virus envelope antigens. *J. Virol.,* 14:773–781.

Lilly, F. (1972): Mouse leukemia: A model of a multiple-gene disease. *J. Natl. Cancer Inst.,* 49:927–934.

Lowry, O. H., Rosenbrough, M. J., and Farr, A. L. (1951): Protein measurement with the folin phenol reagent. *J. Biol. Chem.,* 193:265–275.

Nowinski, R. C., and Kaehler, S. L. (1974): Antibody to leukemia virus: Widespread occurrence in inbred mice. *Science,* 185:869–871.

Oldstone, M., Aoki, T., and Dixon, F. (1972): The antibody response of mice to murine leukemia virus in spontaneous infections: Absence of classical immunological tolerance. *Proc. Natl. Acad. Sci. USA,* 69:134–138.

Rowe, W. P., Hartley, J. W., Lander, M. R., Pugh, W. E., and Jeich, N. (1971): Noninfectious AKR mouse embryo cell lines in which each cell has the capacity to be activated to produce infectious murine leukemia virus. *Virology,* 46:866–876.

Strand, M., and August, T. J. (1974): Structural proteins of mammalian oncogenic RNA viruses: Multiple antigenic determinants of the major internal protein and envelope glycoprotein. *J. Virol.,* 13:171–180.

Waldmann, T. A., and Strober, W. (1969): Metabolism of immunoglobulins. In: *Progress in Allergy,* Vol. 13, edited by P. Kallos and B. H. Waksman, pp. 1–92. S. Karger, New York.

Weber, K., and Osborn, M. (1969): The reliability of molecular weight determinations by dodecyl-sulfate polyacrylamide gel electrophoresis. *J. Biol. Chem.,* 244:4406–4412.

Biology of Radiation Carcinogenesis, edited by
J. M. Yuhas, R. W. Tennant, and J. D. Regan.
Raven Press, New York © 1976.

On the Mechanism of Infectivity of a Murine Leukemia Virus in Adult Mice

Richard L. Levy, Margaret H. Barrington, Richard A. Lerner, and Frank J. Dixon

Department of Immunopathology, Scripps Clinic and Research Foundation, La Jolla, California 92037

For some time after Gross's demonstration in 1950 that murine leukemia could be transmitted with a filterable agent, it was widely held that newborn animals were uniquely susceptible to infection by murine leukemia virus (MuLV) (Gross, 1974). But Moloney (1960) observed that a cell-free concentrate prepared from pooled spleens, livers, and lymph nodes of leukemic BALB/c mice induced generalized lymphatic leukemia in 94% of BALB/c mice injected between the ages of 42 and 67 days.

Since the immune response of a newborn animal might be different from that of an adult, we were interested in a model of oncornavirus infection in which factors unique to the newborn could be excluded. With the development of sensitive and quantitative radioimmunoassays for the measurement of virion polypeptides, it is now possible to monitor the expression of a virus accurately and to design experiments that more closely define the conditions necessary to permit infection of adult mice. The studies presented here demonstrate that otherwise unmanipulated adult mice become infected when injected with a particular MuLV and that infection and tumors are detected much earlier if the animals are given sublethal X-irradiation before or after inoculation of virus. Infection of adult mice is followed by development of lymphomas in the majority of animals.

MATERIALS AND METHODS

Cells and Virus

The virus, MuLV (Scripps), henceforth referred to as MuLV-S, was used in these experiments. It is a typical murine C-type virus (Lerner et al., 1972) of the FMR group and shares many properties with MuLV, Moloney strain. The highly type-specific P-12 antigen of MuLV-S cannot be distinguished from the P-12 of MuLV, Moloney by radioimmunassay (Aaronson and Stephenson, 1975), and at least 90% of their genomes are homologous (Fan and Baltimore, 1973).

The MuLV-S was provided by Dr. B. C. Del Villano. It was purified from the supernatant of lymphocyte line SCRF 60-A cultures (Lerner et al., 1972) grown in suspension as previously described (Kennel and Lerner, 1973). The culture medium was clarified by centrifugation at 10,000 × g in a Sorvall KSB continuous flow rotor at a flow rate of 100 ml/min at 4°C in a Sorvall RC2B centrifuge. Virus was concentrated from the clarified supernatant by sedimentation to its isopycnic density in a linear sucrose gradient in a Beckman CF32 continuous flow rotor. The material at a density of 1.14 to 1.18 g/cm³ was diluted in STE (0.1 M NaCl, 0.01 M Tris, 0.001 M EDTA, pH = 7.4) to a final sucrose concentration of 22% (w/w), and the virus was concentrated by centrifugation onto a cushion of 42% sucrose in STE. The virus preparation contained 1.4 mg/ml of the P-30 antigen. The virus was frozen in aliquots (−195°C) until use.

The Moloney strain of the murine sarcoma virus (MSV) was provided by Dr. Alexander Fefer (Department of Medicine, University of Washington, Seattle, Washington).

Animals

The BALB/c mice (L. C. Strong Foundation, San Diego, California) selected for this experiment have no detectable P-30 in their circulation, and they have a low incidence of spontaneous lymphoid tumors. Adult mice were eight to twelve weeks old at the start of the experiment. The mice were housed six (or fewer) per cage with food and water provided ad libitum. Mice were examined at least weekly, and the mice appearing near death were killed and an autopsy performed.

Mice were bled from the retroorbital fossa. Following overnight clot retraction, blood samples were centrifuged, and the sera removed. Plasma was obtained in a similar manner, except that heparinized capillary tubes were used (Sherwood Medical Industries, St. Louis, Missouri). All mice were anesthetized with ether for bleeding, except those mice from which plasma for the sucrose gradient analysis was obtained. In this case, the mice were given sodium pentobarbital (0.01 mg/g of body weight) in order to avoid possible ether disruption of the virus.

X-irradiation and Cell Reconstitution

All X-irradiation was performed on a Gamma Cell 40 (Atomic Energy of Canada, Ltd.) at a dose rate of 120 rads/min.

The BALB/c spleens and thymuses were removed, placed in cold phosphate buffered saline (PBS) (0.01 M PO₄³⁻ + 0.15 M NaCl, pH = 7.4), teased through stainless steel cloth (140 μm² pore size), and then filtered through nylon bolting cloth (110 μm² pore size). The cells were centrifuged (250 × g for 10 min at 4°C) and gently resuspended in cold PBS. A 20-μl aliquot was added to 1.98 ml of 3% glacial acetic acid, and the lymphocytes were counted in a hemocytometer. After recentrifugation, the cells were again suspended, at a concentration of 2.5×10^8 lymphocytes/ml. Each mouse received 5×10^7 lymphocytes (0.2 ml) via the tail vein.

Determination of P-30

Our P-30 was quantitated by radioimmunassay (RIA). Briefly, the sample was serially diluted in 0.01% Tween 80 in borate buffer (0.1 M boric acid, 0.025 M sodium tetraborate, 0.075 M NaCl, pH = 8.3). Tween 80 disrupts the virions so that all of the P-30 is available for assay. The serially diluted samples were incubated with a standardized amount of antibody, and then a known amount of ^{125}I-labeled P-30 was added. After incubation, the antigen–antibody complexes were precipitated by the addition of ammonium sulfate to a final concentration of 47.5%. The precipitate was removed by centrifugation ($11,000 \times g$ for 5 min), and the radioactivity in the pellet was counted. The degree to which ^{125}I-labeled antigen precipitation was inhibited by various dilutions of the sample permitted us to determine the amount of P-30 in the sample. This test detects 0.05 μg of P-30/ml.

Sedimentation Analysis of P-30

Fresh plasma was obtained from five mice with high circulating levels of P-30. The pool of their plasma contained 6.5 μg of P-30/ml. A 16-ml linear sucrose gradient in STE, with a density range of 1.230 to 1.068 $g \times cm^{-3}$, was used. Fresh plasma (0.8 ml) was layered on the top of the gradient and centrifuged at $201,000 \times g$ (average) in a SW-41 rotor for 3.5 hr, and 0.6 ml fractions were collected; the refractive index of fractions was then determined, with RIA for P-30 was performed on each fraction.

Inoculation of Animals

Adult Mice

Frozen MuLV-S was quickly thawed at 37°C and diluted with cold PBS to a final concentration of 15 μg of P-30/ml; this dilution contained 5×10^3 TCID$_{50}$ units/ml (assay kindly performed by Dr. B. C. Del Villano) as determined by the XC plaque assay (Klement et al., 1969), and 0.2 ml was injected into the tail vein of each recipient. The MSV was diluted 1:10 in PBS, and 0.05 ml was injected into the quadriceps femoris muscle of each recipient.

Newborn Mice

Newborn mice received approximately 50 μl of serum obtained from mice with MuLV-S viremia by subcutaneous injection. Slight leakage always occurred, so the exact injection volume was not known.

RESULTS

Infection of Adult BALB/c Mice with MuLV-S

Twelve normal adult BALB/c mice were given MuLV-S and 17 days later, the mice were bled and the serum P-30 was determined. As shown in Table 1 (Group 1) these normal adult mice given MuLV-S have a low, but significant viremia. Since the thymus is thought to be a target organ for MuLV infections (Davis et al., 1973), we wanted to determine if the thymus of a newborn animal might be a favored target. Adult BALB/c mice were used as recipients, and syngeneic tissues were the source of donor cells. Ten mice

TABLE 1. *Infection of adult BALB/c mice with MuLV*

Group number		Treatment	Micrograms P-30/ml serum[a]		
			17–21 days after treatment		
			Average	SD[b]	Range
1		MuLV-S	0.3	0.2	<0.05–0.7
2		MuLV-S; neonatal thymocytes	0.2	0.2	<0.05–0.6
3	600 r	MuLV-S; neonatal thymocytes; adult spleen	1.6	0.3	0.9–2.0
4	600 r	MuLV-S; adult spleen	1.3	0.4	0.8–2.1
5	600 r	neonatal thymocytes	0.07	0.05	<0.05–0.2
6		MuLV-S; intrathymic injection	<0.05		<0.05

[a] Normal BALB/c mice have <0.05 µg P-30/ml serum.
[b] SD, Standard deviation.

received neonatal thymocytes and MuLV-S (Group 2). Three groups of mice were irradiated with 600 rads to provide room for the growth of adoptively transferred lymphoid cells. On the same day the mice were X-irradiated, they were injected intravenously with neonatal thymocytes, adult spleen cells, and MuLV-S (Group 3); adult spleen cells and MuLV-S (Group 4); or neonatal thymocytes and adult spleen cells (Group 5). In addition, MuLV-S was injected directly into the thymus of otherwise normal adult BALB/c. The results of these experiments are summarized in Table 1. Several facts are clear from these data, in addition to the aforementioned low but significant viremia in Group 1: the addition of neonatal thymocytes alone does not seem to enhance the infectivity of MuLV-S, and X-irradiation prior to virus administration permits early expression of high levels of virus in these adult mice.

The Effect of X-Irradiation on Virus Expression in Adult Mice

Since X-irradiation prior to virus injection enhanced virus expression (see Table 1) we decided to study this further. The first experiment was designed

TABLE 2. *Relation of dose of X-irradiation to viral expression*

Treatment		P-30 μg/ml serum 17–21 days after treatment		
Radiation dose (rads)	Cellular reconstitution (5×10^7)	Average	SD[a]	Range
600	None	2.7	0.8	1.7–4.1
600	spleen cells	1.3	0.4	0.8–2.1
400	None	2.2	0.3	1.8–3.0
400	spleen cells	1.9	1.1	0.1–3.2
150	None	1.9	2.2	<0.05–7.9
50	None	0.3	0.2	<0.05–1.1
0	None	0.3	0.2	<0.05–0.7

[a] SD, Standard deviation.

to determine the dose of X-rays necessary to permit this high level of virus expression. Groups of mice were exposed to graded doses of X-rays and 6 hr later were given MuLV-S. The data presented in Table 2 show that the level of virus expression after X-irradiation is dependent on the radiation dose.

We also wished to determine if X-irradiated adult mice were protected from the effect of X-rays by cellular reconstitution with syngeneic adult spleen cells. Mice were exposed to 400 or 600 rads and given 5×10^7 adult spleen cells after exposure, but before virus injection. As can be seen in Table 2, adoptive transfer of spleen cells appears to lower the level of virus expression regularly in the group given 600 rads, and in two out of ten mice given 400 rads.

Kinetics of Virus Expression after X-Irradiation and Infection

Adult BALB/c mice were irradiated (400 rads), injected with virus the same day, and then exsanguinated at various intervals. Thirty minutes after the intravenous administration of MuLV-S, no P-30 was detectable in the circulation. This was taken as proof that shortly after injection virus cannot

TABLE 3. *Kinetics of virus expression after infection of X-irradiated adult mice*

Time (days) after injection of MuLV-S	P-30 (μg/ml serum)
0.02	<0.05
0.33	<0.05
3.0	<0.05
5	<0.05
10	<0.05
14	0.25
19	1.6

TABLE 4. *Virus expression as a function of the relationship between time of X-irradiation and time of virus injection*

| Time of X-irradiation[a] (hr) | Serum P-30 (μg/ml) 17–21 days after MuLV-S administration | | |
	Average	SD[b]	Range
− 168	1.5	0.3	1.1 −1.6
− 72	2.1	0.4	1.6 −2.8
− 24	1.7	0.2	1.5 −2.1
+ 0.5	1.1	0.5	0.08−2.4
+ 8	2.1	0.4	1.2 −2.4
+ 24	1.7	0.6	0.9 −2.4

[a] MuLV-S was injected at time 0. Minus (−) sign, X-irradiation was administered before virus; plus (+) sign, X-irradiation was administered after virus.
[b] SD, Standard deviation.

be detected in the circulation. As can be seen from Table 3, P-30 was first detected at low levels on day 14 and by day 19, reached very high levels.

To explore the temporal relationship between X-irradiation and enhanced expression, mice were given 600 rads at 168 hr, 72 hr, or 24 hr before injection of MuLV-S and 0.5 hr, 8 hr, or 24 hr after injection of MuLV-S. Eighteen days after virus injection, the mice were bled and the amount of serum P-30 assayed. It can be seen from Table 4 that within this 8-day time-span, the level of serum P-30 was essentially independent of the temporal relationship between X-irradiation and inoculation of virus.

Growth Characteristics of MSV-Induced Sarcomas after X-Irradiation

To examine the possibility that X-irradiation had a permissive effect because of its immunosuppressive effects, seven mice were given 600 rads 1 week before administration of MSV; six nonirradiated mice were given similar virus injections. The time of appearance, rate of growth, and size of tumors was similar in both groups. In both groups, the tumors regressed in an identical manner. From these experiments, we conclude that the immune response in our mice given 600 rads, was sufficiently intact 1 week later, even in the absence of cellular reconstitution, to complete the complicated process of rejection of a virus-induced sarcoma.

Effect of X-Irradiation on the Expression of Intact Infectious Oncogenic Virus in Adult Mice

It was important to determine that, in adult mice, the P-30 we measured was associated with intact virus. Plasma from mice with high levels of P-30 was centrifuged through a linear sucrose gradient. Thirty percent of the P-30 in the plasma sedimented between the densities of 1.13 and 1.16 g/cm^3, and

it very likely represented intact MuLV-S virions (Fig. 1). Sixty percent of
the P-30 failed to enter the gradient and represented "free viral protein." We
can conclude from these data that a significant portion of the circulating P-30
that we measured reflects intact virus. Since a non-infectious or defective
virus could still have the same density, it was important to demonstrate that
the virus we identified was infectious and oncogenic. Fresh plasma from mice
with high levels of viremia induced by 600 rads and MuLV-S were pooled
(P-30 in pool = 1.4 µg/ml), and about 50 µl of plasma were injected subcutaneously into each of 13 newborn mice. One month later, all the newborns
had serum P-30 levels above 2 µg/ml, and by four months, 12 of the 13 had
developed lymphomas. This was taken as proof that each 50 µl of plasma
contains enough infectious virus particles to regularly infect a newborn
mouse.

It has been reported that there are at least three different endogenous
BALB oncornaviruses (Stephenson et al., 1974a), so it was important to
demonstrate that the virus we were measuring was the same virus we had
injected, rather than a host virus induced by X-irradiation or MuLV-S acting
as a "helper" or both. Dr. Stuart Aaronson (Viral Carcinogenesis Branch,
National Cancer Institute) kindly performed a radioimmunassay for murine
P-12 (Stephenson et al., 1974b), a type-specific viral antigen, on a pool of
serum from our viremic mice. The P-12 in the serum blocks the precipitation

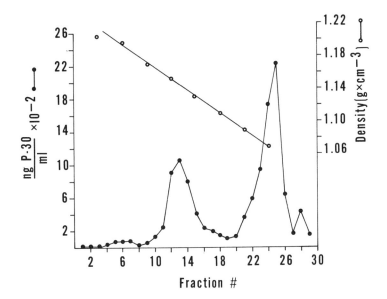

FIG. 1. Sedimentation analysis of P-30. Plasma obtained from MuLV viremic mice was pooled and layered
on the top of a 16-ml linear sucrose gradient (densities 1.068 to 1.230 g × cm⁻³). The gradient was
centrifuged at 201,000 × g(avg.) in a Beckman SW41 rotor for 3.5 hr, and 0.6 ml fractions were collected and individually assayed for P-30.

of MuLV(Moloney) P-12, but not of MuLV(Rauscher) P-12 or MuLV (AKR) P-12. As mentioned above, the type-specific antigen P-12 found in MuLV-S and in MuLV(Moloney) react identically in radioimmunassay. Therefore, the P-12 found in the MuLV circulating in these mice is identical to the P-12 of the MuLV-S with which they were infected and different from any endogenous BALB/c virus. Although minor contamination by an endogenous BALB/c virus cannot be excluded, this assay demonstrated that the bulk of replicating virus was the progeny of the virus we introduced into the animal.

Oncogenicity of MuLV-S in Adult Mice

From the above studies, it was clear that MuLV-S could infect adult mice, but it was not clear that MuLV-S was necessarily oncogenic. But, most adult mice given MuLV-S developed lymphomas later. These tumors regularly involved the thymus and frequently the spleen and lymph nodes. Twelve animals received only MuLV-S. Three months after its administration, all the animals were normal in appearance. By 6 months, 9 of these 12 animals appeared ill and were sacrificed and autopsied or died. All seven of the mice upon which autopsies were performed had lymphoma. These lymphomas cannot be distinguished histologically from those induced by MuLV-S in newborn mice. Fifty-three animals received a combination of X-irradiation and MuLV-S. These mice were also all healthy at three months. By 6 months, 42 of the 53 had died. Twenty-five of these were autopsied, and all but two mice, which died during bleeding, had lymphomas.

At 4.5 months, the adults given only MuLV-S were all healthy. Of the nine mice that died by 6 months, the average time-span from virus administration to evidence of malignancy was 5.6 months. In contrast, 50% of the adult mice given MuLV-S and X-irradiated developed lymphomas by 4.5 months. The average time span between MuLV-S administration with X-irradiation and evidence of tumors was 4.3 months.

There was no difference in time of tumor development between mice given neonatal thymocytes and splenocytes in addition to MuLV-S and X-irradiation and mice not receiving those cells.

DISCUSSION

These studies confirm the report of Moloney that MuLV can be infectious and oncogenic in adult BALB/c mice. In addition, we report that expression of virus and oncogenicity are accelerated by X-irradiation. It is important to put these results into perspective with the extensive work of Kaplan and his colleagues who also utilized X-irradiation to study leukemia (Kaplan, 1967). Despite the utilization of similar materials, their experiments address fundamentally different questions; they are interested in the mechanism of inducing expression of an *endogenous* virus, whereas we are focusing on the conditions necessary to permit infection by an *exogenous* virus. With this in view, we considered the possibility that we had simply induced one of the endogenous viruses of BALB/c mice in our experiments. This was ruled out as the major event by quantitative studies, in which the highly type-specific antigen P-12 found in the sera of our mice was identical to that of MuLV-S and did not cross react in RIA with the P-12 of any of the endogenous BALB/c viruses. Thus, the overwhelming majority of the circulating virus we evaluated was the same exogenous virus we had administered.

It is important to understand the mechanism by which X-irradiation combined with virus administration to increase the rate of appearance of virion proteins in the circulation. Although it is tempting to invoke as an explanation the well-known immunosuppressive effects of X-irradiation, three observations we have made suggest that immunosuppression is not the most likely explanation. First, the more rapid appearance of virion proteins induced by X-irradiation was observed even in mice reconstituted with 5×10^7 syngeneic spleen cells, which should render them immunocompetent. Second, our results show that X-irradiation enhanced the expression of viral P-30 in the serum independent of the temporal relationship between X-irradiation and virus challenge, at least within an 8-day span. By contrast, Dixon and McConahey (1963) showed that the temporal relationship between X-irradiation and antigen challenge is critical in determining the immunologic outcome. If the effect were due to simple immunosuppression, we would have expected to find some variation in our results. Third, since a replicating antigen might be quite different from inanimate antigens, we addressed the issue of immunosuppression in another way. We utilized regression of an MSV-induced tumor as an index of host immunocompetence. In normal adult mice, this tumor grows and then regresses, whereas in immunosuppressed mice, it grows and kills the host (Fefer et al., 1967; Zisblatt and Lilly, 1972). Mice irradiated one week prior to MSV injection rejected an MSV-induced sarcoma in the same way normal mice did, whereas X-irradiation given a week prior to MuLV-S injection permitted adult BALB/c mice to express a high level of virus. Although there are surely differences between these two systems, the ability to reject the tumor induced by MSV given a week after X-irradiation would speak against immunosuppression as the primary consequence of the X-irradiation that permits MuLV-S expression and later tumor development.

It is likely that the magnitude of MuLV-S infection depends on the number of dividing cells in newborns and in adults. It is well known that most oncornaviruses require cellular DNA synthesis for replication *in vitro* (Humphries and Temin, 1972). An increased incidence of cell division thus could result in an increase in production of virus, allowing horizontal infection within the animal. In addition, the progeny of infected cells are of course infected. Although other interpretations are certainly possible, we think that X-irradiation causes adult mice to closely resemble newborn mice with respect to infectivity and oncogenicity of MuLV-S by increasing the frequency of cell division.

In the present studies, cellular reconstitution appears to lower the expression of virus following X-irradiation and MuLV-S injection. Adoptively transferred cells might fill some of the space in lymphoid tissues that is present after X-irradiation and thereby decrease the stimulus for cell proliferation. The longer time necessary for the detection of virus expression in unmanipulated adult mice may be explained by the fact that normal adults have fewer susceptible cells.

Interesting parallels to the present studies have been described. If MuLV (Rauscher) is inoculated into anemic adult mice, the number of infected cells is increased (Weitz-Hamburger, 1973). Anemia stimulates erythrocyte precursors; at least one target for Rauscher virus is thought to be the erythroid stem cell. Lagerlöf (1971) stimulated the myeloid cells of newborn chicks by using a controlled infection by staphylococci. This increases susceptibility to the BAI strain chicken myeloid leukemia virus.

Since we are attempting to understand control of oncornavirus infection quantitatively, it is important to understand the limitations of our methods. Even with our sensitive RIA, a large amount of virus is required for detection. The P-30 contributes approximately 30% of the mass of an intact virion (Fleissner, 1971). Even assuming that only one-fourth of the P-30 is virion associated, and given that the sensitivity of our RIA is 0.05 μg P-30/ml, we calculate that a viremia of about 10^8 particles/ml is required for detection. Because of this, animals with low levels of virus expression would be scored as not infected.

Although our results pertain to only one virus and one strain of mice, we think that this model can be more generally applied. With this quantitative background, we can begin to study those immunologic parameters that follow virus infection. Studies of infection by oncornaviruses were previously hampered by the difficulties imposed by utilizing infected newborns. Aside from technical difficulties, the phenomenon of neonatal tolerance renders newborn animals unsuited to the study of the mechanisms of coping with the immunologic and oncogenic challenge of oncornavirus infection. What already seems clear is that with the amount of virus used in these experiments, the immune response is insufficient, since high levels of virion antigens persist throughout the life-span of the mice.

SUMMARY

Infection of adult BALB/c mice with murine leukemia virus (MuLV) induces typical thymic lymphomas. The MuLV (Scripps), or MuLV-S, which shares many properties of MuLV (Moloney, 1960), was used in these experiments. Expression of virus was measured by using a radioimmunoassay for murine P-30, a virion core protein.

Nineteen days after injection of MuLV-S into adult mice, there were 0.3 μg P-30/ml of serum. X-irradiation permitted the early expression of high levels of viremia, when given before or after MuLV-S administration, and it also hastened the development of lymphomas. Seventeen to 21 days after injection of MuLV-S into X-irradiated (600 rads) adult mice, there were 2.7 μg of P-30/ml of serum. The virus produced by infected adult mice was infectious and oncogenic when given to newborn mice.

Several lines of evidence are presented that suggest the mechanism by which X-irradiation permits early expression of virion proteins and lymphomas is not immunosuppression.

ACKNOWLEDGMENTS

The authors thank Ms. Patricia McConahey for performing the radioimmunoassays for P-30, Dr. Stuart Aaronson for performing the radioimmunoassays for P-12, Dr. Bert C. Del Villano and Dr. Alexander Fefer for providing virus, and Dr. Frank Lilly for valuable discussion. This is publication number 969 from the Department of Immunopathology, Scripps and Research Foundation, La Jolla, California, 92037. This research was supported by USPHS Grant A1-07007, AEC Contract AT (04–3) 410, Council for Tobacco Research Grant CTR 766 AR1, National Foundation Grant CRBS 274, and National Cancer Institute Contract NIH-NC1-E-72-3264. R.L.L. was supported by USPHS Training Grant 5T1GM-683. RAL is the recipient of the National Institutes of Health Career Development Award AA-46372.

REFERENCES

Aaronson, S. A., and Stephenson, J. R. (1975): *Personal communication.*

Davis, B. D., Dulbecco, R., Eisen, H. M., Ginsberg, H. S., and Wood, B. (1973): *Microbiology,* 2nd Ed., Medical Department, Harper & Row, Hagerstown, Maryland, p. 1433.

Dixon, F. J., and McConahey, P. J. (1963): Enhancement of antibody formation by whole body X-irradiation. *J. Exp. Med.,* 117:833–847.

Fan, H., and Baltimore, D. (1973): RNA metabolism of murine leukemia virus: Detection of virus specific RNA sequences in infected and unifected cells and identification of virus specific messenger RNA. *J. Mol. Biol.,* 80:93–117.

Fefer, A., McCoy, J. L., and Glynn, J. P. (1967): Induction and regression of primary Moloney sarcoma virus-induced tumors in mice. *Cancer Res.,* 27:1626–1631.

Fleissner, E. (1971): Chromatographic separation and antigenic analysis of proteins of the oncornaviruses. *J. Virol.,* 8:778–785.

Gross, L. (1974): Facts and theories on viruses causing cancer and leukemia. *Proc. Natl. Acad. Sci. USA,* 71:2013–2017.

Humphries, E. H., and Temin, H. (1972): Cell-cycle dependent activation of Rous Sarcoma Virus-infected stationary chick cells: Avian leukosis virus group specific antigens and ribonucleic acid. *J. Virol.,* 10:82–87.

Kaplan, H. S. (1967): On the natural history of murine leukemias: Presidential Address. *Cancer Res.,* 27:1325–1340.

Kennel, S. J., and Lerner, R. A. (1973): Isolation and characterization of plasma membrane associated immunoglobulin from cultured human diploid lymphocytes. *J. Mol. Biol.,* 76:485–502.

Klement, V., Rowe, W. P., Hartley, J., and Pugh, W. E. (1969): Mixed culture cytopathogenicity. A new test for growth of murine leukemia viruses in tissue culture. *Proc. Natl. Acad. Sci. USA,* 63:753–758.

Lagerlöf, B. (1971): Enhancing the susceptibility of chicks to myeloid leukemia virus by myeloid-cell stimulation. *Acta Pathol. Microbiol. Scand. [A],* 79:208–209.

Lerner, R. A., Jensen, F. C., Kennel, S. J., Dixon, F. J., DesRoches, G., and Francke, U. (1972): Karyotypic and virologic and immunologic analyses of two continuous lymphocyte lines established from New Zealand Black Mice: Possible relationship of chromosomal mosaicism to autoimmunity. *Proc. Natl. Acad. Sci. USA,* 69:2965–2969.

Moloney, J. B. (1960): Biological studies on a lymphoma-leukemia virus extracted from Sarcoma 37. I. Origin and introductory investigations. *J. Natl. Cancer Inst.,* 24:933–947.

Stephenson, J. R., Aaronson, S. A., Arnstein, P., Huebner, R. J., and Tonick, S. T. (1974a): Demonstration of two immunologically distinct xenotropic type-C RNA viruses of mouse cells. *Virology,* 61:56–63.

Stephenson, J. R., Tonick, S. R., and Aaronson, S. A. (1974b): Analysis of type specific antigenic determinants of two structural polypeptides of mouse RNA C-type viruses. *Virology,* 58:1–8.

Weitz-Hamburger, A., Frederickson, T. N., LoBue, J., Hardy, W. D. Ferdinand, P., and Gordon, A. S. (1973): Inhibition of erythroleukemia in mice by induction of hemolytic anemia prior to infection with Rauscher leukemia virus. *Cancer Res.,* 33:104–111.

Zisblatt, M., and Lilly, F. (1972): The effect of immunosuppression on oncogenesis by murine sarcoma virus. *Proc. Soc. Expt. Biol. Med.,* 141:1036–1040.

Biology of Radiation Carcinogenesis, edited by
J. M. Yuhas, R. W. Tennant, and J. D. Regan.
Raven Press, New York © 1976.

Death and Transformation

Robert G. Martin and Jeffrey L. Anderson

Laboratory of Molecular Biology, National Institute of Arthritis, Metabolism, and Digestive Diseases
National Institutes of Health, Bethesda, Maryland 20014

PROPERTIES OF SV40-TRANSFORMED CELLS

Many criteria have been used to define the phenomenon of transformation by SV40 in tissue culture, although none is universally accepted. Included are the ability of "transformed" cells:

1. to form multilayered clones under conditions where normal cells remain as a monolayer (Todaro et al., 1964)
2. to form clones on a monolayer of normal cells (Temin and Rubin, 1958)
3. to reach high cell densities at "saturation" (Todaro et al., 1964)
4. to grow in low concentrations of serum (Smith et al., 1971)
5. to grow more rapidly than nontransformed cells, particularly in low concentrations of serum (Risser and Pollack, 1974)
6. to grow in agar or methyl cellulose suspension (Macpherson and Montagnier, 1964; Stoker et al., 1968)
7. to clone at high efficiency, particularly in low concentrations of serum or Aγ-depleted serum (Smith et al., 1971; Scher and Nelson-Rees, 1971; Tegtmeyer, 1975; Martin and Chou, 1975)
8. to transport 2-deoxyglucose with high efficiency (Isselbacher, 1972)
9. to exhibit altered membrane properties including lectin binding and lectin-induced agglutination (Burger, 1969; Inbar and Sachs, 1969)
10. to overcome topoinhibition (Dulbecco, 1970)
11. to express viral specific T-antigen (Black et al., 1963; Pope and Rowe, 1964; Black, 1966)
12. to survive under conditions where normal cells tend to senesce and die, i.e., "immortalization" (Shein and Enders, 1962; Koprowski et al., 1962; Risser et al., 1974; Osborn and Weber, 1975)
13. to release plasminogen activator (Unkeless et al., 1973)
14. to exhibit morphologic changes (Shein and Enders, 1962; Kimura and Dulbecco, 1973)
15. and of course, to produce tumors in test animals (Freedman and Shin, 1974).

Many, if not all, of these manifestations of transformation are interrelated, and many are clearly nonspecific manifestations of rapidly growing cells, whether normal or transformed (Burger, 1969; Romano and Colby, 1973; Arndt-Jovin and Berg, 1971). But precisely what the role of SV40 is in inducing these changes remains a subject of considerable debate.

EXPRESSION OF AN INTEGRATED SV40 IS SUFFICIENT FOR TRANSFORMATION

The DNA of the SV40 virus is only 3.6×10^6 daltons (Crawford and Black, 1964; Tai et al., 1972). Transformed cells contain an integrated SV40 genome (Sambrook et al., 1968). Only about one-half of the genome, the early region (see Fig. 1) is generally expressed in transformed cells (Khoury et al., 1973; Sambrook et al., 1972; Khoury et al., 1975). The SV40 variants that are completely deleted for the late region can transform (Brockman and Scott, 1975). Therefore, the molecular weight of the protein(s) responsible for transformation by SV40 is at most approximately 100,000 daltons. It has been proposed that the T-antigen is an early protein of SV40, with a molecular weight of 70,000 or greater (Del Villano and Defendi, 1973; Tegtmeyer, 1974). Furthermore, only one early viral cistron has been described (Tegtmeyer and Ozer, 1971; Chou and Martin, 1974). Thus, it may be assumed that SV40 is capable of inducing transformation simply by virtue of the synthesis of active T-antigen and that most if not all of the manifestations of transformation must be interrelated. An alternate explanation would require that T-antigen is necessary but not sufficient for full transformation by SV40, e.g., that SV40 induces some initial event(s), but that full transformation requires some secondary genetic alteration(s).

In general, it is not possible to test simultaneously for each of the phenotypes outlined. Rather, "transformants" are isolated by one or another technique and then assayed for the separate phenotypes. A theoretical difficulty in deducing, from such experiments, that all the various phenotypes are the

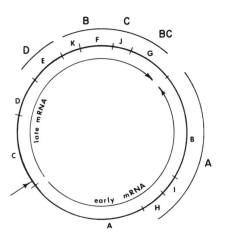

FIG. 1. Physical and genetic map of the SV40 genome. The full circle represents SV40 DNA divided into the various *Haemophilus influenzae* restriction fragments, A through K (Danna et al., 1973). The inner arrows indicate the direction of early (previral-DNA replication) and late mRNA synthesis (Sambrook et al., 1972; Khoury et al., 1973; Khoury et al., 1975). The arrow indicates the point at which DNA replication starts (Fareed et al., 1972). Three genes have been identified (see review of Martin et al., 1974); A, D, and a complex locus divided into complementation groups B, C, and BC (Chou and Martin 1974). Mutants in these genes have been mapped by marker rescue (Lai and Nathans, 1974, 1975), and their approximate positions are indicated by the outer arcs.

direct result of SV40 integration and expression is that multiple passages of the cells are required after the initial event to obtain sufficient numbers of cells to carry out the tests. It is possible, therefore, that transformation by SV40 is a multi-staged process. It is possible, for example, that SV40 acts as a mutator gene (Treffers et al., 1954) and, following integration, induces mutations (Marshak et al., 1973) that give the cells selective growth advantages in tissue culture.

Two types of experiments suggest that full transformation does not require multiple mutagenic or rare physiologic events following the initial expression of an integrated SV40. Risser and Pollack (1974) have shown that when *random* clones are picked following treatment of 3T3 cells by SV40 at multiplicities of 2×10^3 PFU/cell, at least two, and possibly three different types of transformed clones can be obtained. They called those T-antigen negative clones with modestly enhanced ability to grow in low serum (but without definitive proof that SV40 was integrated), "minimal transformants." Those clones able to express T-antigen partially and to grow to intermediate saturation densities were designated "intermediate transformants." And those clones whose cells were all T-antigen positive and were able to overgrow a monolayer of nontransformed cells and also to grow in soft agar or methycellulose were called "full transformants." If transformation by SV40 were a multi-staged phenomenon, there should be many more nontransformed and minimally transformed clones than intermediate transformants and fewer still of the fully transformed phenotype. Instead, roughly equal numbers of each class were found. A second argument against the thesis that transformation by SV40 requires multiple events comes from the study of transformants induced by temperature-sensitive mutants of SV40. Using the appropriate temperature-sensitive mutants, it is possible to obtain transformants by any of several different criteria and show that the phenotype by which the transformants were selected and most other phenotypic properties of transformation are lost on shifting to the nonpermissive temperature.

CONTINUED EXPRESSION OF THE SV40 A FUNCTION IS REQUIRED FOR THE MAINTENANCE OF TRANSFORMATION

Several groups (Martin and Chou, 1975; Tegtmeyer, 1975; Osborn and Weber, 1975; Brugge and Butel, 1975; Kimura and Itagaki, 1975) have independently concluded that the continued expression of the early region of the SV40 genome, the *A* gene product (see Fig. 1), is required for maintenance of the transformed state. In our studies, transformed clones of secondary Chinese hamster lung (CHL) cells were selected on the basis of their ability to overgrow a monolayer and to form clones with higher than normal efficiency (Martin and Chou, 1975). Whereas transformants induced at 33°C by *B, C, BC,* or *D* mutants remained transformed at 40°C by both of these criteria (see for example Fig. 2), clones transformed by *A* mutants

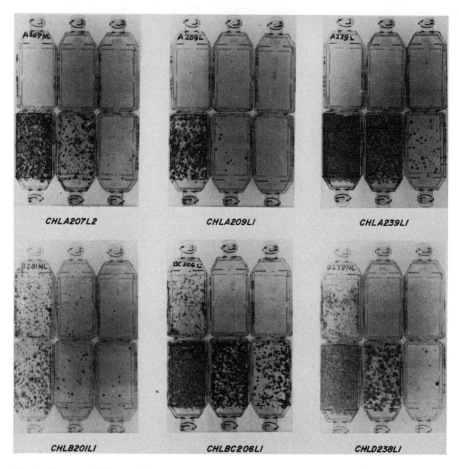

FIG. 2. Cloning at 33° and 40°C of Chinese hamster lung cells transformed by various temperature-sensitive mutants of SV40. Transformed clones induced at 33°C by the temperature-sensitive mutants (upper sets of six flasks, left to right) A207, A209, A239 and (lower sets left to right) B201, BC206, and D238 were purified by recloning (Martin and Chou, 1975). In each set illustrated, the left-hand flasks received 10⁵ cells, the middle flasks 2.5 × 10⁴ cells, and the right-hand flasks 6 × 10³ cells. The upper three of each set were incubated at 40°C for two weeks, the lower three at 33°C for three weeks. The DV medium supplemented with 5% fetal calf serum was changed weekly. Note that in each set, cloning is more efficient at 33° than at 40°C. But, only the A mutant-induced transformants failed to clone at the highest cell densities at 40°C.

lost these phenotypes at 40°C. We have now extended our analyses to some of the other criteria outlined above, using either transformed Chinese hamster lung cells or mouse brain cells.

Table 1 shows the effect of temperature and serum concentration on the generation time of different lines of Chinese hamster lung cells in the relatively rich medium of Dulbecco and Vogt (DV). In 10% serum, the generation times of the transformed and normal cells are nearly indistinguishable from one another at either 33° or 40°C. But, differences become apparent in cells growing in 2.5% serum. At the permissive temperature (33°C), all of the transformants behave like the wild-type transformed control but very differently from the normal, uninfected CHL cells. At the nonpermissive temperature (40°C), however, cell lines transformed by the temperature-sensitive mutants, A207 and A239, behave more nearly like normal cells.

TABLE 1. Generation times of normal and transformed CHL cells in DV medium[a]

Serum concentration (%)	Growth temperature (°C)	Generation time (hours)				
			SV40-tranformed cells			
		Normal CHL[b]	Wild type	BC245	A207	A239
2.5	33	80	44	32	34	36
2.5	40	≥ 80	48	43	82	58
10	33	22	17	17	19	17
10	40	∼ 24	16	20	21	18

[a]Cells growing in DV medium supplemented with 10% serum at 33°C or twice passaged at 40°C were pre-adapted to 2.5% serum medium for at least 48 hr for the experiments in rows 1 and 2. Cells were then trypsinized and plated at 1 to 2 × 10⁴ cells/cm² in 2 cm² wells (Linbro) and reincubated (5 to 6% CO_2). The DV medium (supplemented with 2.5% or 10% serum, No. American Biol.) was replaced every other day. Individual wells were trypsinized daily and the number of cells determined in a Celloscope 101 cell counter. Growth was followed for ten days (well into confluence); generation times were determined graphically.

[b] Average of parent line and two subclones.

Thus, expression of the A function appears to be required for rapid growth in low serum. Similar results with rat embryo cells were obtained by Osborn and Weber (1975).

Next, we have examined the expression of T-antigen in the transformed CHL cell lines. When assayed by the indirect immunofluorescence technique, normal CHL cells contained no T-antigen, whereas cell lines transformed by wild-type virus or by mutants A207, A209, A239, A241, B201, BC245, C219, and D202, all exhibited T-antigen at both 33° and 40°C. Even on continued passage for over a month at 40°C, the A mutant-transformed CHL lines continued to express T-antigen. Similarly, it has been reported that all Syrian hamster, human, rabbit kidney, and mouse cells transformed by temperature-sensitive A mutants remained T-antigen positive at the non-permissive temperature for a week (Tegtmeyer, 1975) or an unspecified time (Brugge and Butel, 1975). Some rat embryo cell lines, however, partially lose T-antigen after 4 days at the nonpermissive temperature (Osborn and Weber, 1975). Although the difference between the rat embryo and other cell types is of interest, the continued expression of T-antigen at the nonpermissive temperature is not necessarily surprising. Most bacterial "missense" mutations make immunologically cross-reacting material (Whitfield et al., 1966; Martin and Talal, 1968), i.e., most enzymatically inactive proteins that result from the substitution of a single amino acid (which is the case for most temperature-sensitive mutants) remain antigenically active.

The transport of 2-deoxyglucose in normal and transformed CHL cell lines has been compared (Table 2). Cell growth in DV-10 at 33° and 40°C was followed over 14 days from subconfluence to early confluence and finally to late confluence in depleted medium. With normal CHL cells (1) uptake at 40°C was about one-third greater than at 33°C, consistent with an increased metabolic rate at the higher temperature; and (2) 2-deoxyglucose uptake was not a parameter particularly sensitive to cell density inhibition. Significant changes in uptake at either 33° or 40°C occurred only when cells were allowed to continue into late confluence under depleted nutrient conditions. Furthermore, hexose transport in the transformed cell lines, SV-16, *A207*, and *A239,* was similar to that for normal CHL cells. We extended these observations to growth in both high (10%) and low (2.5%) serum concentrations and found that 2-deoxyglucose uptake was not helpful in distinguishing between normal mouse brain cells and wild-type or *A239* transformed mouse brain cells at either 33° or 40°C (unpublished results). Thus, 2-deoxyglucose uptake does not appear to be related to other manifestations of transforma-

TABLE 2. 2-Deoxyglucose uptake in Chinese hamster cells[a]

Cell line	Culture Conditions			
	Temperature (°C)	Subconfluent	Confluent	Late confluence (depleted)
CHL	33°	6[b]	5	0.2
	40°	10	6	2
A207	33°	12	8	0.8
	40°	17	10	0.9
A239	33°	7	6	0[c]
	40°	10	6	0[c]
Wild-type	33°	7	6	0[c]
(SV-16)	40°	10	9	0[c]

[a] Cells were plated at about $2 \times 10^4/cm^2$ in 25 cm^2 plastic flasks (Falcon) and grown in 6% CO_2 at the indicated temperatures in DV medium supplemented with 10% serum (Flow). Determinations of deoxyglucose uptake per milligram protein and parallel cell counts were made daily. The experimental protocol was modified after Bose and Zlotnick (1973): cell layers were washed three times with PBS, incubated with [^{3}H]dG in PBS (4 μCi/ml, 4 ml/flask) for 20 min in waterbaths at 33° or 40°C, and washed thoroughly with PBS, solubilized in Lowry's C; aliquots were used for determinations of radioactivity and protein content. Points were taken daily through day 7, the medium was changed a final time and left until day 14 when the last point was taken. Results could be pooled into three groups: subconfluent cultures (days 1 to 3 or 4), confluent cultures (days 4 to 6 or 7), and "late" confluent cultures (day 14). Under depleted nutrient conditions (day 14), various degrees of cell injury and death were observed in the order of SV16 >239 >207 >CHL. The drop in hexose uptake on day 14 is therefore interpreted as predominantly a nonspecific manifestation of cell injury. Not shown: 2-deoxyglucose uptake as a function of cell number gave similar results. A somewhat greater terminal fall in counts per cell was seen as cells became smaller and more densely packed.
[b] Numbers represent [^{3}H]dG counts $\times 10^{-6}$/min/mg cell protein and were reproducible to $\pm$ 10%.
[c] Cell layer lysed.

tion at least in Chinese hamster lung and mouse brain cells. And in other cell types, the correlation between uptake and transformation is also weak. Brugge and Butel (1975) reported that Syrian hamster/A30 transformants transported *less* 2-deoxyglucose at the permissive temperature than untransformed (HEF) cells and that a human, temperature-sensitive transformant (HuF/A28) actually transported more 2-deoxyglucose at the nonpermissive temperature. In contrast, Bose and Zlotnick (1973) found transport of 2-deoxyglucose to be the earliest parameter of density-dependent growth inhibition in Balb 3T3 cells; the rate of transport began declining late in exponential growth, reaching a 10-fold lower level at saturation. These observations confirmed earlier results that SV40-transformed mouse cells transport 2-deoxyglucose at a threefold greater rate than normal Balb 3T3 cells (Issel-

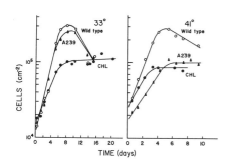

FIG. 3. Growth curves of normal, wild-type, and A239-transformed Chinese hamster lung cells at 33° and 40°C. Equal aliquots of cells were dispensed into 1.6-cm diam 24 well-plates (Linbro Chemical Co., New Haven, Conn.), in Hams' F12 medium supplemented with 5% fetal calf serum. The medium was changed every other day for the plates incubated at 33°C and every day for the plates incubated at 40°C. Cells were removed from the plastic by treatment with trypsin-EDTA and counted in a Celloscope 101 cell counter. The cloned transformed cell lines CHLA239L1 (▲) and CHLWT16 (○) and the uncloned parental CHL cells (●) have been described (Martin and Chou, 1975).

bacher, 1972). And Brugge and Butel (1975) reported a four- to tenfold decrease in 2-deoxyglucose uptake at the nonpermissive temperature in Balb 3T3 cells transformed by the temperature-sensitive A7 mutant. On the basis of further studies, however, Romano and Colby (1973) have argued that enhanced hexose transport is in fact not a specific consequence of the SV40 genome even in 3T3 transformation.

The effect of temperature on the saturation density of normal and transformed CHL cells in relatively poor medium (Ham's F-12) has also been examined (Fig. 3). At 33°C, under the conditions employed, wild-type and A239-transformed CHL cells grow more rapidly than normal CHL cells, and continue growing beyond a cell density of 10^5 cells/cm². A curious property of transformed cells noted previously (Dulbecco and Elkington, 1973; Oey et al., 1974) is that they frequently slough and die after reaching high cell densities. The death and sloughing of CHL-transformed cells (discussed in more detail below) is seen after densities of approximately 3×10^5 cells/cm² are reached. Figure 3 further illustrates that cells transformed by mutant A239 behave more nearly like normal CHL cells at 40°C: their growth rate is reduced and they reach a saturation cell density comparable to that of the normal cells.

Changes in chromosome number frequently accompany both SV40 transformation and phenotypic reversion from the transformed state. For example, Pollack et al. (1970) found phenotypic revertants of SV40-transformed mouse cells to show a striking increase in chromosome number, whereas malignant back revertants returned to the original subtetraploid mode. We therefore examined the karyotypes of the temperature-sensitive transformed CHL cell lines. Cells growing in DV-10 at 33° or 40°C were incubated in colcemid (0.3 μg/cc) for 3 hr, allowed to swell in hypotonic buffer (1% sodium citrate), fixed with methanol acetic acid (3:1), spread on clear, chilled glass slides, and stained with Giemsa. Many well-spread mitotic figures were counted for each cell line. The following lines had the diploid number of chromosomes (i.e., 22 ± 2): CHL, *A207, A209, A239, A241* (33°C). In addition, *A207* and *A239* were karyotyped after growth at 40°C for a week, and there was no change in chromosome number. A wild-type (SV-16) and three representative "late mutant" transformants, *BC245, C219,* and *D202,* displayed average chromosome numbers of 32 ± 5, 36 ± 5, 20 ± 3, and 22 ± 2, respectively. It is clear from these data, therefore, that neither fully transformed growth at 33°C nor temperature-sensitive "revertant" behavior at 40°C is dependent on accompanying changes in chromosome number and that mechanisms at a more subtle level of growth control than chromosome dosage must be sought.

We have recently examined a number of characteristics of mouse brain cells transformed by SV40 (unpublished results). Here the criteria for transformation were immortalization and rapid growth (our normal mouse brain cells had a generation time of about a week and could not be cloned or even successfully subcultured at low cell densities). Cells transformed by wild-type and *A239* have been obtained and analyzed. Their growth behavior is similar to that shown in Fig. 3. The wild-type transformed cells grow to high density with a reduced generation time in medium with low concentrations of serum at both permissive and nonpermissive temperatures, whereas the *A239*-transformed cells have a prolonged generation time and reduced saturation density at the nonpermissive temperature. The cells are T-antigen positive at both temperatures, and show no significant difference in 2-deoxyglucose transport under any condition examined. Whereas wild-type and *A239* transformed cells clone equally efficiently at the permissive temperature, at 40°C, cloning of *A239* is sharply reduced relative to wild-type. The wild-type transformed cells overgrow a monolayer of normal cells at both temperatures, but the *A239* cells overgrow only at 33°C. In soft agar, cloning is observed at both temperatures with the wild-type transformed cells, but it is greatly reduced at 40°C with the *A239*-transformed cells.

As shown above, many of the parameters of cell growth associated with transformation are temperature sensitive in CHL and mouse brain cells transformed by temperature-sensitive *A* mutants of SV40. Similar results have been obtained by others with Syrian hamster cells (Tegtmeyer, 1975; Brugge and Butel, 1975), human cells (Brugge and Butel, 1975), rat embryo cells (Osborn and Weber, 1975), and a contact-inhibited rat cell line (Kimura and Itagaki, 1975). Indeed, with the exceptions of the readily understood discrepancy in T-antigen expression and questionable inclusion of hexose transport as a criterion of transformation, all of the phenotypes discussed in this section are temperature sensitive in *A* mutant transformants of the cell types indicated. However, somewhat conflicting data have been obtained with mouse 3T3 lines and rabbit kidney cells (Tegtmeyer, 1972; Tegtmeyer, 1975; Brugge and Butel, 1975), which suggests that host functions may also be important in the maintenance of transformation or, more likely, that some hosts are capable of suppressing the *A* mutant phenotype. One criterion of transformation, cell morphology, appears to yield the most conflicting data with regard to temperature sensitivity. In fact, Kimura and Dulbecco (1973) first argued that *A* function was not required for the maintenance of transformation in rat cells because they observed no morphologic differences at 33° and 40°C. Similarly, Tegtmeyer (1972, 1975) has observed no morphologic changes at the two temperatures, whereas Brugge and Butel (1975) and Osborn and Weber (1975) have. We find morphologic criteria to be of little assistance. Despite these discrepancies we conclude that SV40 *A* function is required for the maintenance of transformation.

A MECHANISM FOR SV40 TRANSFORMATION

Since it has been demonstrated (Tegtmeyer, 1972; Chou et al., 1974) that the *A* function is required for the initiation of viral DNA replication, and since it appears that the *A* function is required for the maintenance of many if not all of the phenotypic manifestations of transformation, it has been generally proposed that transformation by SV40 is a consequence of aberrant DNA synthesis (Brockman et al., 1974; Martin and Chou, 1975; Brugge and Butel, 1975; Tegtmeyer, 1975; Osborn and Weber, 1975). A detailed model has been proposed (Martin et al., 1974), which suggests that SV40 acts by providing a new initiator protein, the *A* gene product (Tegtmeyer, 1972), which is presumably identical to the T-antigen (Tegtmeyer, 1974). This initiator protein might then drive host DNA replication either (1) by recognizing only the replicator site of the integrated SV40 (in which case some mechanism for cascading host DNA synthesis from one to many sites would be required) or (2) by recognizing host nucleotide sequences, which, fortuitously, are identical to the replicator site of SV40 (for terminology see Jacob et al., 1963). The phenotypic properties of transformed cells are considered to be the properties of any "normal" cell unable to enter a resting phase. Different degrees of transformation would be explained by position effects on the expression of the SV40 genome, e.g., when SV40 was integrated in regions of the chromosome that were normally "turned off," the cells would be minimally transformed, whereas SV40 integrated in regions of the chromosome expressed constitutively would be fully transformed because the *A* gene product would constantly drive the host to enter *S* phase (DNA synthesis).

DEATH AS A MANIFESTATION OF TRANSFORMATION

Animal Cells

One of the predictions of such a model is that cells fully transformed by SV40 should not be capable of entering a resting stage [variously referred to as G_0 or R (Pardee, 1974)]. This prediction is consistent with earlier results (Oey et al., 1974; Pardee, 1974). What then might be the effect of amino acid or serum deprivation on such cells? Obviously, such cells might stop growth at whatever point in the growth cycle the deprivation became manifest. If, however, deprivation at other than G_0 or R of *any* cell were a lethal event, transformed cells should die at very high cell densities and normal or transformed cells should die when nutrient became limiting by "shift down" to depleted medium (provided the normal cells were not able to return to G_0). The death of transformed cells by nutrient depletion or after achieving high cell density has been noted previously (Studzinski and Gierthy, 1973; Paul, 1973) and is illustrated for CHL cells in Fig. 3.

Bacterial Analogies

This observation led us to examine the possibility that the inhibition of nascent DNA strand elongation is a lethal event. Although we have not yet examined this hypothesis in animal cells, we have studied the effect of sudden cessation of DNA synthesis in bacteria. Our study was facilitated by the availability of temperature-sensitive mutants of DNA synthesis in *Escherichia coli* (Wechsler and Gross, 1971). Figure 4 shows that in rich medium (LB broth) *dnaE, dnaF,* and *lig* mutants rapidly die upon shifting the cells from 33 to 43°C. Similar results are obtained with *dnaB, dnaC,* and *dnaG* mutants. All of these mutants are blocked (directly or indirectly) in the elongation of nascent DNA chains (Wechsler and Gross, 1971). The *dnaA* mutants, which are capable of finishing a round of replication because they are blocked in the initiation but not elongation of DNA strands (Wechsler and Gross, 1971), are considerably less prone to die at 43°C. This same result can be seen more dramatically when minimal medium is employed (Fig. 5). Not shown in Fig. 5 is the fact that when mutants blocked in elongation—*dnaB, dnaE, dnaF, dnaG* or *lig*—are first starved for amino acids for 90 min prior to shifting the cultures to 43°C, the cells become immune and do not die (i.e., they behave like *dnaA* in Fig. 5).

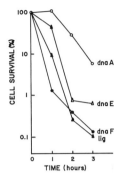

FIG. 4. Survival in LB broth at 43°C of temperature-sensitive *E. coli* mutants defective in DNA synthesis. Logarithmically growing cultures in LB broth supplemented with 20 μg/ml thymine were shifted at zero time to 43°C, and aliquots were taken at the indicated times into LB broth in soft agar. Colony counts were made after growth on LB plates. The mutant stains are: N1554, dnaA508 *thr⁻ leu⁻ B⁻ thy⁻ lac⁻ str^R*; JG55, dnaE486, *thr⁻ leu⁻ thy⁻ B₁⁻ met⁻ str^r*; N1543, dnaF10i *thr⁻ leu⁻ B₁⁻ thy⁻ lac⁻ str^R* [Wechsler and Gross, 1971]; and N2677, lig7 *ilv⁻ his⁻* [Gottesman et al., 1973].

These results are, of course, very similar to the classic observations of Maaløe and Hanawalt (1961) on thymineless death (Cohen and Barner, 1951). Namely, logarithmically growing cells suddenly deprived of thymine die. Amino acid starvation allows such cells to complete a round of DNA synthesis, but not to reinitiate, and renders the cells immune to thymineless death. One of many proposals to explain why thymine deprivation leads to cell death is that thymine deprivation leads to irreparable fragmentation of the DNA (Mennigmann and Szybalski, 1962; Freifelder, 1969). The creation of single-strand breaks might be a normal part of DNA replication and explain the greater susceptibility of growing cells to thymineless death (Nakayama and Hanawalt, 1975). The accumulation of irreparable single-strand breaks could also be the explanation for the death of *dnaB, dnaE, dnaF, dnaG,* and *lig* mutants at 43°C, since all of these genes are probably necessary for repair as well as for replication. It is a curious, but not necessarily

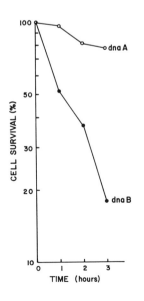

FIG. 5. Survival in minimal medium at 43°C of temperature-sensitive *E. coli* mutants defective in DNA synthesis. Logarithmically growing cultures in minimal medium M56 supplemented with 0.2% gluose, 20 μg/ml thymine, 0.01% methionine, 0.01% histidine, 0.01% isoleucine, 0.01% valine, 0.01% threonine, 0.01% leucine, and 10⁻⁴% B₁ were shifted to 43°C, and aliquots were taken and plated at various times as in Fig. 4. The strains are N1554 and T473, dnaB279, *thr⁻ leu⁻ B₁⁻ endI⁻*.

related fact, that the DNA of transformed CHL cells is more highly fragmented than that of normal cells (Avila and Martin, unpub.).

SUMMARY

Many of the properties of SV40-induced transformants, including the death of transformed cells at high density, can be accounted for by the following postulates:

1. An integrated SV40 genome directly induces the initiation of aberrant host DNA synthesis as a consequence of its production of the A gene product (presumably the T-antigen). The level of A gene expression determines the extent of transformation (see Martin et al., 1974, for further details).

2. Normal cells deprived of serum factors enter a resting stage (G_o or R), whereas because of (1) above, SV40-transformed cells cannot.

3. Cells engaged in DNA synthesis are highly susceptible to nutrient deprivation and die when deprived of serum factors.

REFERENCES

Arndt-Jovin, D. J., and Berg, P. (1971): Quantitative binding of ^{125}I-Concanavalin A to normal and transformed cells. *J. Virol.*, 8:716–721.

Black, P. H. (1966): Transformation of mouse cell line 3T3 by SV40: Dose response relationship and correlation with SV40 tumor antigen production. *Virology*, 28:760–763.

Black, P. H., Rowe, W. P., Turner, H. C., and Huebner, R. J. (1963): A specific complementation fixing antigen present in SV40 tumor and transformed cells. *Proc. Natl. Acad. Sci. USA*, 50:1148–1156.

Bose, S., and Zlotnick, B. (1973): Growth- and density-dependent inhibition of deoxyglucose transport in Balb 3T3 cells and its absence in cells transformed by murine sarcoma virus. *Proc. Natl. Acad. Sci. USA*, 70:2374–2378.

Brockman, W. W., Lee. T. N. H., and Nathans, D. (1974): Characterization of cloned evolutionary variants of simian virus 40. *Cold Spr. Harb. Symp. Quant. Biol.*, 39:119–127.

Brockman, W. W., and Scott, W. A. (1975): Biological activities of cloned evolutionary variants of simian virus 40. *Fed. Proc.*, 34:526.

Brugge, J. S., and Butel, J. S. (1975): Role of Simian virus 40 gene A function in maintenance of transformation. *J. Virol.*, 15:619–635.

Burger, M. M. (1969): A difference in the architecture of the surface membrane of normal and virally transformed cells. *Proc. Natl. Acad. Sci. USA*, 62:994–1001.

Chou, J. Y., Avila, J., and Martin, R. G. (1974): Viral DNA synthesis in temperature-sensitive mutants of simian virus 40. *J. Virol.*, 14:116–124.

Chou, J. Y., and Martin, R. G. (1974): Complementation analysis of simian virus 40 mutants. *J. Virol.*, 13:1101–1109.

Cohen, S. S., and Barner, H. D. (1954): Studies on unbalanced growth in *E. coli. Proc. Natl. Acad. Sci. USA*, 40:885–893.

Crawford, L. V., and Black, P. H. (1964): The nucleic acid of simian virus 40. *Virology*, 24:388–392.

Danna, K. J., Sack, Jr., G. H., and Nathans, D. (1973): A cleavage map of the SV40 genome. *J. Mol. Biol.*, 78:363–376.

Del Villano, B. C., and Defendi, V. (1973): Characterization of the SV40 T-antigen. *Virology*, 51:34–46.

Dulbecco, R. (1970): Topoinhibition and serum requirement of transformed and untransformed cells. *Nature*, 227:802–806.

Dulbecco, R., and Elkington, J. (1973): Conditions limiting multiplication of fibroblastic and epithelial cells in dense cultures. *Nature*, 246:197–199.

Fareed, G. C., Garon, C. F., and Salzman, N. P. (1972): Origin and direction of SV40 DNA replication. *J. Virol.*, 10:484–491.

Freedman, V. H., and Shin, S. (1974): Cellular tumorigenicity in *nude* mice: Correlation with cell growth in semi-solid medium. *Cell*, 3:355–359.

Freifelder, D. (1969). Single-strand breaks in bacterial DNA associated with thymine starvation. *J. Mol. Biol.*, 45:1–7.

Gottesman, M. M., Hicks, M. L., and Gellert, M. (1973): Genetics and function of DNA ligase in *Escherichia coli*. *J. Mol. Biol.*, 77:531–547.

Inbar, M. and Sachs, L. (1969): Structural difference in sites on the surface membrane of normal and transformed cells. *Nature*, 223:710–712.

Isselbacher, K. J. (1972): Increased uptake of amino acids and 2-deoxy D glucose by virus-transformed cells in culture. *Proc. Natl. Acad. Sci. USA*, 69:585–589.

Jacob, F., Brenner, S., and Cuzin, F. (1963): On the regulation of DNA replication in bacteria. *Cold Spr. Harb. Symp. Quant. Biol.*, 28:329–348.

Khoury, G., Byrne, J. C., Takemoto, K. K., and Martin, M. A. (1973): Patterns of simian virus 40 deoxyribonucleic acid transcription. II. In transformed cells. *J. Virol.*, 11:54–60.

Khoury, G., Martin, M. A., Lee, T. N. H., and Nathans, D. (1975): A transcriptional map of the SV40 genome in transformed cell lines. *Virology*, 63:263–272.

Kimura, G., and Dulbecco, R. (1973): A temperature sensitive mutant of simian virus 40 affecting transforming ability. *Virology*, 52:529–534.

Kimura, G., and Itagaki, A. (1975): Initiation and maintenance of cell transformation by simian virus 40: A viral genetic property. *Proc. Natl. Acad. Sci. USA*, 72:673–677.

Koprowski, H., Ponten, J. R., Jensen, F., Ravdin, R. G., Moorehead, P. S., and Saksela, E. (1962): Transformation of cultures of human tissue infected with simian virus SV40. *J. Cell. Comp. Physiol.*, 58:281–292.

Lai, C-J., and Nathans, D. (1974): Mapping temperature-sensitive mutants of simian virus 40: Rescue of mutants by fragments of viral DNA. *Virology*, 60:466–475.

Lai, C-J., and Nathans, D. (1975): A map of temperature-sensitive mutants of simian virus 40. *Virology*, 66:70–81.

Maaløe, O., and Hanawalt, P. C. (1961): Thymine deficiency and the normal DNA replication cycle. I. *J. Mol. Biol.*, 3:144–155.

Macpherson, I., and Montagnier, L. (1964): Agar suspension culture for the selective assay of cells transformed by polyoma virus. *Virology*, 23:291–294.

Marshak, M. I., Varshaver, N. B., and Shapiro, N. I. (1973): Mutagenic action of simian vacuolating virus 40 on mammalian cells *in vitro*. (Induction of mutagenic resistance to 8-azaguanine and 6-mercaptopurine.) *Genetika*, IX, 12:1–6.

Martin, R. G., and Chou, J. Y. (1975): Simian virus 40 functions required for the establishment and maintenance of malignant transformation. *J. Virol.*, 15:599–612.

Martin, R. G., Chou, J. Y., Avila, J., and Saral, R. (1974): The semiautonomous replicon: A molecular model for the oncogenicity of SV40. *Cold Spr. Harb. Symp. Quant. Biol.*, 39:17–24.

Martin, R. G., and Talal, N. (1968): Translation and polarity in the histidine operon. IV. Relation of polarity to map position in *hisC*. *J. Mol. Biol.*, 36:219–229.

Mennigmann, H. D., and Szybalski, W. (1962): Molecular mechanism of thymineless death. *Biochem. Biophys. Res. Commun.*, 9:398–404.

Nakayama, H., and Hanawalt, P. (1975): Sedimentation analysis of deoxyribonucleic acid from thymine-starved *Escherichia coli*. *J. Bacteriol.*, 121:537–547.

Oey, J., Vogel, A., and Pollack, R. (1974): Intracellular cyclic AMP concentration responds specifically to growth regulation by serum. *Proc. Natl. Acad. Sci. USA*, 71:694–698.

Osborn, M., and Weber, K. (1975): Simian virus 40 gene *A* function and maintenance of transformation. *J. Virol.*, 15:636–644.

Pardee, A. B. (1974): A restriction point for control of normal animal cell proliferation. *Proc. Natl. Acad. Sci. USA*, 71:1286–1290.

Paul, D. (1973): Quiescent SV40 virus transformed 3T3 cells in culture. *Biochem. Biophys. Res. Commun.*, 53:745–753.

Pollack, R., Wolman, S., and Vogel, A. (1970): Reversion of virus-transformed cell lines: Hyperploidy accompanies retention of viral genes. *Nature*, 238:938, 967–970.

Pope, J. H., and Rowe, W. P. (1964): Detection of specific antigen in SV40 transformed cells by immunofluorescence. *J. Exp. Med.*, 120:121–128.

Risser, R., and Pollack, R. (1974): A nonselective analysis of SV40 transformation of mouse 3T3 cells. *Virology*, 59:477–489.

Risser, R., Rifkin, D., and Pollack, R. (1974): The stable classes of transformed cells induced by SV40 infection of established 3T3 cells and primary rat embryonic cells. *Cold Spr. Harb. Symp. Quant. Biol.*, 39:317–324.

Romano, A. H., and Colby, C. (1973): SV40 virus transformation of mouse 3T3 cells does not specifically enhance sugar transport. *Science*, 176:1238–1240.

Sambrook, J., Westphal, H., Srinivasan, P. R., and Dulbecco, R. (1968): The integrated state of DNA in SV40 transformed cells. *Proc. Natl. Acad. Sci. USA*, 60:1288–1295.

Sambrook, J., Sharp, P. A., and Keller, W. (1972): Transcription of simian virus 40. I. Separation of the strands of SV40 DNA and hybridization of the separated strands to RNA extracted from lytically infected and transformed cells. *J. Mol. Biol.*, 70:57–71.

Scher, C. D., and Nelson-Rees, W. A. (1971): Direct isolation and characterization of "flat" SV40 transformed cells. *Nature [New Biol.]*, 233:263–265.

Shein, H. M., and Enders, J. F. (1962): Transformation induced by simian virus 40 in human renal cell cultures. I. Morphology and growth characteristics. *Proc. Natl. Acad. Sci. USA*, 48:1164–1172.

Smith, H., Scher, C., and Todaro, G. (1971): Induction of cell division in medium lacking serum growth factor by SV40. *Virology*, 44:359–370.

Stoker, M., O'Neill, C., Berryman, S., and Waxman, J. (1968): Anchorage and growth regulation in normal and virus-transformed cells. *Int. J. Cancer*, 3:683–693.

Studzinski, G. P., and Gierthy, J. F. (1973): Selective inhibition of the cell cycle of cultured human diploid fibroblasts by aminonucleoside of puromycin. *J. Cell. Physiol.*, 81:71–84.

Tai, H. T., Smith, C. A., Sharp, P. A., and Vinograd, J. (1972): Sequence heterogeneity in closed SV40 DNA. *J. Virol.*, 9:317–325.

Tegtmeyer, P. (1972): Simian virus 40 deoxyribonucleic acid synthesis: the viral replicon. *J. Virol.*, 10:591–598.

Tegtmeyer, P. (1974): Altered patterns of protein synthesis in infection by SV40 mutants. *Cold Spr. Harb. Symp. Quant. Biol.*, 39:9–15.

Tegtmeyer, P. (1975): Function of simian virus 40 gene *A* in transforming infection. *J. Virol.*, 15:613–618.

Temin, H. M., and Rubin, H. (1958): Characteristics of an assay for Rous Sarcoma virus and Rous Sarcoma cells in tissue culture. *Virology*, 6:669–688.

Todaro, G., Green, H., and Goldberg, B. (1964): Transformation of properties of an established cell line by SV40 and polyoma virus. *Proc. Natl. Acad. Sci. USA*, 51:66–73.

Treffers, H. P., Spinelli, V., and Belser, N. O. (1954): A factor (or mutator gene) influencing mutation rate in *Escherichia coli*. *Proc. Natl. Acad. Sci. USA*, 40:1064–1071.

Unkeless, J. C., Tobia, A., Ossowski, L., Quigley, J. P., Rifkin, D. B., and Reich, E. (1973): An enzymatic function associated with transformation of fibroblasts by oncogenic viruses. *J. Exp. Med.*, 137:85–111.

Wechsler, J. A., and Gross, J. D. (1971): *Escherichia coli* mutants temperature sensitive for DNA synthesis. *Molec. Gen. Genet.*, 113:273–284.

Whitfield, Jr., H. J., Martin, R. G., and Ames, B. N. (1966): Classification of aminotransferase (C gene) mutants in the histidine operon. *J. Mol. Biol.*, 21:335–355.

Biology of Radiation Carcinogenesis, edited by
J. M. Yuhas, R. W. Tennant, and J. D. Regan.
Raven Press, New York © 1976.

The Use of *In Vitro* Methods for the Study of X-Ray-Induced Transformation

Joosje C. Klein

Radiobiological Institute TNO, Lange Kleiweg 151, RIJSWIJK (ZH), The Netherlands

At present, only a few investigators use *in vitro* methods to study X-ray-induced transformation. This is unfortunate, because cell culture systems can be used to investigate malignant transformation directly at the cellular level with the exclusion of the interfering factors operating in whole animals.

With these *in vitro* methods, it is possible to establish dose-response relationships for malignant transformations induced by single and split doses of X-rays and also for other types of radiation. This offers the possibility of obtaining better insight into the potentially carcinogenic effect of very low doses of radiation.

Another important advantage of *in vitro* systems is that chemical and viral carcinogens can be introduced and investigated in the same system. This makes these systems suitable for the exploration of the fundamental mechanism of carcinogenesis.

But, in spite of these many advantages, *in vitro* systems also have disadvantages. One drawback becomes very clear if one tries to summarize the experiments in this field. All investigators use the best system, their own. Everyone uses his own recipe and knows how to handle it and what it is worth. This adds a lot of flavor to the overall cooking, but makes it difficult to compare the dishes.

Despite this variety, the data as a whole point in the same direction. Radiation induces malignant transformation in cells *in vitro*. The expression of malignancy depends not only on the radiation and radiation dose, but also the condition of the culture and last but not least, on the cells that are irradiated.

For the correct interpretation of the results of an experiment, it is of prime importance to be sure that a malignant transformation is induced by the irradiation. This implies: first, the target cell must be at least nonmalignant; second, the malignant potency of a cell or a group of cells after the treatment has been demonstrated; and third, other factors that could influence the transformation process are excluded or known.

Target cells

The most suitable culture technique for transformation experiments is the monolayer culture. Detailed information on the difficulties and possibilities of this culture technique is presented in the proceedings of a symposium held in the National Cancer Institute in December 1973 under the title "New Horizons for Tissue culture in Cancer Research" (1974).

Investigators of radiation carcinogenesis *in vitro* have made use of the following target cells (Klein, 1975). Borek and Sachs (1966, 1967, 1968) and Borek and Hall (1974) used primary and secondary, and DiPaolo et al. (1971) secondary and tertiary cell cultures of minced whole hamster embryo as target cells. Established cell strains with a high passage number were employed by Stoker, namely the BHK21 line of hamster fibroblasts (1963, 1964), whereas we have used cloned mouse spleen sublines (1966, 1969, 1974). The BALB 3T3 line was used by Pollock (1968), and a C3H mouse embryo-derived cell line (10T½ clone 8) by Terzaghi and Little (1975). Stoker (1963, 1964) added polyoma virus to his irradiated cultures; Di Paolo et al. (1971) added benz(α)pyrene (BP).

Malignancy tests

These tests can be performed either *in vivo* or *in vitro*. The *in vivo* test is mainly qualitative and best approximates the clinical situation. A culture is defined as malignant if 10^6 or more cells injected subcutaneously into an isologous host give rise within six months to a progressive infiltrative growth that ultimately kills the host. The number of cells that can give rise to a tumor and the length of the latent period give some quantitative information. Disadvantages of the *in vivo* test are (a) the cells must be derived from inbred strains; (b) testing in immunologically depressed animals, such as nude mice or irradiated or ALS-treated animals, or at protected sites, such as the hamster pouch can lead to false-negative and sometimes even to false-positive tests. Further drawbacks are that the test conditions must be arbitrarily chosen; they are time-consuming, and hardly quantitative.

The *in vitro* malignancy test introduced by Sachs and Medina (1961) and Vogt and Dulbecco (1969) and employed by Borek (1966–1968, 1973, 1974 uses the cloning technique in which transformed piled-up colonies can be distinguished from nonmalignant colonies and scored. It provides quantitative information at the cellular level. The technique itself is laborious and takes some weeks. The scoring is not difficult. Malignantly transformed fibroblasts form clearly piled-up colonies, provided they have enough time to develop. Transformed epithelial cell colonies also show multilayer formation, but no crisscrossing; the overlaying cells mostly form relatively dark clusters known as domes. This *in vitro* technique is now widely accepted. But, the malignancy of the cells in colonies of a particular system should be confirmed qualitatively at least once with the *in vivo* test.

A number of other *in vitro* tests are said to be specific for the detection of malignant cells. Some of these are growth in agar, in suspension culture, or in medium with a low serum content, and others include agglutinability by low concentrations of plant lectins (Sanford, 1974). In my opinion, these tests are not conclusive, but they are indicative of malignancy, especially if a number of such tests are positive for a particular cell population. The reason I am suspicious of such tests is that unsuspected normal cells can express the same capacities in these tests; for instance, freshly drawn normal bone marrow cells grow well in agar and stimulated lymphocytes proliferate in suspension culture.

For an accurate score, the colonies should be allowed time enough to develop fully. The reason for stressing this point is twofold. Firstly, working with Borek's system, we found rather large variations in transformation rates, probably due to a too short culture time after seeding of the cells for the cloning experiment. To determine the optimal time for fixation, parallel cultures should be fixed after different culture periods. The same method is used to establish survival curves after irradiation. Here, parallel colonies that are fixed on successive days show an initial increase in the number of colonies with 50 cells or more. This is followed by a plateau, during which the number is constant. After approximately 4 more days, there is again an increase in the number of colonies grown from cells derived from the already present colonies. I should expect that radiation-induced transformed colonies would show the same pattern. The second reason for stressing the importance of the culture period is the finding of Mondal and Heidelberger (1970), who investigated malignant transformation in single cells of a cell line derived from C3H mouse ventral prostate following methylcholanthrene (MC) treatment. In the progeny of these treated cells, malignant conversion occurred at quite varied ages in culture; the average number of days for transformation to take place was approximately 60 and the transformation was from 33 to 100%, depending on the treatment. My own experiment with chemical carcinogens (MC and urethane) agreed with Mondal and Heidelberger's findings (1969). Whether radiation-induced transformants show the same late effect has not been investigated.

Exclusion of Carcinogenic Factors

Attention to the equipment used as well as to the constituents of the medium is important. Samples of the serum should be tested on control cultures. The cells should be kept in the exponential growth phase and tested for virus or indications of the presence of virus (Todaro and Green, 1963; Klein, 1966, 1969).

Evaluation Methods

In reviewing (Klein, 1975) the target cells used in the *in vitro* radiation induced transformation experiments, it is clear that a number of the target cells and some of the culture conditions do not satisfy the standard conditions of the experiment.

The first objection concerns those experiments in which oncogenic chemicals and viruses (SV40 or BP) are introduced. The cells in such experiments, in fact, received a combined treatment. Radiation could have had an enhancing effect in this situation.

A second objection concerns the answer to a question: Can cells of established cell lines qualify as nonmalignant, normal cells? The test system for malignancy of cells *in vitro* determines whether a cell is malignant. Can nonmalignant cells also qualify as normal? Reasoning along the same lines as we do for malignant cells, all cells are judged as normal as they exist *in vivo*. In a recent article, Finckh (1974) presented a good description of the various cell types and transitional forms that occur *in vivo*. There are cells under normal (undisturbed) conditions, but there are also cells under less "normal" conditions. The animal may have had an infection, hyperplasia, metaplasia, and even dysplasia. Many of these conditions are thought to be reversible. The animal may have even been confronted with carcinogenic agents. In comparing the effect of radiation *in vitro* and *in vivo,* it seems worthwhile to keep in mind that not all cells exist under an "undisturbed" condition *in vivo*.

In a way, cell lines present the same picture. For example, in our radiation experiments, we found (Klein, 1974) that some of the sublines could be malignantly transformed and others could not. This is one of the reasons to conclude that there exists a series of cells between completely nonmalignant and highly malignant. The other reason is that the culture technique used can influence the place of the culture in this series. To maintain a culture in a nonmalignant condition, the cells should be kept in the exponential growth phase. Cell overcrowding and conditions in the stationary phase tend to lead to malignancy; low inocula and slow growth favor nonmalignancy. It is possible that the same transitional forms are present in the living animal. In practice, this would imply that there are cells *in vivo* that are more at risk and more easily transformed than are other cells, as is the case with the various target cells used in the *in vitro* experiments.

In discussing the use of *in vitro* methods for radiation carcinogenesis, it is tempting to also say something about the results of the experiments. Perhaps, it is worthwhile to mention some of the general findings (Klein, 1975). Borek (1966) has mentioned that a crucial factor in the process of neoplastic transformation by ionizing radiation is that the cells must undergo one or probably two divisions shortly after radiation, so that the transforming event will become a hereditary property of the cell. The same factor is found in the other test systems used in this area. This implies that, whatever test system is used for radiation carcinogenesis, the target cells must be allowed to divide shortly after treatment (Terzaghi and Little, 1975). The implications for the clinical situation are also obvious; for example, the effectiveness of very low doses of radiation *in vivo* and the risk involved could be less than expected, because there is hardly any cell loss and therefore no compensating cell divisions can be expected. On the other hand, actively growing tissues are probably more at risk, especially if damaged cells and cell debris are present.

Another striking observation is the sharp drop in transformation incidence after a maximum of around 250 and sometimes up to 500 rad of X-rays. In this respect, there is a striking discrepancy as compared with the *in vivo* situation (Van Putten, 1973). Borek (1972) suggests that this *in vitro* drop is due to reproductive death caused by the extra damage produced by the additional "hits" received at doses higher than 400 rad. Perhaps this is part of the explanation, but it is still an unexpected finding, because most transformations *in vivo* occur after doses much higher than 500 rad.

Also the point can be made that by no means can all cells be transformed by irradiation. Such negative results often are not reported.

A last remark concerning my own radiation experiments. I use sublines of a cloned mouse spleen cell line as target cells. The cells are hypotetraploid, have a passage number higher than 57, and are cultured as a monolayer culture in the exponential growth phase with a passage time of 1 week (Klein, 1966). In the first experiment, four cell lines were started from a cell pool; cells of three lines were irradiated with 100, 200, or 300 rad (X-rays) on every second day of the weekly passage up to a total accumulated dosage of 16,800 rad. Cells of these groups were regularly tested by the *in vivo* malignancy test. Cloning experiments were also performed. All these tests were negative; no signs of malignant transformation were found. The experiments of Borek and Sachs (1966) at that time indicated that their target cells (embryonic cells) were only sensitive for radiation carcinogenesis in the first two passages. The cells from the high passage number we used should have lost this capacity. Because of the differences between early and higher passages, for example, in plating efficiency (about 1 and 80%, respectively), we tried to reproduce the conditions used by Borek for cells of a number of our cell lines (Klein, 1974). What we did was to irradiate cells at a concentration of 10^6 cells/ml with a single dose of 300 rad of X-rays. According to the survival curve, this dose kills about 80% of the cells. Subsequently, the irradiated cell suspension was centrifuged, and 10^6 or 10^7 of the cells, based on the preirradiation counts, were subcutaneously injected in 0.1 ml of medium into the test animals for *in vivo* malignancy testing. Malignancy tests with cells of two out of three sublines were positive. Because transformation was indeed found in irradiated cultures under these conditions, the experiments were extended, and an extra control was introduced, based on the fact that high cell density (10^6 cells/ml) along with many (about 80%) damaged cells and much cell debris might influence the transformation process. To this end, 80% (the same amount killed by the irradiation with 300 rads of X-rays) of the cell suspension was removed, and the cells contained were killed by freezing and thawing 10 times. Subsequently, the untreated 20% of the suspension containing living cells was mixed with the treated cell suspension and centrifuged. Based on the pretreatment counts, 10^6 or 10^7 cells were injected subcutaneously into the test animals for *in vivo* malignancy testing. The result was that the sublines that could be transformed by the irradiation could also be transformed by killing part of the cell population, lines that could not be transformed by irradiation also gave negative tests after freezing and thawing. In conclusion, under these specific experimental conditions, the malignant transformation of established cell strains could be induced, and this was shown to be due to a combination of crowding and cell killing but not to any specific effect of the radiation (Klein, 1974). An extensive search for carcinogenic mouse viruses that might have been involved gave totally negative results. It also became clear that not all strains are susceptible to malignant transformation either by irradiation or by killing part of the cell population in another way. This seems to imply that material from damaged normal cells is involved in malignant transformation; in other words, that normal cells contain all the genetic information required for a malignant transformation (Klein, 1974). Experiments to determine the trigger in this system are underway.

CONCLUSION

In conclusion, *in vitro* methods for the investigation of radiation carcinogenesis are very useful, but they have pitfalls. The biggest pitfall is that many cells cannot be transformed by irradiation.

REFERENCES

Borek, C. (1972): Neoplastic transformation *in vitro* of a clone of adult live epithelial cells into differentiated hepatoma-like cells under conditions of nutritional stress. *Proc. Natl. Acad. Sci. USA,* 69:956–959.

Borek, C., and Hall, E. J. (1973): Transformation of mammalian cells *in vitro* by low doses of X-rays. *Nature,* 243:450–453.

Borek, C., and Hall, E. J. (1974): Effect of split doses of X rays on neoplastic transformation of single cells. *Nature,* 252:499–501.

Borek, C., and Sachs, L. (1966): *In vitro* cell transformation by X-irradiation. *Nature,* 210:276–278.

Borek, C., and Sachs, L. (1967): Cell susceptibility to transformation by X-irradiation and fixation of the transformed state. *Proc. Natl. Acad. Sci. USA,* 57:1522–1527.

Borek, C., and Sachs, L. (1968): The number of cell generations required to fix the transformed state in X-ray-induced transformation. *Proc. Natl. Acad. Sci. USA,* 59:83–85.

DiPaolo, J. A., Donovan, P. J., and Nelson, R. L. (1971): X-irradiation enhancement of transformation by Benzo(α)Pyrene in hamster embryo cells. *Proc. Natl. Acad. Sci. USA,* 68:1734–1737.

Finckh, E. S. (1974): The genesis of tumours–Mutation or abnormal differentiation? *Med. J. Aust.,* 1:438–441.

Klein, J. C. (1966): Absence of malignant transformation after weekly irradiation of a mouse spleen in culture. *J. Natl. Cancer Inst.,* 37:655–661.

Klein, J. C. (1969): An *in vitro* system for radiocarcinogenesis. In: *Proceedings Series 118/18,* International Atomic Energy Agency, pp. 57–66.

Klein, J. C. (1974): Evidence against a direct carcinogenic effect of X-rays *in vitro*. *J. Natl. Cancer Inst.*, 52:1111–1115.

Klein, J. C. (1975): Ionizing radiation experimental; radiation carcinogenesis *in vitro*. (*Proceedings XI International Cancer Congress, Florence 1974.*) *Excerpta Medica. Int. Congr. Ser. 351* (3):125–130.

Mondal, S., and Heidelberger, Ch. (1970): *In vitro* malignant transformation by methylcholanthrene of the progeny of single cells derived from C3H mouse prostate. *Proc. Natl. Acad. Sci. USA,* 65:219–225.

New Horizons for Tissue Culture in Cancer Research (1974): In: Proc. Symp. at Mazur Auditorium, Natl. Cancer Inst., NIH, Bethesda, Maryland, December 3 and 4, 1973. *J. Natl. Cancer Inst.*, 53:1427–1519.

Pollock, E. J., and Todaro, G. J. (1968): Radiation enhancement of SV 40 transformation in 3T3 and human cells. *Nature,* 219:520–521.

Sachs, L., and Medina, D. (1961): *In vitro* transformation of normal cells by polyoma virus. *Nature,* 189:457–458.

Sanford, K. K. (1974): Biologic manifestations of oncogenesis *in vitro:* A critique. *J. Natl. Cancer Inst.*, 53:1481–1485.

Stoker, M. (1963): Effect of X-irradiation on susceptibility of cells to transformation by polyoma virus. *Nature,* 200:756–758.

Stoker, M. (1964): Further studies on radiation-induced sensitivity of hamster cells to transformation by polyoma virus. *Virology,* 24:123–125.

Terzaghi, M., and Little, J. B. (1975): Repair of potentially lethal radiation damage in mammalian cells is associated with enhancement of malignant transformation. *Nature,* 253:548–549.

Todaro, G. J., and Green, H. (1963): Quantitative studies of the growth of mouse embryo cells in culture and their development into established lines. *J. Cell Biol.,* 17:299–313.

Van Putten, L. M. (1973): Het risico van het ontstaan van tumoren na kleine stralingsdoses. *Atoomenergie en haar toepassingen,* 15(7–8):176–182.

Vogt, M., and Dulbecco, R. (1969): Virus-cell interaction with a tumor-producing virus. *Proc. Natl. Acad. Sci. USA,* 46:365–370.

Biology of Radiation Carcinogenesis, edited by
J. M. Yuhas, R. W. Tennant, and J. D. Regan.
Raven Press, New York © 1976.

In Vitro Cell Transformation by Low Doses of X-Irradiation and Neutrons

Carmia Borek

Radiological Research Laboratories, Columbia University, New York 10032

One of the basic questions in radiation carcinogenesis has been whether ionizing radiation produces neoplasms directly by inducing heritable changes in a single cell or indirectly by activating a virus (Kaplan, 1949) or changing homeostatic mechanisms (Furth and Lorenz, 1954). The complexity of *in vivo* systems and the inordinate number of animals required for whole-body studies greatly hinder investigators who are trying to elucidate the mechanism(s) of radiation carcinogenesis. Our approach has been to use an *in vitro* system, in which cells are irradiated either in mass cultures or as cloned single cells (Ham and Puck, 1952). These cells are maintained *in vitro* under defined conditions before and after treatment and therefore are not subject to homeostatic mechanisms that could modify their behavior.

In the work described here, we set out to study whether X-rays could directly induce a hereditary conversion of normal cells into neoplastic cells, a process referred to as transformation. Following the successful completion of this first stage, we attempted to characterize some of the conditions required for this transformation and to study the biologic properties of the cells. A logical extension of this work was to determine a dose-response relationship between absorbed dose and transformation and to investigate the ability of other types of ionizing radiation to produce this transformation.

IN VITRO CELL TRANSFORMATION BY X-IRRADIATION

We chose short-term cultures of midterm golden hamster embryos as the source of normal cells (Borek and Sachs, 1966a; Borek and Hall, 1973). Hamster cells have a very low rate of spontaneous transformation. The variety of cell types derived from an embryo supplied a diverse population of fast replicating diploid cells in various stages of differentiation as target cells for irradiation.

Methods

Primary cultures were established by progressive dissociation of the minced fresh tissue (Borek, 1972), and the cells were cultured and maintained in

Petri dishes in Dulbecco modified Eagle's medium (EM) fortified with 10% fetal calf serum. In experiments carried out with mass cultures, primary cultures were used unless otherwise noted. Cloned cultures were prepared directly from the original primary cell suspension on feeder layers or by dissociating primaries. When cloning, 10^3 to 10^4 cells were seeded, depending on the experiment. Feeder cells were used at a concentration of $3 \times 10^4/60$ mm dish of X-irradiated (4,000 rad) cells.

In earlier experiments (Borek and Sachs, 1966a, 1967, 1968), we used rat embryo cells as feeder cells, whereas in later ones (Borek and Hall, 1973, 1974) these were replaced by hamster embryo cells from the same pool of cells used in that experiment. Scoring and assay of transformed clones were carried out by fixing and staining 10- to 12-day-old clones with Giemsa (Borek and Sachs, 1966a). Clonal isolation was carried out using the reported methods (Ham and Puck, 1952). Transformed clones were distinguished morphologically by their piled up morphology and lack of contact inhibition (Abercrombie and Ambrose, 1962). In the transformation-study experiments, cells were irradiated at room temperature 24 hr after seeding primary cultures or after cloning. We used X-ray sources of 250 kVp and 56 kVp with a dose rate of 60 rad/min and 280 rad/min, respectively (Borek and Sachs, 1966, 1967, 1968) or 210 kVp (Borek and Hall, 1973, 1974) with a dose rate of 70.6 rad/min for doses of 75 to 600 and 4.25 rad/min for the range of 1 to 10 rad.

Direct Transformation In Vitro of Mass Cultures and of Cloned Cultures

One-day-old semiconfluent primary cultures were irradiated with a dose of 300 rad and continuously subcultured at low density. Within 40 to 60 days, controls were in a state of degeneration, although in several of the experimental plates, there began to appear foci of fusiform cells growing randomly on a background of flat cells (Borek and Sachs, 1966a). Within 20 days, these cells invaded the culture, showing a piled up random pattern of growth, loss of contact inhibition, increased acid production in the medium, resistance to benzpyrene toxicity, a lower serum requirement for growth; and upon injection into 2- to 6-week-old hamsters, they gave rise to fibrosarcomas. In this way, several transformed cell lines were established.

A quantitative assay of the rate of transformation in mass cultures was carried out by cloning the irradiated cells onto feeder layers and scoring for colonies that had a piled up morphology and random cell orientation; these morphologic features were similar to those observed in the mass cultures and quite different from the controls. Representative clones of both normal and transformed cells are shown in Fig. 1. The total number of colonies and the number of transformed colonies were obtained by direct count. The percent of transformed colonies was determined as percent of total colonies. In this way, it was established that when semiconfluent primary cultures were ir-

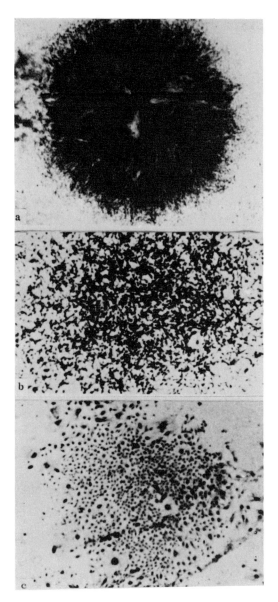

FIG. 1. a: A 10-day-old clone of hamster embryo cells transformed by 300 rad of X-rays. Note the piled up multilayer pattern of growth. Giemsa ×13. b: A ten-day-old clone of hamster embryo cells transformed by 300 rad of X-rays. Note the random crisscross orientation of the cells. ×13. c: A 10-day-old clone of normal hamster embryo cells, in control cultures. Note the flat "contact inhibited" pattern of growth. ×13.

radiated with 300 rad about 1 to 1.5% of the cells transformed. The same frequency of transformation was observed when confluent stationary cultures were irradiated and cloned 0 to 2 hr after radiation and when single cells were cloned directly from the dissociated fresh mince, irradiated as single cells with 300 rad, and allowed to grow into clones. Transformation was not observed in the controls, could not be induced by incubating normal cultures with sonicated irradiated cells, and occurred whether or not there had been a change of medium before and after irradiation. No transformation was observed in stationary cultures, which were cloned 2 to 5 days after irradiation.

The fact that the percent transformation in mass cultures and in clones were similar, that no transformation was found in control cultures, and that the percent transformation was too high to be considered a random event, strongly suggested that X-rays induced transformation *in vitro* by a direct action on the single cells. These experiments further suggested that in order to fix transformation as a hereditary event, the irradiated cells must replicate shortly after exposure to radiation. The hereditary susceptibility of the cells to transformation by radiation was indicated by the fact that cells irradiated from 1 to 9 days after they had been cloned showed the same percent of transformation following a total of 13 days incubation (Borek and Sachs, 1967).

Irradiation of cells cloned directly from the animal, as compared to cells cloned from subsequent passages as mass cultures, indicated that the percent transformation decreased with an increased number of passages (Borek and Sachs, 1967). This suggests that, within the diploid cell population in the mixed embryo cultures, only some cells are susceptible to radiation transformation and that passaging in culture selected against these cells.

Fixation of Transformation

As mentioned above, transformation was fixed and expressed when single cells were irradiated and grown into clones, when semiconfluent cultures were irradiated and allowed to replicate before cloning, or when confluent cultures were irradiated and cloned 0 to 2 hr after irradiation. We found no transformation in parallel confluent cultures, which were not dissociated immediately but incubated after irradiation for 3 to 5 days at 37°C and only then cloned, indicating that a loss of the transformed state had occurred (Borek and Sachs, 1966a, 1967) (Fig. 2).

In order to determine the time required for this loss of fixation, confluent cultures were irradiated and cloned at daily intervals after irradiation. We found that the incubation of stationary cultures at 37°C for more than 2 days following irradiation resulted in a loss of fixation of the transformed state. But, if the same cultures were incubated at 24°C for 5 days, loss of fixation was inhibited. This suggested that an error-correcting mechanism, which may be active before the cells are able to replicate, is inhibited at 24°C.

Recent data by Terzaghi and Little (1975) demonstrated that when con-

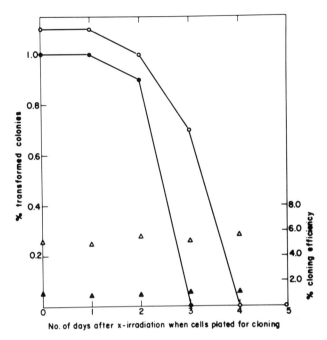

FIG. 2. Transformation in confluent cultures cloned at daily intervals after irradiation. Confluent primary cultures grown in EM with nonfetal calf serum were irradiated 3 or 4 days after seeding, and the cells cloned at daily intervals with fetal or nonfetal serum. Each point represents an average of at least three experiments: Percent transformed colonies (○, ●); percent cloning efficiency (△, ▲); cells cloned in fetal calf serum (○, △); cells cloned in nonfetal calf serum (●, ▲). (Borek and Sachs, 1967.)

fluent cells were irradiated and dissociated less than 24 hr after irradiation transformation was observed.

The number of cell replications required to fix the transformed state was determined by allowing the cells to undergo one to three divisions after irradiation before reaching stationary phase and then assaying for transformation (Borek and Sachs, 1968). The results indicate that an average of twice the population doubling time was required after irradiation. Since the cell population in the embryonic cultures is extremely diverse, this would allow one to two generations to take place depending on the cell type.

It therefore appears that similar to transformation by SV40 (Todaro and Green, 1966) there is a requirement for DNA synthesis for fixation of X-ray-induced transformation. Cellular DNA must replicate after irradiation to form a strand which codes for transformation and that the transformed state is fixed in cells containing this new type of DNA.

Dose-Response Curve

A comprehensive study of the carcinogenic action of radiation must include a knowledge at a cellular level of the relationship between absorbed dose and the probability of neoplastic conversion. One of the principal assets of the *in vitro* system is that a very low frequency of transformation can be detected by irradiating large numbers of isolated single cells and scoring thousands of clones. This is in contrast to the *in vivo* situation, in which inordinately large numbers of animals would be required. Using the system of cloned cells described previously in which primary cultures were dissociated and cloned on feeder cells (Borek and Sachs, 1966a) we designed experiments to elucidate the dose-response relationship for transformation over a range of doses from 600 rad down to 1 rad (Borek and Hall, 1973).

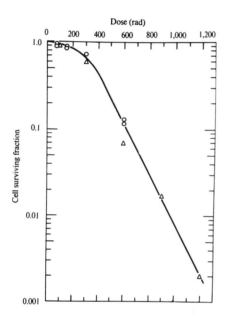

FIG. 3. Survival of reproductive integrity of hamster embryo cells as a function of X-ray dose. Points calculated from the transformation experiments are shown (○) (Borek and Hall, 1966); also points established from a separate cell survival experiment (△) (see text); the extrapolation number ($N = 6$) is defined as the point in the surviving curve extrapolates; the dose required to reduce the population to a fraction of 37% ($D_o = 147$ rad) is used as a measure of the slope in the linear portion of the survival curve. (Borek and Hall, 1973.)

After a postirradiation period of 9 to 11 days, the clones were fixed and stained and scored for transformation as in our earlier experiments. In several experiments, transformed clones were isolated and grown into mass cultures. The ability of the cells to form colonies in semisolid agar (Sanders and Burford, 1964), their agglutinability by 50 μg/ml Concanavalin A and wheat germ agglutinins (Borek et al., 1973), and their tumorigenicity *in vivo* served as additional criteria to determine if the cells were transformed, as compared with control cultures.

The data for cell survival is seen in Fig. 3 and is characteristic for mammalian cells exposed to sparsely ionizing radiation. A broad initial shoulder at lower doses implies that X-rays are relatively inefficient in killing cells in this region, whereas, for larger doses, the survival curve becomes a straight line on a semilog plot; from these data, it can be implied that over this dose range cell survival is an exponential function of dose.

The data presented in Fig. 4 indicate that neoplastic transformation can be induced in single cells with doses of X-rays as low as 1 rad. At any of the doses used, the fraction of the cells killed is small, and this observation, along with the fact that no transformation was observed in the controls, strongly reaffirms our earlier view that transformation is induced directly by the ionizing radiation and is not a result of selection of spontaneously occurring transformed cells. The shape of the dose-response curve is not unlike the shapes reported by others (Bond et al., 1960; Upton, 1961) in the human and in the experimental animal. It consists of an ascending limb between 1 and 150 rad, in which a linear dependence of induction on dose cannot be ruled out, and a flat-topped maximum between 150 and 300 rad, similar to that reported in *in vivo* experiments (Upton, 1961), in which a change in dose by a factor of two does not alter the frequency of transformation. A

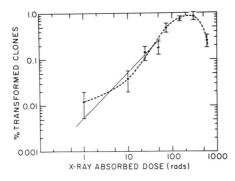

FIG. 4. Incidence of hamster embryo cell transformation following exposure *in vitro* to X-irradiation. For doses at which more than one experiment was performed, data were pooled; the mean value, together with the standard deviation, is plotted in the figure [see Borek and Hall (1974) for the results of individual experiments]. One curve is drawn by eye to the mean data points (– – –); the other has a slope of +1 and passes through the error bars of each datum point (—). (Borek and Hall, 1973.)

further increase in dose above 300 rad results in a marked decrease in transformation rate. Similar observations in humans and animals (Bond et al., 1960; Upton, 1961) have resulted in speculation that cell killing occurring in these multihit dose ranges is responsible for the sharp decline in the capacity to induce tumors.

Although our data do support the idea that above 300 rad cell reproductive death begins to be an important factor, they also suggest that there is a preferential killing of potentially transformed cells, since our system inherently accounts for cell killing, i.e., we score the transformed clones from among the survivors. If normal and potentially transformed cells were equally sensitive to radiation, then a decline in the proportion of transformed cells at higher doses would not be expected. The data support the ideas proposed by Gray (1965) in that they suggest that the potentially transformed cells never have a chance to form a colony because they die a reproductive death due to the cummulative damage produced by larger doses.

SPLIT-DOSE EXPERIMENTS

In addition to the observations described in the dose-response relationship for transformation, we have found a strong correlation between the proportion of cells killed and cells transformed in experiments designed to study the effect of dose fractionation (Borek and Hall, 1974).

A single dose of 50 rad was compared with two doses of 25 rad, and similarly, 75 rad was compared with two doses of 37.5 rad. The interval between the split doses was 5 hr, long enough to allow repair of sublethal radiation damage but short enough to minimize the probability of cell division between exposures.

The results, summarized in Fig. 5, indicate that there was a clear *increase* in the proportion of clones transformed for doses delivered in two fractions as compared with the same total dose given as a single exposure. Survival was slightly higher in cells treated with split doses. These results indicate that when a dose of radiation is delivered as two fractions fewer cells are injured

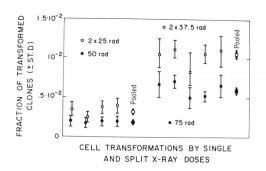

CELL TRANSFORMATIONS BY SINGLE
AND SPLIT X-RAY DOSES

FIG. 5. Incidence of cell transformation in cloned cultures of hamster embryo cells. Four replicate experiments were performed in which the effect of a single dose of 50 rad (●) was compared with that of two doses of 25 rad (○). The results of the individual experiments are shown, together with the pooled data; vertical bars are standard deviations. The consequence of a single dose of 75 rad (□) compared with two doses of 37.5 rad (□) are shown. (Borek and Hall, 1974.)

lethally, and consequently, more cells sustain sublethal damage. As transformation by radiation presumably involves sublethal events, it is not surprising that splitting the dose leads to less killing but enhanced transformation.

BIOLOGICAL PROPERTIES OF X-RAY TRANSFORMED CELLS

Characterization of the cells transformed by X-irradiation has been carried out on transformed cell lines derived by treating mass cultures with X-rays and on genetically homogeneous cultures grown for several generations from transformed clones. Within our range of studies, transformed lines derived in mass culture did not differ from the lines of cloned cultures. In contrast to the normal diploid cells of the controls with a limited life-span, in culture the transformed cells can be propagated indefinitely.

TABLE 1. *Some biologic properties of hamster embryo cells transformed in vitro by X-irradiation*

Property	Transformed cells	Control
Growth in culture	Multilayers	Monolayers
Serum requirement for growth	Low	High
Agglutination by low concentrations of some plant lectins	+	−
Colony formation in semi-solid agar	+ (varies)	−
Ion communication at intercellular permeable junctions	+ −	+
Surface structure as seen by scanning electron microscopy	Multiple surface features: blebs and microvilli, lack of contact inhibition	Smooth surfaces except in mitosis Smooth intercellular junction formation and contact inhibition
Karyotype using quinacrine fluorescence	Aneuploid No obvious chromosomal aberrations	Diploid
C-type virus particles	−	−
Tumorogenicity	+ (varies)	−
Heterogencity of surface properties in cells independently transformed by X-irradiation	+	−

Table 1 summarizes some of the various biologic characteristics we have studied.

The transformation of normal cells into neoplastic cells involves a change in the control of cell replication, which is manifested phenotypically by alterations in the cell surface and in social interactions among neighboring cells.

Karyotype

Chromosomal analysis was carried out shortly after transformation in five transformed cell lines grown from isolated clones, using the quinacrine fluorescence banding method (Miller et al., 1972). We found that within the limitations of this method no gross chromosomal aberrations were observed. The transformed cells were aneuploid with no apparent consistency from one cell to another.

CELL-TO-CELL INTERACTION AND SCANNING ELECTRON MICROSCOPY

In contrast to the normal control cells, which grow into monolayers, the X-ray transformed cells were able to multilayer in culture. Their general growth pattern, however, was less random than that found in some chemically and virally transformed cells (Borek and Sachs, 1966a).

Cells were examined with a scanning electron microscope (Borek and Fengolio, *in press*). The normal cells have relatively flat smooth surfaces, except during mitosis and demonstrate close, smooth cell-to-cell contacts at high

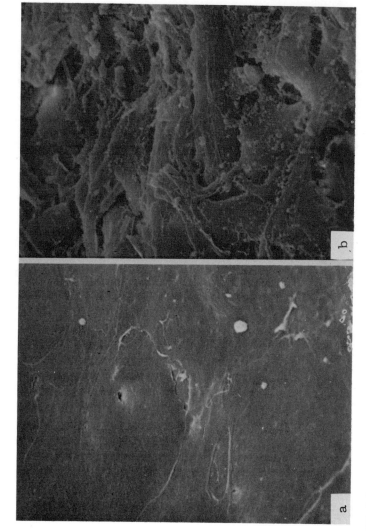

FIG. 6. Scanning electron microscopy of hamster embryo cells, cultured at high density. a: A population of control cells. Note the tight intercellular contacts, the flatness of the cells, and their smooth surfaces. b: A population of cells transformed by 300 rad of X-rays; they are tumorigenic. Note the extensive features on the surfaces of the cells and their ability to pile up in culture.

densities (Fig. 6). By contrast, the transformed cells at all times exhibited a variety of extensive surface features, including blebs and microvilli, which varied from one transformed cell line to another. Following transformation, the cells lost their flatness. They clearly pile up in a manner that suggests a lack of response to their social environment and possibly a loss of cell-to-cell recognition (Fig. 6).

Intercellular Communication Between Cells

Cytoplasmic communication, as monitored by the movement of small ions, exists between normal cells in culture and is lost in some epithelial tumors and epitheloid cells transformed *in vitro*. In the case of X-ray transformed cells, which were mainly fibroblasts (Borek et al., 1969) as in the case of a variety of cells transformed by viruses and chemicals (Borek et al., 1969), the slight differences seen between the normal and the transformed cells depended on the environment, and especially the serum content. These slight differences could not explain the loss of cell-to-cell recognition that occurs under a variety of conditions.

Change in Surface Structure

Change in the distribution of certain sugar-containing receptor sites on the cell membrane following neoplastic transformation can be detected by agglutination with plant lectins (Inbar and Sachs, 1969; Burger, 1969; Borek et al., 1973). Whereas the normal cells were not agglutinable by 50 μg/ml of Concanavalin A and wheat germ agglutinin, the X-ray transformed cells of all cell lines tested were.

Growth in Agar

The ability of cells of solid tissue to grow in suspension or in a semisolid medium, such as agar, is confined to tumor cells or cells that have been transformed *in vitro* and have lost "anchorage dependence" (Stoker, 1972).

In the case of the X-ray transformed cells we have found that although some cells did not acquire this ability to replicate in agar yet gave rise to tumors *in vivo* (Borek and Sachs, 1966a), other cell lines were able to form colonies (Borek and Hall, 1973).

Contact Inhibition and Cell Interaction Between Cells Independently Transformed by X-Irradiation

A series of experiments were undertaken to determine the contact relationship between normal cells and cells transformed by various carcinogens (Borek and Sachs, 1966b). In these experiments, the ability of cells of one cell type marked by India ink to replicate upon their own kind or upon cells of another line was used as a measure of cell recognition and loss of contact inhibition. We found that, in contrast to the lack of inhibition of replication between cells of different lines that were transformed by the same tumor virus, cells of lines independently transformed by X-rays inhibited one another, but they were still able to replicate each one upon themselves. These results suggest that following transformation by X-rays, newly acquired surface properties, possibly antigenicity, were specific for each transformed cell line.

TUMORIGENICITY

The ability of *in vitro* transformed cells to produce tumors *in vivo* varied among the cell lines studied. In all cases, tumors were fibrosarcomata. In some cases, transformed cells injected subcutaneously into 2- to 3-week-old hamsters gave rise to fibrosarcomas, which regressed after 3 to 4 weeks (Borek and Sachs, 1966a). These tumors were transplantable, and cells taken from them before regression and transplanted into adult hamsters either with or without further growth *in vitro* gave rise to fibrosarcomata.

When animals in which tumor growth had regressed were inoculated a second time with the same number of cells (2 to 6 × 10⁶) from the same transformed line, the second inoculation gave rise to smaller tumors, which regressed more rapidly. These results suggest that regression was partly or wholly due to an immune reaction as a result of the acquisition of a new antigen by the transformed cells. If however, the second inoculation was with *another* cell line independently transformed by X-rays, we observed in three separate instances an enhancement of tumor growth, with the tumors growing progressively until they killed the animal (Borek and Sachs, *unpublished*). Recently, we have induced tumors by inoculating cells from several transformed cell lines derived from clones that have given rise to progressively growing tumors (Borek and Hall, 1973) (Fig. 7).

VIRUSES

Using reported methods (Weinstein et al., 1972) we have found no C-type virus particles in cell lines transformed by X-rays. The presence of other virus cannot yet be excluded, in view of some types of leukemias that have been found to be associated with the presence of virus (Upton, 1961; Lieberman and Kaplan, 1959).

CELL TRANSFORMATION BY 430-keV NEUTRONS

In contrast to X-rays, neutrons are a densely ionizing radiation. X-ray photons interact with the orbital electrons of atoms of the absorbing material

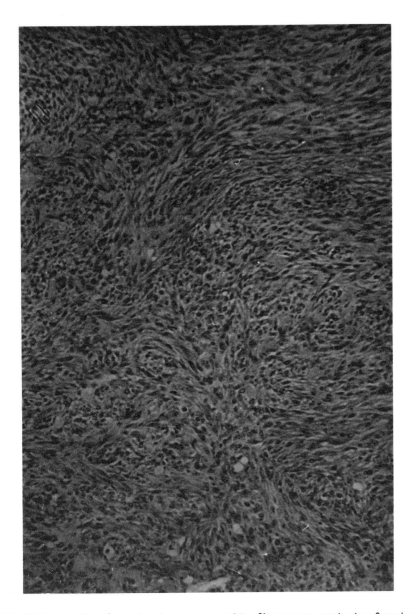

FIG. 7. Histologic section of a noninvasive, non-metastasizing fibrosarcoma growing in a 3-week-old-hamster 10 days after a subcutaneous injection of 10^6 transformed cells obtained as follows: A transformed clone, of the type illustrated in Figure 1(b), produced by X-irradiation of single cells, was isolated and grown through 30 passages before inoculation. Haemotoxylin and eosin $\times$100. (Borek and Hall, 1974.)

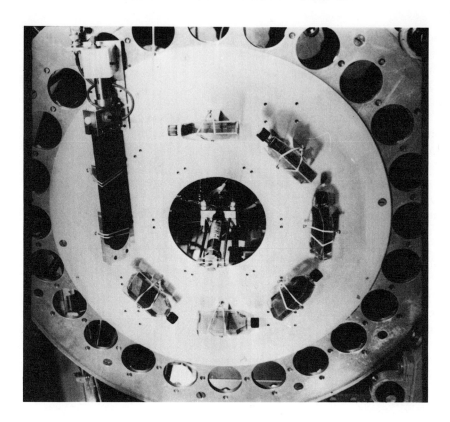

FIG. 8. Irradiation of adherent single cells by 430-keV neutrons from the van de Graaff accelerator in Brookhaven. The flasks are arranged around the tritium source, which emits a spectrum of neutrons. The angle of the cells with respect to the source determines the energy of radiation received by the cells.

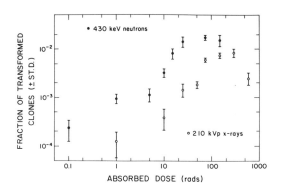

FIG. 9. A comparison of the incidence of transformation in vitro induced by 430-keV neutrons and by 210-kV X-rays. For doses at which more than one experiment was performed, the mean value together with the standard deviation is plotted. Additional data are required to establish the exact shapes of the curves.

and set in motion fast electrons, whereas neutrons interact with the nuclei of atoms of the absorbing material and set in motion fast recoil photons and other nuclear fragments.

Neutrons are available over a wide range of different energies. We elected to use 430-keV monoenergetic neutrons because this energy has been found to be the most effective producer of such biologic effects as cell killing and somatic mutations. Using the hamster embryo cloned cell system, we set out to determine whether 430-keV neutrons would induce *in vitro* transformation of single cells, in the range of 150 rad down to 0.1 rad.

A 4-million-volt van de Graaff accelerator was used to produce the neutrons. Protons (H_2 gas) are accelerated onto a tritium source, which then emits a spectrum of neutrons. The angle of the cells with respect to the source determines the neutron energy they receive (Fig. 8).

A partial dose-response relationship is presented in Fig. 9 and is compared with the X-ray data. The neutrons appear to have a significantly higher capacity to produce transformation. A scorable number of transformations is obtained with doses as low as 0.1 rad. Additional data are required to determine the exact shape of the curve. Neutron induced, transformed colonies have been found to be similar to X-ray-induced transformants.

DISCUSSION

The results of the investigations presented above demonstrate that low doses of X-rays and neutrons, in the range of 1 to 600 rad of X-rays, and 0.1 rad to 150 rad of 430-keV neutrons, can induce neoplastic transformation *in vitro* in diploid short-term cultures of hamster embryo cells. Although we cannot yet exclude the presence of viruses, we have found no C-type particle virus in the transformed cells.

The frequency of neoplastic transformation in mass cultures was found to be similar to that induced in single cells plated at low density. Although the presence of low concentrations of feeder cells increased the plating efficiency in the cloned cultures, the same rate of transformation was observed with or without feeder cells (Borek and Hall, 1974). Replacement of medium before or after irradiation, as well as incubation of both mass cultures and cloned cells with sonicated irradiated cells and sonicated transformed cells, had no influence on the rate of the transformation.

In the course of several hundred experiments carried out with X-rays, we have not observed spontaneous transformation in the control cultures despite the fact that over one-half a million clones have been scanned. Recently, in one out of 70 neutron experiments, we found two spontaneous transformed clones in control dishes. This was associated with an unusually high frequency of radiation-induced transformation in that same experiment. But, the frequency of transformed cells found in the irradiated cells is too high to be considered a random mutation or a selection of spontaneously transformed cells; it suggests a direct interaction of the ionizing radiation with the target cells *in vitro*.

Although we found aneuploidy in the transformed cells, no obvious alterations were observed in the chromosomal structure. This is not surprising, since it is likely that the event that leads to transformation is a subtle genetic alteration. Whatever the nature of the initial event, cell replication is required to fix the transformed state as a hereditary property of the cell. Cell lines independently transformed by X-rays are heterogeneous as far as their surface properties are concerned, as well as in their ability to produce tumors. Although in some cases we found regression, in others progressive growth was observed.

The use of short-term embryonic cultures has its advantage in the fact that we have a varied population of fast replicating normal diploid cells in which different cell types serve as target cells. This, however, is also a drawback, for the mixed population from the whole embryo is asynchronous, so that the cells exposed to radiation are in different phases of the cell cycle.

Our data for X-rays suggest that within the diverse cell population derived from the hamster embryos, cells *potentially* transformed by radiation are more susceptible to being killed by high doses of radiation than are normal cells. In other words, due to cumulative damage produced by larger doses, the *potentially* transformed cells die a reproductive death more readily than do the normal cells and never have a chance to form a colony. This is illustrated by the observation that at doses above 300 rad, a level at which cell killing becomes more significant, less transformation was observed in spite of the fact that transformed colonies are scored from among the survivors, a technique that inherently accounts for cell killing. The same conclusion is also suggested by the split-dose experiments, in which two equal doses of radiation resulted in higher cell survival and *increased* transformation, as compared with a single acute dose. Our data with neutrons are still incomplete. It appears that at the level of 75 to 150 rad of 430-keV neutrons the transformation rate reaches a plateau. Technically, it is impossible to obtain sufficient data per experiment at doses higher than 150 rad.

When considering the relationship between cells transformed by radiation *in vitro* and cancer *in vivo,* we find a similarity in cell behavior. Both tumor cells and transformed cells fail to respond to the social environment and grow under conditions in which normal cells do not. A discrepancy appears in the rate of transformation. At 300 rad, transformation frequency *in vitro* is around 1%.

In vivo, however, it is nowhere near this rate. It may be that *in vitro* transformation in the hamster system is artifically high because culturing cells from various organs exposes cells that are genetically susceptible to transformation but are in resting phase *in vivo* to conditions *in vitro* under which they can proliferate rapidly and become more vulnerable to transformation. An alternative explanation is that *in vivo,* in the intact animal, immunologic surveillance mechanisms prevail to inhibit transformation *in vivo,* and in cells, once removed from these metabolic defenses and cultured *in vitro,* the transformation rate by radiation is increased.

ACKNOWLEDGMENTS

These investigations were supported in part by USPHS Research Grant CA-12536 from the National Cancer Institute and by USAEC grant AT-(11–1)-3243.

REFERENCES

Abercrombie, M., and Ambrose, E. J. (1962): The surface properties of cancer cells: A review. *Cancer Res.,* 22:525–548.

Bond, V. P., Cronkite, E. P., Lippincott, S. W., and Shellabarger, C. J. (1960): Studies on radiation-induced mammary gland neoplasia in the rat. III. Relation of the neoplastic response to dose of total-body radiation. *Radiat. Res.,* 12:276–285.

Borek, C., and Sachs, L. (1966*a*): *In vitro* cell transformation by x-irradiation. *Nature,* 210:276–278.

Borek, C., and Sachs, L. (1966*b*): The difference in contact inhibition of cell replication between normal cells and cells transformed by different carcinogens. *Proc. Nat. Acad. Sci. USA,* 56:1705–1711.

Borek, C., and Sachs, L. (1967): Cell susceptibility to transformation by X-irradiation and fixation of the transformed state. *Proc. Natl. Acad. Sci. USA,* 57:1522–1527.

Borek, C., and Sachs, L. (1968): The number of cell generations required to fix the transformed state in X-ray-induced transformation. *Proc. Natl. Acad. Sci. USA,* 59:83–85.

Borek, C. (1972): Neoplastic transformation *in vitro* of a clone of adult liver epithelial cells into differentiated hepatoma-like cells under conditions of nutritional stress. *Proc. Natl. Acad. Sci. USA,* 69:956–959.

Borek, C., and Hall, E. J. (1973): Transformation of mammalian cells *in vitro* by low doses of X-rays. *Nature,* 243:450–453.

Borek, C., and Hall, E. J. (1974): Effect of split doses of X-rays on neoplastic transformation of single cells. *Nature,* 252:499–501.

Borek, C., and Fengolio, C. (*In preparation.*)

Borek, C., Grob, M., and Burger, M. M. (1973): Surface alterations in transformed epithelial and fibroblastic cells in culture: A disturbance of membrane degradation versus biosynthesis? *Expt. Cell Res.,* 77:207–215.

Borek, C., Higashino, S., and Lowenstein, W. R. (1969): Intercellular communication and tissue growth. IV. Conductance of membrane junctions of normal and cancerous cells in culture. *J. Membr. Biol.,* 1:274–293.

Burger, M. M. (1969): A difference in the architecture of the surface membrane of normal and virally transformed cells. *Proc. Natl. Acad. Sci. USA,* 62:994–1001.

Furth, J., and Lorenz, E. (1954): Carcinogenesis by ionizing radiations. In: *Radiation Biology,* Vol. 4, edited by A. Hollander, pp. 1145–1201. McGraw-Hill Book Co., New York.

Gray, L. H. (1965): Radiation biology and cancer. In: *Cellular Radiation Biology,* pp. 7–25. William & Wilkins, Baltimore.

Ham, R. G., and Puck, T. T. (1952): Quantitative colonial growth of isolated mammalian cells. In: *Methods in Enzymology,* Vol. 5, edited by S. P. Colowick and M. D. Kaplan, pp. 90–119. Academic Press, New York.

Inbar, M. S., and Sachs, L. (1969): Interaction of the carbohydrate-binding protein concanavalin A with normal and transformed cells. *Proc. Natl. Acad. Sci. USA,* 63:1418–1425.

Kaplan, H. S. (1949): Preliminary studies of the effectiveness of local irradiation in the induction of lymphoid tumors in mice. *J. Natl. Cancer Inst.* 10:267–270.

Lieberman, M., and Kaplan, H. J. (1959): Leukemogenic activity of filtrates from radiation-induced lymphoid tumors of mice. *Science,* 130:387–388.

Miller, D. A., Dev, D. G., Borek, C., and Miller, O. J. (1972): The quinacrine fluorescent and Giemsa banding karyotype of the rat, *Rattus norvegicus,* and banded chromosome analysis of transformed and malignant rat liver cell lines. *Cancer Res.,* 32:2375–2382.

Sanders, F. K., and Burford, B. O. (1964): Ascites tumors from BHK. 21 cells transformed *in vitro* by polyoma virus. *Nature,* 201:786–789.

Stoker, M. G. P. (1972): Tumor viruses and the sociology of fibroblasts. *Proc. Ry. Soc.* [*Biol.*], 181:1–17.

Terzakghi, M., and Little, J. B. (1975): Repair of potentially lethal radiation damage in mammalian cells is associated with enhancement of malignant transformation. *Nature,* 253:548–549.

Todaro, G. J., and Green, H. (1966): Cell growth and the initiation of transformation by SV40. *Proc. Natl. Acad. Sci. USA,* 55:302–308.

Upton, A. C. (1961): The dose-response relation in radiation-induced cancer. *Cancer Res.,* 21:717–729.

Weinstein, I. B., Gerbert, R., Stadler, U. C., Ornstein, J. M., and Axel, R. (1972): Type C virus from cell cultures of chemically induced rat hepatomas. *Science,* 178:1098–1100.

Biology of Radiation Carcinogenesis, edited by
J. M. Yuhas, R. W. Tennant, and J. D. Regan.
Raven Press, New York © 1976.

Oncogenic Transformation *In Vitro* by X-rays: Influence of Repair Processes

Margaret Terzaghi and John B. Little

Department of Physiology, Harvard School of Public Health, Boston, Massachusetts 02115

Reports in the literature of X-ray-induced oncogenic transformation *in vitro* (Borek and Sachs, 1966; Borek and Hall, 1973) are far outnumbered by reports of failure to induce transformation following irradiation of a variety of cell cultures (Coggin, 1969; DiPaolo et al., 1971; Klein, 1966; Pollock and Todaro, 1968; Stoker, 1963). Klein (1974) observed transformation in an established line of mouse spleen cells. The techniques used were analogous to those used by Borek and Sachs (1966). Similar transformation was obtained by Klein (1974), however, when the same proportion of the cell population was killed by mechanical means. The question of whether oncogenic transformation (in contradistinction to morphologic transformation) occurs *in vitro* as a specific radiation induced phenomenon has thus remained ambiguous. In the experiments initially reported by Borek and Sachs (1966) with primary hamster embryo cells, the problem of demonstrating nonregressing malignant tumors is frequently cited. The need for more data bearing on the process of radiation-induced transformation *in vitro* is clear.

The cell line used in the present experiments offers several advantages over other cell systems. The cells are derived from a highly inbred strain of mouse, thereby facilitating tumorigenicity testing of transformed clones. The high plating efficiency characteristic of this established cell line obviates the use of high density cultures. Previously described quantitative and qualitative data on methylcholanthrene-induced transformation (Reznikoff et al., 1973a) and MNNG-induced transformation (Bertram and Heidelberger, 1974) make possible parallel comparison of chemical induced and radiation induced transformations in the same cell line.

MATERIALS AND METHODS

Cell Cultures

A C3H mouse embryo-derived cell line (10T½ clone 8) was used. This cell line was originally developed and described by Reznikoff et al. (1973b) as a stable, highly contact-inhibited, aneuploid line (hypertetraploid), with no spontaneous background transformation and no evidence of spontane-

327

ous production of C-type viral particles. Stock cultures were maintained in Eagle's basal medium supplemented with 10% heat-inactivated fetal calf serum in accordance with the protocol outlined by Reznikoff et al. (1973b) and Terzaghi and Little (1974). Experiments were carried out with cells from cultures at the 8th to 15th passages. Irradiation was carried out with a Phillips industrial X-ray unit operating at 100 kVp and 10 mA yielding a dose rate of 83.5 rad/min with 0.795-mm Al filtration.

Exponential Cultures: Survival Curves and Transformation Assays

Cells were initially seeded at a density such that, regardless of dose used, 50 to 75 viable cells were obtained on each 100-mm Petri dish used for survival assays, and 250 to 350 cells on each 100-mm dish to be used for transformation assays. Dishes were irradiated 12 to 15 hr after seeding. Survival assay experiments were terminated about two weeks after seeding, but transformation assay plates were maintained for 6 weeks. Culture medium was changed twice weekly until the cells were confluent and then at weekly intervals until termination of the experiment. All plates were fixed in Bouin's solution, and stained with trypan blue.

Density Inhibited Plateau Phase Cultures: Survival Curves and Transformation Assay

Dishes were seeded several days in advance of irradiation with approximately 10^5 cells/100-mm Petri dish. When confluency was attained, the culture medium was changed. Twenty-four hours later, the medium was changed a second time. Irradiation of the cultures was carried out 24 hr after the second medium change. At specified time intervals after irradiation, cells were subcultured by exposure to 0.05% trypsin for 5 min and suspended in complete media; the appropriate dilutions were made, and the cells seeded to assay for survival or transformation frequency as described for exponentially growing cultures (vide supra).

Scoring and Tumorigencity Testing

Scoring for transformants was carried out as described by Reznikoff et al. (1973a) and Terzaghi and Little (1974, 1975). Type I foci were not scored as transformants. Types II and III were scored as transformants. Transformation frequency is expressed as the total number of transformed foci divided by the total number of surviving (colony-forming) cells (i.e., cells at risk to transformation). Clones derived from transformed foci were tested for tumorigenicity in syngeneic C3H mice pre-irradiated with 350 rad (Reznikoff et al., 1973b; Terzaghi and Little, 1974). Clones were considered tumorigenic when 10^6 cells injected subcutaneously resulted in a non-regressing tumor.

Tumorigenicity data on radiation-transformed clones of 10T½ cells have been previously reported by Terzaghi and Little (1974, 1975). Types II and III transformed foci were found to be tumorigenic in syngeneic mice upon inoculation of 1 to 5 × 10⁶ cells. Type I foci and normal cells have not been found to be tumorigenic when up to 10⁷ cells were injected subcutaneously.

RESULTS

Survival Curves

Figure 1 shows the typical survival curves obtained following irradiation of cells in the exponential phase of growth (lower curve), and when irradiated

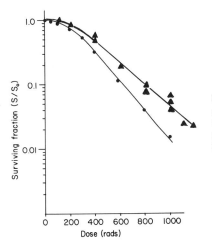

FIG. 1. Survival curves. Cells irradiated as exponentially growing cultures (●—●), $D_o = 180$ rad, and cells irradiated as density-inhibited plateau-phase cultures with subculture delayed 3 hr post-irradiation (▲—▲), $D_o = 250$ rad.

in a density-inhibited plateau phase of growth with subculture to lower cell density 3 hr after irradiation (upper points). The D_o (inverse of the slope) for exponentially growing cells was 180 rad. A similar D_o was found for cells irradiated in the plateau phase and subcultured immediately afterward. When subculture was delayed, however, the D_o increased to 250 rad. The effect of holding cells in plateau phase for 3 hr post-irradiation was thus to enhance survival as reflected by a decrease in the slope of the survival curve. This effect has been demonstrated in a number of mammalian cell lines, and has been interpreted as resulting from the repair of potentially lethal radiation damage (Little, 1969, 1973).

Survival and Transformation in Density Inhibited Cultures

The upper curve in Figure 2 represents the change seen in ultimate survival following a single radiation dose (1,200 rad) when the time interval between

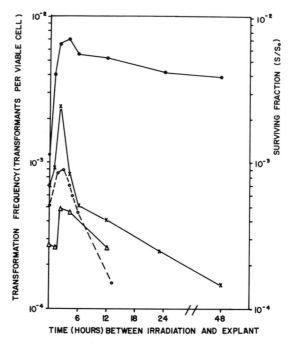

FIG. 2. Survival and transformation frequency. Cells irradiated in the density-inhibited plateau phase of growth and subculture delayed various times thereafter. Surviving fraction after 1,200 rad (○); transformation frequency after 200 rad (△); 300 rad (○); 400 rad (X). (Terzaghi and Little, 1975a.)

irradiation and subculture was varied between 0 and 24 hr. The lower three curves demonstrate the changes in transformation frequency under similar conditions. Both survival and transformation frequency rose in parallel to a maximum when subculture was delayed (cells were held in the plateau phase) for about 3 hr after irradiation. With longer time intervals before subculture, the transformation frequency declined while survival remained essentially constant.

Transformation Dose-Response Curves

The curves drawn in Figure 3 illustrate the change in transformation frequency we observed with increasing doses of radiation when cells were irradiated during exponential growth. The individual datum points are for cultures irradiated in the plateau phase of growth and subcultured 3 hr after irradiation to a lower cell density. Note that the transformation frequency (lower curve) in exponential cells irradiated with doses greater than 400 rad did not change significantly. When cells were irradiated in plateau-phase growth and subculture delayed for 3 hr, on the other hand, the transformation frequency continued to increase exponentially at doses greater than 400 rad.

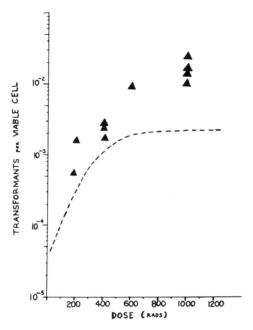

FIG. 3. Dose-transformation frequency response. Cells irradiated as exponentially growing cultures (---); cells irradiated as density-inhibited plateau phase cultures with subculture delayed for 3 hr after irradiation (▲).

Effect of Lethally Pre-irradiated Cells on Observed Transformation Frequencies

The addition of 10^3 to 10^4 cells pre-irradiated with 1,500 to 2,000 rad to control (untreated) and experimental dishes did not affect either the behavior of the normal untreated cells or the transformation frequencies observed in the experimental groups.

DISCUSSION

The morphology and corresponding tumorigenicity of the transformed clones induced by radiation appear to be analogous to those previously reported following treatment with MCA (Reznikoff et al., 1973a). This observation tends to support the hypothesis that radiation is capable of inducing oncogenic transformation *in vitro*. The suggestion by Klein (1974) that such a process may be related solely to cell killing and the consequent release of a transformation factor did not appear to be the case in 10T½ cells. The addition of lethally pre-irradiated cells to normal cells did not result in spontaneous transformation nor in any enhancement of radiation-induced transformation. Furthermore, we have found that an increase in the density of cells used for any given dose of radiation results in a decrease in the transformation frequency. (Terzaghi and Little, 1976). This observation is contrary to expectation if the number of dead or dying cells play a critical role in the transformation process. Also, if the quantity of dead and dying cells present were critical, one would not expect to find the observed leveling off of the transformation frequency with increased dose as seen in 10T½ cells or a decline in transformation as reported by Borek and Hall (1973).

A comparison of our transformation frequency–dose-response data obtained with 10T½ cells (Fig. 3) with those obtained by Borek and Hall (1973) with primary hamster embryo cells indicates two important differences. First, the transformation frequencies reported by Borek and Hall (1973) are higher. The maximum transformation frequency they reported following 300 rad was 9.2×10^{-3} transformants/surviving cell. In the 10T½ cell system, the maximum transformation frequency observed when cells were irradiated in exponentially growing cultures was 2×10^{-3} transformants/surviving cell. This difference could be related to the type of cells used, variations in culture conditions, and possible differences in the criteria used in scoring for transformants. A second difference between the two systems relates to the slopes of the exponential portions of the transformation dose-response curves. In the Borek and Hall (1973) experiments, a dose of roughly 10 rad yielded a doubling in the observed transformation frequency. In the 10T½ cell system, a dose of about 100 rad was necessary to double the transformation frequency.

These results suggest that the damage a cell is capable of accumulating or repairing at low doses of radiation (as reflected in the shoulder of the survival curve) may be linked to the transformation process. We have further investigated the relationship between processes involved in cell survival and those involved in oncogenic transformation by observing the changes in transformation frequency associated with the repair of potentially lethal damage in irradiated plateau phase cells. It has been previously shown (Little, 1969, 1973) that survival in plateau phase cultures can be considerably enhanced if a stimulus-to-cell proliferation, such as subculture to low cell density, is delayed following irradiation. As can be seen in Fig. 2, a peak in survival occurred when the subculture of density-inhibited 10T½ cells was delayed for 3 hr after irradiation. Interestingly, this enhancement in survival was associated with a parallel *increase* in the transformation frequency (Fig. 2) also with a peak at 3 hr. Figure 3 demonstrates the change that occurred in the dose-transformation frequency relationship when cells were irradiated under these conditions rather than during exponential growth. One hypothesis that would explain these results is that errors that eventuate in the transformed state are inserted during the early post-irradiation repair period by some mechanism, such as error-prone repair.

These observations clearly indicate that a relationship exists between processes controlling cell survival and transformation, and they suggest that molecular repair mechanisms may be intimately involved in both effects. Further examination of possible cell-cycle effects and of molecular events associated with alterations in susceptibility to transformation may increase our understanding of the mechanisms of oncogenic transformation. If indeed repair, or misrepair, is a critical aspect of the transformation process, care must be taken in the extrapolation of data between different cell systems, since significant differences have been demonstrated among species in their DNA repair capacities (Regan, 1975, *this volume*).

SUMMARY

X-Ray induced oncogenic transformation has been demonstrated in a C3H mouse embryo derived cell line. The transformation appears to be produced by a specific effect of the radiation on the cells rather than by an effect mediated by nonspecific cell killing. An exponential increase in transformants per surviving cell with doses of radiation between 50 and 400 rad was observed. At doses above 400 rad delivered to exponentially growing cells, the transformation frequency remained at approximately two transformants/10^3 surviving cells. Little decline in survival occurred at doses below 300 rad. Survival declined exponentially at higher doses with a D_0 of 180 rad. When cells were irradiated in density-inhibited plateau-phase growth and allowed to repair potentially lethal radiation damage by delaying subculture for 3 hr post-irradiation, the D_0 of the survival curve increased to 250 rad. Under these conditions, the transformation frequency continued to increase exponentially with doses up to 1,000 rad. Analogous trends in the kinetics of cell survival and oncogenic cell transformation make possible a preliminary examination of the possible role of repair or misrepair in the process of oncogenic transformation *in vitro*.

ACKNOWLEDGMENTS

Research supported by grants CA-11751 and ES-00002 and Contract CP-33273 from the National Institutes of Health.

REFERENCES

Bertram, J. S., and Heidelberger, C. (1974): Cell cycle dependency of oncogenic transformation induced by *n*-methyl-N'-nitro-N-nitrosoguanidine in culture. *Cancer Res.,* 34:526.

Borek, C., and Hall, E. J. (1973): Transformation of mammalian cells *in vitro* by low doses of X-rays. *Nature,* 243:450.

Borek, C., and Sachs, L. (1966): *In vitro* cell transformation by X-irradiation. *Nature,* 210:276.

Coggin, J. H. (1969): Enhanced virus transformation of hamster embryo cells *in vitro*. *J. Virol.,* 3:458.

Di Paolo, J. A., Donovan, P. J., and Nelson, R. L. (1971): X-irradiation enhancement of transformation by benzo(a)pyrene in hamster embryo cells. *Proc. Natl. Acad. Sci. USA,* 68:1734.

Klein, J. A. (1966): Absence of malignant transformation after weekly irradiation of a mouse spleen in culture. *J. Natl. Cancer Inst.*, 37:655–661.

Klein, J. C. (1974): Evidence against a direct carcinogenic effect of X-rays *in vitro*. *J. Natl. Cancer Inst.*, 52:1111–1116.

Little, J. B. (1969): Repair of sub-lethal and potentially lethal radiation damage in plateau phase cultures of human cells. *Nature*, 224:804.

Little, J. B. (1973): Factors influencing the repair of potentially lethal radiation damage in growth-inhibited human cells. *Radiat. Res.*, 56:320.

Pollock, E. J., and Todaro, G. J. (1968): Radiation enhancement of SV-40 transformation in 3T3 and human cells. *Nature*, 219:520.

Reznikoff, C. A., Bertram, J. S., Brankow, D. W., and Heidelberger, C. (1973a): Quantitative and qualitative studies of chemical transformation of cloned C3H mouse embryo cells sensitive to postconfluence inhibition of cell division. *Cancer Res.*, 33:3238.

Reznikoff, C. A., Brankow, D. W., and Heidelberger, C. (1973b): Establishment and characterization of a cloned line of C3H mouse embryo cells sensitive to postconfluence inhibition of division. *Cancer Res.*, 33:3231.

Stoker, M. (1963): Effect of X-irradiation on susceptibility of cells to transformation by polyoma virus. *Nature*, 200:756.

Terzaghi, M., and Little, J. B. (1974): Interactions between radiation and benzo-(a)pyrene in an *in vitro* model for malignant transformation. In: *Experimental Lung Cancer. Carcinogenesis and Bioassays,* edited by E. Karbe and J. Park, pp. 467–506. Springer-Verlag, New York.

Terzaghi, M., and Little, J. B. (1975): Repair of potentially lethal radiation damage in mammalian cells is associated with enhancement of malignant transformation. *Nature*, 253:548.

Terzaghi, M., and Little, J. B. (1976): Radiation-induced oncogenic transformation in a C3H mouse embryo-derived cell line. *Cancer Res. (In press.)*

Biology of Radiation Carcinogenesis, edited by
J. M. Yuhas, R. W. Tennant, and J. D. Regan.
Raven Press, New York © 1976.

In Vitro Transformation:
Interactions of Chemical Carcinogens and Radiation

J. A. DiPaolo

Biology Branch, Carcinogenesis Program, National Cancer Institute, Bethesda, Maryland 20014

As part of a program to determine the factors that influence transformation and the degree to which any agent acts alone or interacts with another agent from the same or a different category of carcinogen, we have been studying the interaction of potent chemical carcinogens in combination with either weak chemical carcinogens, such as alkylating agents, or physical agents, such as X-irradiation (X-ray) and ultraviolet irradiation (UV). The interactions of various agents may be responsible for an increased risk of cancer in laboratory animals and human populations. The use of multiple agents may lead to different but specific new types of assay for surveillance of our environment for carcinogenic agents and should give us an insight as to their possible mode of action.

The etiologic role of X-ray and UV in human cancer formation has been recognized practically from the discovery of ionizing and non-ionizing radiation (Upton, 1974). Quantitative studies on the relationship of radiation to carcinogenesis of man, particularly for leukemia, has been the subject of a presentation by Dr. R. W. Miller (*this volume*). Experiments in laboratory animals have shown conclusively that radiobiologic insult, in conjunction with chemicals, influences the incidence of cancer (Furth and Boon, 1943; Berenblum and Trainin, 1960; Shellabarger, 1967; Cole and Foley, 1969; Vogel and Zaldivar, 1971). Cancer incidence is found to vary with the type of neoplasm, with radiologic variables, host-factor, and the interval between exposure to the two types of agents as well as with the nature of the radiation. Thus, the frequency of the type of cancer produced may be unaffected, decreased, additive, or synergistic. The direct treatment of cells with X-ray or UV irradiation followed by virus results in the enhancement of the transformation associated with the virus (Stoker, 1963; Pollock and Todaro, 1968; Coggin, 1969; Lytle et al., 1970; Casto, 1973). Analysis of some of the experiments indicated that the mechanism for enhancement of transformation was an actual increase in transformation susceptability of the cells. This conclusion was suggested by the increase in the absolute number of transformants with radiation exposure. Our *in vitro* results show that the interaction between carcinogenic agents leads to increased transformation by known potent chemical carcinogens when the cells are pretreated with X-irradiation or alkylating agents (DiPaolo et al., 1971*b;* DiPaolo et al., 1974). Maximum enhancement was obtained when cells were pretreated 48 hr prior to administration of chemical carcinogens.

MATERIALS AND METHODS

The brilliant studies of Puck and Marcus (1956) and Puck et al. (1956), which established techniques for quantitative procedures utilizing mammalian cells in culture, have made possible the foundation for both radiation biology and quantitative studies in chemical carcinogenesis. Approximately a decade later, Berwald and Sachs (1965), followed by other groups (Huberman and Sachs, 1966; DiPaolo et al., 1969; Chen and Heidelberger, 1969; DiPaolo et al., 1972), reported quantitative studies dealing with transformation of cultured fibroblasts by chemicals. Our published procedure (DiPaolo et al., 1969) used as a standard transformation assay is outlined in Fig. 1. Usually, tertiary Syrian hamster cell strains 2 to 4 days old were used. Cells in Dulbecco's medium, with 10% fetal bovine serum, were added to each Petri dish containing an irradiated feeder cell layer. Cells were exposed to chemicals dis-

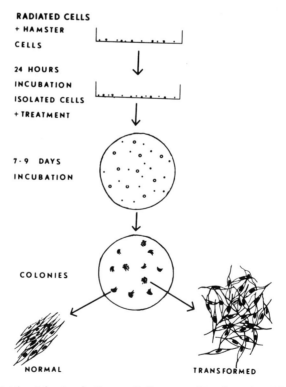

RADIATED CELLS
+ HAMSTER
CELLS

24 HOURS
INCUBATION
ISOLATED CELLS
+ TREATMENT

7-9 DAYS
INCUBATION

COLONIES

NORMAL   TRANSFORMED

FIG. 1. Standard experimental system for the quantitative assay of transformation of Syrian hamster cell strains by carcinogenic chemicals or physical agents.

solved in acetone or balanced salt solution and diluted with complete medium from 6 to 24 hr after the hamster embryo cells had been seeded for colony formation. Feeder layers, usually composed of secondary culture of hamster fetal cells, were irradiated as confluent monolayer cultures in 2 ml of medium with a Picker Portable X-ray apparatus at 100 kV and 5 mA; a total of 4,500 R in air was delivered to a distance of 22.2 cm. Cells to be at risk in the combination carcinogenesis experiments were X-irradiated with a two-tube Westinghouse Quandrocondex machine, 200 kV and 15 mA (output of 139 R/min). Irradiation with UV was done with a GE germicidal lamp (15T8) at a distance of 160 cm with a fluence of 1.5 erg/mm^2/s (DiPaolo and Donovan, 1975). Variations of this model have been utilized to demonstrate that transformation can be quantitated with fibroblasts, that it follows a linear relationship with dose, that transformed colonies do produce transformed lines with attributes of neoplastic cells, including the production of tumors, and that *in vivo* activity correlates with *in vitro* activity, thereby providing the evidence that chemically induced carcinogenesis can be studied *in vitro*.

From a series of studies combining X-irradiation, UV irradiation, or methylmethane sulfate (MMS), an alkylating agent, with known potent chemical carcinogens, an enhancement of transformation normally associated with the chemical carcinogen was obtained if the cells were first X-irradiated (DiPaolo et al., 1971*b*) or treated with the alkylating agent methyl methane sulfonate (DiPaolo et al., 1974). A combination of the chemical carcinogens with UV-irradiation did not have this effect (DiPaolo and Donovan, 1975). Under the conditions of these experiments, no transformation was observed following X-irradiation only; rare transformants were obtained with the alkylating agents, and significant numbers of transformants were obtained subsequent to UV-irradiation.

The X-ray sensitivity of irradiated hamster cells increased with increasing doses as determined by the criterion of colony formation. A typical curve measuring post-irradiation growth has a small shoulder followed by a slope indicating a multi-hit type of damage. The addition of a chemical carcinogen, post-insult, by irradiating agents results in similar types of curves. By normalizing the results, superimposable curves may thus be constructed as is shown for irradiation by X-ray and benzo(a)pyrene (BP) (Fig. 2). The combined effect of X-ray and BP with low doses of radiation, such as 150 to 250 R, results in only a 20 to 30% increase in toxicity relative to treatment by BP. Interestingly, a time relationship was found between various doses of X-ray and subsequent treatment with either 2.5 or 10 μg BP/ml of medium. Maximal enhancement was obtained when cells were irradiated 48 hr prior to treatment with this potent chemical carcinogen (DiPaolo et al., 1971*b*). Within the range of concentration of BP used, the maximum enhancement of 8- to 9-fold obtained at 48 hr appears to be independent of the concentration of the carcinogen. The addition of BP at intervals, such as 6, 12 or 24 hr

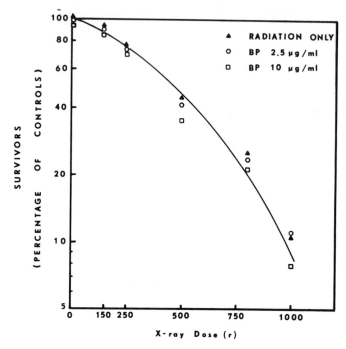

FIG. 2. The reproductive capacity (colony formation) of irradiated hamster fetal cells; the cells were seeded for colony formation and treated with benzo(a)pyrene 24 hr after irradiation. The colonies formed with 0.0 (▲), 2.5 (○), and 10 (□) μg benzo(a)pyrene/ml medium set at 100%.

after irradiation, resulted in at least a threefold enhancement; but, the addition of BP 72 hr after irradiation resulted in no significant enhancement and, with the lower concentration of BP (2.5 μg/ml of medium), the transformation frequency equaled that obtained without irradiation. Decreasing or increasing the X-ray dose also influenced enhancement of transformation. For example, with either 750 or 1,000 R, practically no enhancement of BP transformation occurred regardless of the time interval between irradiation and the addition of the chemical carcinogen. When data obtained from addition of various concentrations of BP at different intervals post-irradiation (250 R) were analyzed, it was found that the average enhancement ratio was 8.6. If the data are plotted on a log-log basis, the result is consistent with a one-hit hypothesis (Fig. 3) and confirms the observation that the increased sensitivity of the cells caused by irradiation is constant. The increase in transformation on a per cell basis that was obtained up to 500 R is an indication that the phenomenon is inductive rather than selective. Similar data, as shown, have also been obtained for transformation by a chemical carcinogen only (DiPaolo et al., 1971a). The highly significant transitory increase of enhancement among irradiated cells can also be taken as evidence that irradiation did not cause a selection of cells more likely to be transformed by BP because of a special radiation-resistant state. Selection of radiation-resistant cells would

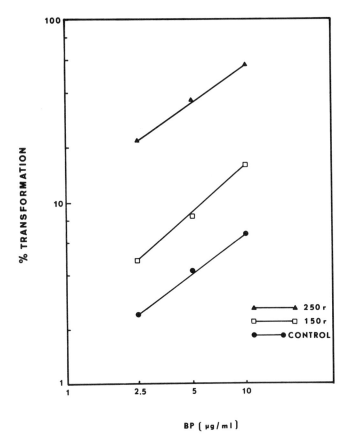

FIG. 3. Pre-X-irradiation of hamster cells with 0 (●), 150 (□), or 250 R (▲); 48 hr after seeding, the cells were treated with benzo(a)pyrene.

have produced a relative increase in the fraction of transformed colonies among the surviving colonies at most of the intervals during which BP was added. Furthermore, the multiplication of resistant cells would have maintained a relatively high enhancement factor.

Experiments in which an alkylating agent was substituted for radiation were carried out in conjunction with chemical carcinogens. From a logistic point of view, our laboratory could treat the hamster embryo cells before or after they were seeded into Petri dishes for colony formation. Because MMS induces physiochemical effects similar to those produced by ionizing radiation in cell DNA, it was considered a logical agent to substitute for irradiation. At 24-hr intervals, BP (2.5 μg/ml) was added to dishes that had been pretreated with 11 or 27.5 μg MMS/ml and to untreated control dishes. Maximum enhancement occurred 48 hr following MMS pretreatment and was greater when the cells were treated with the lower concentration of MMS. Since this enhancement of transformation occurred whether cells were treated before or after being seeded, it cannot be attributed to some alteration in the cell cycle resulting from differences in recovery periods associated with treatment combined with the passage of the cells. One interesting observation is that no significant increase in transformation occurs when the cells are treated with BP 24 hr post-MMS treatment.

Since these studies had been limited to combinations with BP, it could be postulated that the enhancement was due to an effect on microsomal enzymes. Before this possibility was explored, other potent chemical carcinogens belonging to the class of carcinogenic polycylic hydrocarbon, as well as to other classes, were added to cells that had been X-irradiated or treated with MMS, to determine if the enhancement phenomenon could be extended to include a variety of diverse chemical carcinogens (DiPaolo et al., 1974). Transformation by any of the chemicals used was significantly enhanced when the cells were treated with MMS or X-irradiated 48 hr prior to the second treatment. With all carcinogens, the enhancement was slightly greater when pretreatment of cells was by X-irradiation rather than MMS; in both cases, the lethality attributable to the pretreatment was 10 to 20% relative to controls. The cause of the enhancement in transformation resulting from the interaction of these agents is not yet known.

The possibility that the interaction of treatments altered DNA synthesis, or its repair, or caused a specific type of chromosome aberration at the time interval of greatest enhancement, was pursued (DiPaolo, Donovan, and Popescu, 1976). It should be kept in mind, however, that large populations of cells were observed and that the events occurring in these populations might not necessarily reflect the events that occur in the small number of cells that undergo transformation. When the growth rate of 10^5 cells, irradiated or not irradiated, was followed for three days, there was an initial obvious loss of cells due to irradiation but very little change in the growth rate. The addition of carcinogen two days post-irradiation and the recounting of cells 24 hr later showed that the effects attributable to the carcinogen relative to the nonirradiated or irradiated cells, were insignificant. The difference between irradiated and nonirradiated cells 72 hr after treatment was of the same order of magnitude as that observed when colony formation was used as the index of lethality. Therefore, we thought it advisable to examine the mass populations of cells after the various treatments.

When cell populations were examined 48 hr post-irradiation, in terms of changes in cell cycle, no differences from the control were found. Additional studies were carried out on the different aspects of the cycle. Pertinent to this investigation is the observation that no difference was found within the various groups when mitotic accumulations with colcemid were determined for X-irradiation only or X-ray plus BP and compared to the proper controls. Cells exposed to MMS were also examined for disruptions in the cell cycle, for partial synchronization, and analysis of unscheduled DNA synthesis by autoradiography or by alkline sucrose gradients. All evidence indicated that damaged DNA was rapidly repaired after treatment.

When UV was used for the primary treatment, the enhancement of chemical transformation usually associated with such compounds as BP or N-acetoxy-fluorenyl-acetamide did not occur. On the other hand, UV did produce a transformation that was dose related when applied to cells that had been seeded to form colonies. When mass cultures of Syrian hamster cells were X-irradiated with 250 R, as in the other experiments, seeded for colony formation, and treated with UV at 15 or 30 erg/mm^2 48 hr later, enhancement of UV transformation was increased on a colony or on a dish basis.

Thus, combinations of chemical carcinogens with irradiation indicate that enhancement of transformation follows a X-ray–type of insult. In some respects, there are similarities to *in vivo* experimental results in that small or relatively small doses of radiation, when combined with chemical carcinogens, enhance the malignancy, whereas large doses may have opposite effects.

SUMMARY

The development of reproducible quantitative *in vitro* procedures resulting in neoplastic transformation of mammalian cells has made possible the separation of events related to the process leading to transformation from secondary events that interfere with the early recognition of transformation. The use of chemical carcinogens on Syrian hamster cell strains results in a dose-response relation consistent with a Poisson distribution, indicating that the transformation phenomenon is inductive. In some circumstances, the joint action or interaction of chemical carcinogens with other agents results in an increased incidence of transformation. The pretreatment of Syrian hamster cells with ionizing radiation (250 R) or alkylating chemicals enhances the frequency of transformation on a cell or colony basis ordinarily obtained with known chemical carcinogens. Pretreatment with non-ionizing irradiation (UV, 254 nm) did not have a similar effect. The two types of irradiation and the alkylating agents reduced the cloning efficiency of the cells. X-Ray alone produced no transformation; the alkylating chemicals produced transformations infrequently, whereas UV produced a significant number of transformations. The number of transformations associated with UV is increased by pretreatment of the cells by X-irradiation. The enhancement of transformation by X-ray or X-ray–type agents appears to be independent of the type of second carcinogen used.

REFERENCES

Berenblum, I., and Trainin, N. (1960): Possible two-stage mechanism in experimental leukemogenesis. *Science,* 132:40–41.
Berwald, Y., and Sachs, L. (1965): *In vitro* transformation of normal cells to tumor cells by carcinogenic hydrocarbons. *J. Natl. Cancer Inst.,* 35:641–661.

Casto, B. C. (1973): Enhancement of adenovirus transformation by treatment of hamster cells with ultraviolet-irradiation, DNA base analogs, and dibenz(a,h) anthracene. *Cancer Res.,* 33:402–407.

Chen, T. T., and Heidelberger, C. (1969): Quantitative studies on the malignant transformation of mouse prostrate cells by carcinogenic hydrocarbons *in vitro. Int. J. Cancer,* 4:166–178.

Coggin, J. H., Jr. (1969): Enhanced virus transformation of hamster embryo cells *in vitro. J. Virol.,* 3:458–462.

Cole, L. J., and Foley, W. A. (1969): Modification of urethan-lung tumor incidence by low X-radiation doses, cortisone, and transfusion of isogenic lymphocytes. *Radiat. Res.,* 39:391–399.

DiPaolo, J. A., and Donovan, P. J. (1975): *In vitro* transformation of Syrian hamster cells by UV irradiation is enhanced by X-irradiation and unaffected by chemical carcinogens. *Proc. Am. Assoc. Cancer Res.,* 16:75.

DiPaolo, J. A., Donovan, P. J., and Nelson, R. L. (1969): Quantitative studies of *in vitro* transformation by chemical carcinogens. *J. Natl. Cancer Inst.,* 42:867–874.

DiPaolo, J. A., Donovan, P. J., and Nelson, R. L. (1971a): *In vitro* transformation of hamster cells by polycyclic hydrocarbons: Factors influencing the number of cells transformed. *Nature [New Biol.],* 230:240–242.

DiPaolo, J. A., Donovan, P. J., and Nelson, R. L. (1971b): X-irradiation enhancement of transformation by benzo(a)pyrene in hamster embryo cells. *Proc. Natl. Acad. Sci. USA,* 68:1734–1737.

DiPaolo, J. A., Donovan, P. J., and Popescu, N. C. (1976): Kinetics of Syrian hamster cells during X-irradiation enhancement of transformation *in vitro* by chemical carcinogen. *Radiat. Res. (in press).*

DiPaolo, J. A., Takano, K., and Popescu, N. C. (1972): Quantitation of chemically induced neoplastic transformation of BALB/3T3 cloned cell lines. *Cancer Res.,* 32:2686–2695.

DiPaolo, J. A., Donovan, P. J., and Casto, B. C. (1974): Enhancement by alkylating agents of chemical carcinogen transformation of hamster cells in culture. *Chem.-Biol. Interact.,* 9:351–364.

Furth, J., and Boon, M. C. (1943): Enhancement of leukemogenic action of methylcholanthrene by pre-irradiation with X-rays. *Science,* 98:138–139.

Huberman, E., and Sachs, L. (1966): Cell susceptibility to transformation and cytotoxicity by the carcinogenic hydrocarbon benzo(1)pyrene. *Proc. Natl. Acad. Sci. USA,* 56:1123–1129.

Lytle, C. D., Hellman, K. B., and Telles, N. C. (1970): Enhancement of viral transformation by ultra-violet light. *Int. J. Radiat. Biol.,* 18:297–300.

Pollack, E. J., and Todaro, G. J. (1968): Radiation enhancement of SV40 transformation in 3T3 and human cells. *Nature,* 219:520–521.

Puck, T. T., and Marcus, P. I. (1956): Action of X-rays on single mammalian cells. *J. Exp. Med.,* 103:653–666.

Puck, T. T., Marcus, P. I., and Cieciura, S. J. (1956): Clonal growth of mammalian cells *in vitro.* Growth characteristics of colonies from single HeLa cells with and without a "feeder" layer. *J. Exp. Med.,* 103:273–284.

Shellabarger, C. J. (1967): Effect of 3-methylcholanthrene and X-irradiation, given singly or combined, on rat mammary carcinogenesis. *J. Natl. Cancer Inst.,* 38:73–77.

Stoker, M. (1963): Effect of X-irradiation on susceptibility of cells to transformation by polyoma virus. *Nature,* 200:756–758.

Upton, A. C. (1974): Somatic and genetic effects of low-level radiation. In: *Recent Advances in Nuclear Medicine,* Vol. IV, edited by J. H. Lawrence, Grune & Stratton, Inc., New York, pp. 1–40.

Vogel, H. H., Jr., and Zaldivar, R. (1971): Co-carcinogenesis: The interaction of chemical and physical agents. *Radiat. Res.,* 47:644–659.

A

Absorbed dose
  specific energy and, 1-6
  time factor dependence on, 9-10
N-Acetoxy-2-aminofluorene, as car-
    cinogen, 155
2-Acetylaminofluorene (AAF)
  activation to carcinogen, 152-155
  DNA repair after exposure to, in
    normal and xeroderma pigmen-
    tosum cells, 133-142
  effect on nucleic acid, 175-187
  N-hydroxy-, as inhibitor of nucleic
    acid synthesis, 178-179
2-Acetylaminophenanthrene (AAP), DNA
    repair after exposure to, in normal
    and xeroderma pigmentosum cells,
    133-142
4-Acetylaminobiphenyl (AABP), DNA re-
    pair after exposure to, in normal
    and xeroderma pigmentosum cells,
    133-142
4-Acetylaminostilbene (AAS), DNA repair
    after exposure to, in normal and
    xeroderma pigmentosum cells,
    133-142
Acute myelogenous leukemia, chromosomal
    abnormality in, 46, 47
Adenomas, pulmonary, induction of, mis-
    coding in DNA and, 52-56, 172
Adenoviruses, mammary tumor induction
    by, 39
Aflatoxin B_1, metabolic activation of, 157,
    175
AKR mice, genetic aspects of leukemia
    virus in, 195-205
Alkylating agents
  as carcinogens, radiation carcinogenesis
    compared to, 165-174
  as mutagens, 166-168
4-Aminobiphenyl, as carcinogen, 149
Animal studies, on radiation carcinogenesis,
    13-29

Antibodies, natural, to murine leukemia
    virus, 261-273
Arsenic compounds, as carcinogens, 149
Asbestos, as carcinogen, 149
Ataxia telangiectasia
  immunodeficiency in, 46
  leukemia with, 47

B

Base displacement model, for nucleic acid
    changes in chemical carcinogenesis,
    175-187
Benzidine, as carcinogen, 149
Benzo(α)pyrene, as carcinogen, activation
    of, 155-156
Betel nuts, as carcinogens, 149
Bloom's syndrome, leukemia incidence
    with, 45-46
Bone, radionuclides seeking, carcinogenesis
    from, 14-19

C

Carcinogenesis
  chemical, see Chemical carcinogenesis
  epigenetic mechanisms of, 160
  genetic aspects of, 159-160
Carcinogens
  chemical
    interactions with cells, 150-151
    list of, 149
    nuclear mechanisms involving, 159
  definition of, 147-148
  DNA repair after exposure to, in normal
    and xeroderma pigmentosum cells,
    129-145
  mammary tumor induction by, 38-39
  metabolic activation of, 147-164
Cell culture, of leukemia viruses, radiation
    activation of, 217-225